The Epidemiology of Prematurity

Proceedings of a working conference
held at NICHD/NIH, Bethesda, Maryland
November 8–9, 1976

The Epidemiology of Prematurity

Edited by

Dwayne M. Reed, M.D., M.P.H., Ph.D.
and
Fiona J. Stanley, M.B., B.S., M.Sc., M.F.C.M.

Urban & Schwarzenberg • Baltimore-Munich 1977

Urban & Schwarzenberg, Inc.
7 E. Redwood Street
Baltimore, Maryland 21202

Urban & Schwarzenberg
Pettenkoferstrasse 18
D-8000 München 15
Germany

Library of Congress Cataloging in Publication Data
Epidemiology Workshop, National Insitute of Child
    Health and Human Development, 1976.
    The epidemiology of prematurity.
    Includes index.
    1. Infants (Premature)—Congresses. 2. Birth weight, Low—Congresses. 3. Epidemiology—Congresses. I. Reed, Dwayne M. II. Stanley, Fiona J. III. United States. National Institute of Child Health and Human Development. IV. Title. [DNLM: 1. Infant, Premature—Congresses. 2. Infant, Low birth weight—Congresses. 3. Labor, Premature—Occurrence—Congresses. 4. Labor, Premature—Etiology—Congresses. (WS410 E64e 1976]
    RJ250.E64 1976   618.3'97   77-24474

ISBN 0-8067-1611-8   (Baltimore)
ISBN 3-541-71611-8   (Munich)

Printed in the United States of America

Table of Contents

Acknowledgments

We wish to express our special appreciation to Rebecca A. Paytash who worked many long days to help organize the conference and to prepare the manuscripts for publication, and to Robert P. Nugent who provided technical assistance and helpful advice in the work on the manuscripts. We also wish to thank all those who generously helped with the conference.

Preface

Prematurity is a term used to describe various combinations of being born too early, or too small, or both. As infectious diseases have been controlled, prematurity has now become the single most important problem which affects an infant's risk of dying or of being disabled. During the past few years important findings have been reported and we are now able to make strong inferences about some causal factors. In spite of these advances, we have been unable to prevent or even lower the frequency of prematurity.

Epidemiology is chiefly concerned with the patterns of disease in human populations, with a special orientation towards the social and environmental interactions which favor the occurrence of these diseases. This extension of medical concern offers additional ways of preventing disease through modification of environmental causes.

We requested and received the enthusiastic support of the National Institute of Child Health and Human Development to hold a working conference which would stimulate further interest in the epidemiology of prematurity. We thought that the best approach would be to first examine the strength of previous work and to uncover the major gaps of epidemiologic knowledge concerning the causes and prevention of prematurity. Armed with these judgements, we then wanted to focus upon the future needs for epidemiologic research. It is our hope that this forum will provide a resource for those persons who share our belief that the time to control prematurity has come.

Dwayne M. Reed, M.D.
Fiona J. Stanley, M.B.

Contributors

Eva Alberman, M.D.
Reader in Epidemiology
London School of Hygiene and
  Tropical Medicine
Department of Community
  Health
London, England
and
Guys Pediatric Research Unit
Guys Hospital, London, England

Sir Dugald Baird, FRCOG
formerly Regius Professor of
Obstetrics and Gynaecology
University of Aberdeen
and Director, Medical Research
Council, Medical Sociology Unit
Institute of Medical Sociology
Aberdeen, Scotland

Leiv S. Bakketeig, M.D.
University of Trondheim
Department of Community
  Medicine
Eirik Jarls gt. 4
7000 Trondheim, Norway
and
Visiting Scientist
Epidemiology Branch
Epidemiology and Biometry Research
  Program
National Institute of Child Health
  and Human Development
National Institutes of Health
Bethesda, Maryland 20014

Heinz Berendes, M.D.
Chief, Contraceptive Evaluation
  Branch
Center for Population Research
National Institute of Child Health
  and Human Development
National Institutes of Health
Bethesda, Maryland 20014

Bea J. van den Berg, M.D.
Director, Child Health and
  Development Studies
School of Public Health
University of California
Berkeley, California 94611

Rosanne Boldman, M.P.H.
Research Assistant
Epidemiology Branch
Epidemiology and Biometry Research
  Program
National Institute of Child Health
  and Human Development
National Institutes of Health
Bethesda, Maryland 20014

Helen C. Chase, Dr. P.H.
Deputy Chief
Epidemiologic Studies Branch
Division of Biological Effects/Food
  and Drug Administration
Bureau of Radiological Health
Parklawn Building/DHEW/PHS
Rockville, Maryland 20857

Dorothy Edmonds
Infectious Diseases Branch
National Institute of Neurological
   and Communicative Disorders
   and Stroke
National Institutes of Health
Bethesda, Maryland 20014

Jonas H. Ellenberg, Ph.D.
Office of Biometry and Epidemiology
National Institute of Neurological
   and Communicative Disorders
   and Stroke
National Institutes of Health
Bethesda, Maryland 20014

Irvin Emanuel, M.D.
Director, Child Development and
   Mental Retardation Center
University of Washington
Seattle, Washington 98195

Stanley M. Garn, Ph.D.
Fellow of the Center for Human
   Growth and Development
Professor of Human Nutrition and
Professor of Anthropology
University of Michigan
Ann Arbor, Michigan 48109

Janet B. Hardy, M.D. C.M.
Professor of Pediatrics
Director
Office of Continuing Education
The Johns Hopkins University
School of Medicine
Turner Auditorium Building
Baltimore, Maryland 21205

Ernest E. Harley, M.S.
Head, Computer Specialist
Epidemiology and Biometry Research
   Program
National Institute of Child Health
   and Human Development
National Institutes of Health
Bethesda, Maryland 20014

Howard J. Hoffman, M.A.
Mathematical Statistician
Biometry Branch/Epidemiology
   and Biometry Research Program
National Institute of Child Health
   and Human Development
National Institutes of Health
Bethesda, Maryland 20014

Dwight T. Janerich, D.D.S., M.P.H.
Director, Genetic Oncology
State of New York
Department of Health
Tower Building, Empire State Plaza
Albany, New York 12237

Zelda L. Janus
Research Associate
Information Sciences Research
   Institute
Maternal and Child Health Studies
Washington, DC 20006

Norman Kretchmer, M.D., Ph.D.
Director, National Institute of Child
Health and Human Development
National Institutes of Health
Bethesda, Maryland 20014

Frank E. Lundin, Jr., M.D., D.P.H.
Chief, Epidemiologic Studies Branch
Division of Biological Effects/Food
   and Drug Administration
Bureau of Radiologic Health
Parklawn Building/DHEW/PHS
Rockville, Maryland 20857

Kinne D. McCabe, M.D.
The Collaborative Perinatal Project
   of the National Institute of
   Neurological and Communicative
   Disorders and Stroke
National Institutes of Health
Bethesda, Maryland 20014

E. David Mellits, Sc.D.
The Johns Hopkins Hospital
CMSC 804
Baltimore, Maryland 21205

Mary B. Meyer, Sc.M.
Associate Professor of Epidemiology
The Johns Hopkins University
School of Hygiene and Public Health
Department of Epidemiology
Baltimore, Maryland 21205

Newton E. Morton, Ph.D.
Director of the Population Genetics
  Laboratory
University of Hawaii at Manoa
Honolulu, Hawaii 96822

Kenneth R. Niswander, M.D.
Professor and Chairman
Department of Obstetrics and
  Gynecology
School of Medicine
University of California, Davis
Sacramento, California 95817

Paul J. Placek, Ph.D.
Statistician (Demography)
Natality Statistics Branch
Division of Vital Statistics
National Center for Health Statistics
Health Resources Administration
Parklawn Building/DHEW/PHS
Rockville, Maryland 20857

Margaret W. Pratt, B.A.
Senior Research Associate
Director of Maternal and Child
  Health Studies Project
Information Sciences Research
  Institute
Washington, DC 20006

Dwayne M. Reed, M.D., Ph.D.
Chief, Epidemiology Branch
Epidemiology and Biometry Research
  Program
National Institute of Child Health
  and Human Development
National Institutes of Health
Bethesda, Maryland 20014

David Rush, M.D.
Associate Professor of Public Health
(Epidemiology) and Pediatrics
Columbia University
School of Public Health
The Faculty of Medicine
Division of Epidemiology
New York, New York 10032

Naresh C. Sayal
Research Associate
Information Sciences Research
  Institute
Maternal and Child Health Studies
Washington, DC 20006

Helen A. Shaw, B.A.
Center for Human Growth and
  Development
University of Michigan
Ann Arbor, Michigan 48109

Daniel G. Seigel, Sc.D.
Director, Epidemiology and
  Biometry Research Program
National Institute of Child Health
  and Human Development
National Institutes of Health
Bethesda, Maryland 20014

xii

John L. Sever, M.D. Ph.D.
Chief, Infectious Disease Branch
National Institute of Neurological and
Communicative Disorders and Stroke
National Institutes of Health
Bethesda, Maryland 20014

Fiona J. Stanley, M.B., B.S., M.Sc.,
M.F.C.M.
Fellow in Clinical Sciences
(Epidemiology)
Unit of Clinical Epidemiology
University Department of Medicine
Perth Medical Centre
Shenton Park, Western Australia
and
Guest Worker
Epidemiology Branch
Epidemiology and Biometry Research
Program
National Institute of Child Health and
Human Development
National Institutes of Health
Bethesda, Maryland 20014

Zena Stein, M.B.
Professor, Division of Epidemiology
School of Public Health
and Administrative Medicine
Columbia University Faculty of
Medicine and Psychiatric Institute
New York State Department of Mental
Hygiene
New York, New York 10032

Mervyn Susser, M.B.
Professor and Head
Division of Epidemiology
Columbia University,
Faculty of Medicine
School of Public Health and
Administrative Medicine
New York, New York 10029

Milton Terris, M.D.
Professor and Chairman
Department of Community and
Preventive Medicine
New York Medical College
New York, New York 10029

Other Participants

Henry L. Barnett, M.D.
Professor of Pediatrics
Albert Einstein College of Medicine
of Yeshiva University
Department of Pediatrics
Bronx, New York 10461

A. Michael Davies, M.D.
Professor of Medical Ecology
Hebrew University
Hadassah Medical School
Jerusalem, Israel

Sarah Friedman, Ph.D.
Psychologist
Wilson House
National Institute of Mental Health
Component of Alcohol, Drug Abuse
and Mental Health Administration
National Institutes of Health
Bethesda, Maryland 20014

Robert L. Heuser, M.A.
Chief, Natality Statistics Branch
Division of Vital Statistics
National Center for Health Statistics
Health Resources Administration
Parklawn Building/DHEW/PHS
Rockville, Maryland 20857

Edward H. Kass, M.D.
William Ellery Channing
Professor of Medicine
Harvard Medical School
Director of Channing Laboratory
Boston, Massachusetts 02118

Charles R. Stark, M.D.
Medical Officer
Center for Research for Mothers and
Children
Pregnancy and Infancy Branch
National Institute for Child Health
and Human Development
National Institutes of Health
Bethesda, Maryland 20034

Josephine A. C. Weatherall, M.B.
Senior Medical Statistician
Office of Population Census and
Surveys
Medical Statistics Division
St. Catherine's House
London, England

Support Personnel

Rebecca A. Paytash
Medical Secretary
Epidemiology Branch
Epidemiology and Biometry Research
Program
National Institute of Child Health
and Human Development
Bethesda, Maryland 20014

Robert P. Nugent, M.P.H.
Research Assistant
Epidemiology Branch
Epidemiology and Biometry Research
Program
National Institute of Child Health and
Human Development
Bethesda, Maryland 20014

The Epidemiology of Prematurity

Welcome

I would like to welcome all of you to the NIH. Over the past two years the National Institute of Child Health and Human Development has set out certain initiatives that it intends to follow. In fact, NICHD has been given a certain number of initiatives by the Congress of the United States. One of these emphasis areas is high risk pregnancy and high risk infancy. The Institute intends to concentrate its efforts to discover means of preventing or ameliorating problems associated with high risk pregnancy and high risk infancy.

This conference, then, fits very neatly within the Institute's "prejudice"—that is, the prejudice against the high risk infant and the high risk pregnancy. The conference will try to answer certain questions not posed in previous conferences—in particular, questions of epidemiology and questions concerning the risk of prematurity among different populations, both in this country and throughout the world.

We at the Institute look forward to the progress of this conference and its results. I think that all of you would agree that conferences have two purposes, really. The first involves an examination of "the state of the art" among professionals in the field. Those of you at the table and those of you in the audience are certainly professionals in the field, and this kind of a dialogue or "polylogue" between various disciplines is one way to examine the state of an art. The second purpose of a conference —that is, to disseminate information to the public and to those interested in the problems of high risk pregnancy and high risk infancy—will also be accomplished here.

We look forward to great accomplishments over the next two days. Again, I would like to welcome all of you, and I am delighted you braved the vicissitudes of Washington weather to come here.

Norman Kretchmer, M.D., Ph.D.
Director, National Institute of Child
Health and Human Development
National Institutes of Health
Bethesda, Maryland 20014

Epidemiologic Patterns Over Time

Sir Dugald Baird, F.R.C.O.G.

Very few national epidemiologic studies of low birth weight (LBW) have been undertaken because accurate information on birth weight and the many factors to which it is related cannot be guaranteed. Fryer and Ashford (1972), using data collected by local health authorities in England, showed that the incidence of babies weighing 2500 gm. or less decreased between 1960 and 1965 and rose thereafter until 1969. They were of the opinion that "a rise in the incidence is likely to involve an accumulation of many small effects rather than a single dominant factor." In the city of Aberdeen the incidence of LBW fell between 1954 and 1963 and rose thereafter until 1969. Analysis by pregnancy number showed that the incidence fell in first and second births in the years 1954–63 and then rose in all parity groups until 1969 when it fell again. The explanation of these variations in incidence will become clear later.

The mother's height is the most important single factor influencing the birth weight of her baby. Even today in many highly developed countries a proportion of adults have not reached their genetic potential in respect to height, as a result of having been reared from birth to maturity in an unfavorable environment. Thus, the height distribution of young adults gives a convenient, if rather imprecise, measure of the level of health and physique of a population.

The tallest women in Britain have fathers and mothers in professional occupations. The percentage of first babies weighing 2500 gm. or less is

lowest in tall women in social classes I and II (professional and manage-
erial) and highest in short women in classes IV and V (semiskilled and
unskilled). Those who move up in the social scale on marriage have a
lower incidence of LBW than those who remain in their class of origin.
This is one of the reasons why in Britain, despite the advantages of 25
years of the National Health Service, the social class differences in stillbirth and infant mortality rates and in the incidence of LBW have
widened. Women who migrate from depressed to more affluent areas in
the UK tend to be taller, healthier and more able, and to have lower
perinatal mortality (PNM) rates than those in the same social classes
who do not migrate, a fact which tends to maintain the regional differences in mortality. In 1958 the PNM rate was lowest in tall women in
the south of England who lived outside conurbations and highest in
short women in the north who lived in conurbations.

Baird and Thomson (1969) classified the causes of perinatal deaths
into two groups: 1) "environmental," where the deaths resulted from
malformations, especially of the central nervous system, or occurred in
association with LBW of "unexplained" etiology; and 2) "obstetric,"
where the deaths resulted from difficult labor, preeclampsia or other
well-recognized complications of pregnancy or labor. The high PNM
rates in the north of Britain compared to the south were due very largely
to excessive "environmental" causes; in other words, they were related
much more to the poorer health and physique to mothers than to lower
standards of obstetric care.

ENVIRONMENTAL CAUSES

In Caucasians there is probably a genetic predisposition to CNS malformations which is not present in many other ethnic groups. Its incidence is closely related to socioeconomic conditions (Baird, 1974) and,
because the condition can be diagnosed easily and accurately without an
autopsy, it is a very useful tool for national surveys. In Scotland the stillbirth rate from anencephaly rose in 1946 in mothers under the age of
20, in 1951 in those aged 20–24, and in 1956 in those aged 25–29. The
rise in the rate in the oldest age group was relatively small and lasted for
a short period of time because a high proportion of the women of this
group came from classes I and II. In the 15–19 age group, where the rise in
the rate was much higher and remained high for almost 20 years, a
majority of the women were from classes IV and V. The women in all
three age groups had in common the fact that they were born between
the years 1927 and 1934.

In the city of Aberdeen from 1920 to 1926 the stillbirth rate was
approximately 40 per 1000 and rose to 50 between 1927 and 1935.

Between 1948 and 1962 the number of deaths from CNS malformations increased greatly. Between 1948 and 1954 a majority of them were in first and second pregnancies, and between 1958 and 1962 in third and later pregnancies. Most of the mothers giving birth to these malformed babies were born between 1926 and 1932. The findings were therefore in agreement with those obtained in the national survey on the changes in the incidence of anencephaly.

The PNM rate in the city of Aberdeen fell by 50% between 1948 and 1972. It fell steadily in each five year period in the "obstetric" cause group, except in fourth and later births where little reduction in the rate occurred until 1963–67 because, until 1960, more than 50% of the women in this parity group still elected to have a home confinement. The fall in the PNM rate from "environmental" causes was much less and the pattern of change very different. The rate was highest in first births in 1948–52 and in fourth or later births in 1963–67. In first births the rate was highest in those under the age of 20 in 1948–52 and in those over the age of 30 from 1958–62 onward.

These facts suggest that the cohort of women born during the worst of the industrial depression and who started childbearing in 1948–52 had high PNM rates from "environmental" causes in each pregnancy. By 1967 most of them had finished childbearing, hence the fall in the PNM rate from these causes in fourth and later pregnancies in 1968–72. The changes over these years in the incidence of LBW are very similar.

OBSTETRIC CAUSES

Relatively little can be done during the course of pregnancy to lower the PNM rate from "environmental" causes. In the "obstetric" cause group, two of the most important advances in primigravidae have been an increase in the incidence of induction of labor in 1954 and again in 1964, and a steady increase in the cesarean section rate.

In babies weighing more than 2500 gm., a substantial fall in the PNM rate occurred, coinciding in time with the increases in the incidence of induction in 1954 and 1964 (Fig. 1). In babies weighing between 1501–2500 gm., very little reduction in the PNM rate occurred in 1954, but it fell from 7.2 per 1000 in 1958–63 to 3.7 in 1964–75. In babies weighing 1500 gm. or less, no reduction occurred in the PNM rate as a result of the induction policy, nor was there any reduction in the rate from malformations. However, very similar changes in the PNM rate occurred in both of these groups during the course of the 25 years (Fig. 2). For example, in social classes I-IIIa, a rise in the rate occurred in both groups in 1957-60. In social classes IV and V, the rate was high in both groups in the early 1950s and again in the late 1960s and early 1970s.

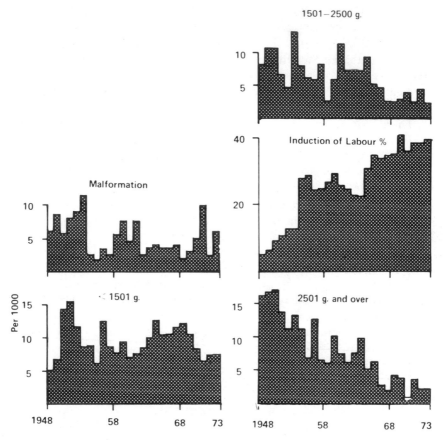

Figure 1. **Perinatal Mortality Rate (First Births) by Birth Rate and Malformations (All Birth Weights), Aberdeen, 1948-73.**

The rise in the rate from both causes in the years 1963-70 occurred in the daughters of the cohort of women who had high death rates from these "environmental" causes between 1946 and 1954.

In the 1501-2500 gm. weight group, no obvious cause for the LBW was found in 40% of the cases, but in another 30% it was attributed to the effect of preeclampsia. The substantial fall in the PNM rate in this weight group in 1964-73 occurred mostly in those due to preeclampsia. It occurred in stillbirths rather than first-week deaths, which points to the beneficial effect of the increased use of induction of labor.

In the 1500 gm. or less weight group, no obvious clinical cause for the LBW could be detected in 60% of cases, except that one-quarter of them resulted from a twin pregnancy. In another 20% of cases the LBW was attributed to preeclampsia. These percentages remained unchanged throughout the 25 years under review.

Scottish statistics show that malformation was the only cause of still-birth which did not fall during the war years. In Scotland and in Aberdeen the PNM rate from CNS malformations and that associated with LBW rose from 1946 onward in mothers who had been born between 1927 and 1935. This suggests that babies born during the worst of the depression sustained damage which, in due course (from 1964 onward), affected their reproductive efficiency and resulted in damage to their babies. This might have come about in several ways. For example, problems may have arisen at the time of implantation of the blastocyst, resulting in faulty development of the neural tube. A second possibility is a poor endometrial response, leading to the development of a small placenta unable to meet the demands on the fetus when it starts to increase in weight, thus resulting in the "unexplained" LBW baby.

Apart from the babies who died, or showed signs of abnormality, others inside the normal weight range may have received damage which in turn could have lowered the reproductive efficiency of mothers of the second generation, as shown by the increase in the incidence of CNS malformations or LBW babies in the late 1960s and early 1970s. This would be more likely to happen if a very unfavorable home en-

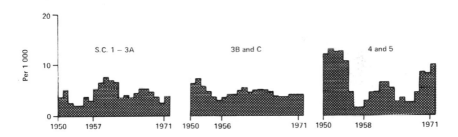

P.N.M. RATES IN ASSOCIATION WITH L.B.W. < 1501 g* BY SOCIAL CLASS ABERDEEN 1948 – 73

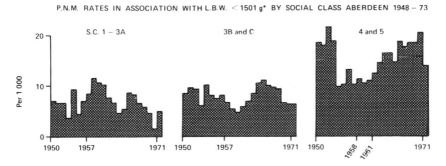

* 5 year moving average

Figure 2. **Perinatal Mortality Rate (First Births) in Association with Low Birth Weight (< 1501 g, per 5-year moving average) by Social Class, Aberdeen, 1948–73.**

vironment persisted in the second generation, as occurred in many cases in social classes IV and V in 1968–72 in Aberdeen. The importance of an optimal intrauterine environment is illustrated by the fact that the stillbirth rate from anencephaly is lowest in social class I and highest in class V. In every social class the rate is 30% less in a second than in a first pregnancy. In social class I the rate does not rise with increasing age of the mother, but it does rise steadily with increasing age in all other social classes, especially class V. The rise in the incidence of LBW in New York state in the early 1960s was postponed until the age of 35 in the wives of farmers, good evidence of their very high level of reproductive efficiency (Fig. 3).

DISCUSSION

Although it is probable that the occurrence of a CNS malformation depends basically on a genetic predisposition, the frequency with which the lesion occurs is very much influenced by the mother's reproductive efficiency, which in turn is greatly influenced by the quality of her environment from birth to maturity. While these factors also apply in the

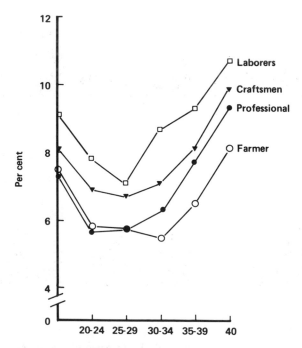

Figure 3.   **Percentage Low Birth Weight Infants by Father's Occupation and Mother's Age, New York (exclusive of New York City), 1960–61.**

case of "unexplained" LBW, the outcome of pregnancy can probably be influenced much more by the events of the pregnancy.

The PNM rate in Britain is considerably higher than in many countries in Europe. This is clearly seen in the case of congenital malformations. For example, in the early 1960s the PNM rate from malformations was twice as high in England and three times as high in Scotland as in the Netherlands.

Britain was the first of these countries to industrialize and obviously made many beginner's mistakes. Not enough consideration was given to the working and living conditions of the men and women who constituted the work force. The changes in the infant mortality rate (IMR) over the last 100 years reflect this clearly. For example, in 1880 the IMR was 120 per 1000 in Norway, Sweden and Scotland; 140 in England; and 180 in the Netherlands. From that date the rate in Norway and Sweden fell steadily and today is less than 12. In the Netherlands in 1880 there was poverty and widespread unemployment, but the infant mortality rate has fallen steadily since then and is now less than 12. Despite the very high population density, the PNM rate is low and the general level of health and physique high. In the Netherlands industrialization occurred later, after its dangers had become apparent. Better techniques were available in factories and legislation existed to protect health.

In England and Scotland, on the other hand, the IMR rose between 1880 and the end of the century. It then fell more rapidly in England than in Scotland and by 1911 the rate in Scotland was higher than in England for the first time. In Glasgow it was 100 per 1000 as late as 1940 and is still more than 20. The extent of the stunting of growth and skeletal deformity seen in many women in large conurbations such as Manchester and Glasgow showed the devastating effect on health and physique. Unemployment, poverty, large families, overcrowding, poor sanitation, a cold and wet climate, little sunshine, pollution of the atmosphere with smoke from factories and open domestic coal fires and, finally, a very poor diet all created an environment more deleterious to health than almost anywhere else in the world.

The very poor health and physique of young recruits to the armed forces during the Boer War at the end of the last century shocked the nation and led to the enactment of much social legislation, including the development of the Public Health Service. In 1926 there was a general strike followed by the worldwide depression of 1928 which caused mass unemployment. From 1936 an increase in employment began in the armaments industries. During the war there was little unemployment and a unique rationing system was introduced which placed mothers and young children in a priority class for milk and other essential foods and vitamins. As is well known, the PNM rate, which had been stationary between 1928 and 1937, fell by over 30% between 1938 and 1947. By 1954 there were many more marriages and at a younger age. Nevertheless, the PNM rate remained almost unchanged between 1948 and 1957. Some were of the opinion that we had almost reached the limit of what could be done to lower the PNM rate by improving the mother's food intake during pregnancy. In some areas the rate continued to fall because of high standards of obstetric care, and a national inquiry in 1958 showed that there was great scope for improving standards of obstetrics throughout the country as a whole.

One of the features of postwar Britain has been the increase in the height of children and their healthier appearance. The mean height and weight of children entering school in Aberdeen at the age of five increased very slowly between 1933 and 1958, but more quickly from 1959 onward (Fig. 4). By 1954, the year in which the 1959 cohort of five-year-old girls was born, the infant mortality had fallen to 20 per 1000 from over 80 twenty years earlier. One might expect these children, reared in more prosperous circumstances, to grow to be taller and healthier than their mothers and to have fewer LBW babies. However,

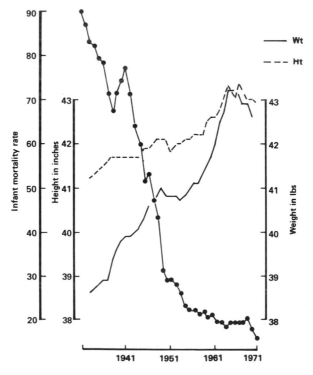

Figure 4. **Infant Mortality Rates, Height and Weight of School Entrants (aged 5 yrs), Aberdeen, 1933–71.**

the situation has been complicated by the changing pattern of sexual mores among the young. In 1961 one percent of all first pregnancies were terminated, and in 1974 twenty-three percent (39% in the 15-19 age group, 18% in the 20-24 age group, and less than 2% in the 25-29 age group). In all age groups, but especially the youngest one, the women who had their pregnancies terminated were considerably taller on the average than those who continued with them. Young mothers today are therefore not representative of their age group in terms of height.

The competing claims of clothes, cosmetics, alcohol, cigarettes and entertainment, together with the increasing cost of food, may have caused some deterioration in the health and nutrition of the most vulnerable groups in our society. The divorce rate after only four years of marriage is rising steadily in those who marry before the age of 20. It may be inferred, therefore, that many marriages among the very young are characterized by serious emotional distress and uncertainty about the future, a state of affairs unlikely to be conducive to the most successful outcome of pregnancy and the care of children.

In Aberdeen in 1968-72 the PNM rate was 20 per 1000 in first births, 50% less than in 1948-52. In 65% of cases the PNM rate was 13 per 1000; in 22% (social classes IV and V) 39 per 1000; and 13% (illegitimate births) 27 per 1000. In 1973-74, 28% of the deaths were from malformations and 39% were in babies weighing 1500 gm. or less at birth.

Great progress has been made in lowering the PNM and LBW rates in other parity groups. For example, the number of fourth or later births has fallen by almost 70% in the last 10 years as a result of oral contraception, sterilization, vasectomy and abortion. This dramatic reduction in the number of children born to women of high parity has occurred in all social classes in most parts of the UK and will result in a substantial reduction in the incidence of LBW and the prevalence of problem families and of mental subnormality.

CONCLUSION

Britain was the first country to industrialize and prosper, but at the same time, this process led to the emergence of cities such as Glasgow where "wealth accumulates and men decay." The emphasis on economic and social justice since the last world war has raised the general level of health and physique of the young people in the population. The emphasis among the young has now shifted to freedom of expression and behavior, unfettered by the conventions of the past. In the field of sex and reproduction, statistics on abortion, illegitimacy and divorce suggest that only a minority of young men and women are able to cope successfully with this new freedom. Changes in the incidence of LBW and PNM rates closely reflect these changes but sometimes only after an interval of 20 years, by which time substantial new changes in society may have taken place.

As with so many facets of the human situation, there is no finality.

TEXT REFERENCES

Baird, D.: Epidemiology of Congenital Malformations of the Central Nervous System in (a) Aberdeen and (b) Scotland. J Biosoc Sci 6(1974)113

Baird, D.; Thomson, A.M.: Perinatal Problems: Second Report of the British Perinatal Mortality Survey. Livingstone, Edinburgh and London, 1969

Fryer, J.G.; Ashford, J.R.: Trends in Perinatal and Neonatal Mortality in England and Wales 1960-1969. Brit J Prev Soc Med 26(1972)1

DISCUSSION

Dr. Susser: A number of analyses of factors in birth weight have been made in the last 10 or 15 years on US data. With regard to maternal height, the relation with birth weight disappears when controlled for maternal weight, which is best seen as an intervening variable between maternal height and birth weight.

Dr. Baird: I have not considered that because it was impossible to quote variations in weight over a 25-year period. It has been shown that in Scotland at least, birth weight of the baby is highest in tall women with a high weight/height ratio who gain more than one pound per week in weight between the 20th and 30th weeks of pregnancy.

Dr. Kass: I think there are some things that one ought to say about Professor Baird's interesting presentation. The first is that correlation between maternal weight and newborn weight at the 20th week of pregnancy is quite uniform in different populations, with an r of about 0.24. The r for maternal height against newborn weight is about 0.16, and all the height effects, as Dr. Susser pointed out, are absorbed into the weight effect, so it does not appear that height offers much useful data as a separate indicator of outcome.

Secondly, although it is often stated that the lower social classes are fatter, the actual analysis of distribution of weight shows something quite different. They are often lighter in weight, but they have a greater tail on the excessively obese, particularly in the wealthier countries.

Dr. Garn: Can I get into the fatness and height fray? Most of our studies measuring fat—subcutaneous fat, not weight—show that there is a remarkably linear, *negative* regression between economic level and fatness. Roughly speaking, the higher the educational level and the higher the per capita income, the leaner the female. From this one could project accurately to the fact that Howard Hughes would have no wife!

So, we have to talk about weight in terms of its components since both the fat-free weight of the mother and her fatness level bear on the size and weight of the conceptus, but again in differing fractions. This is one of the reasons why it is difficult to correct simply by using maternal weight or weight for height alone.

Dr. Baird: Women in the upper social classes have fewer premature babies and fewer weighing less than 2500 gm. after 38 weeks of gestation. The mean height of a representative sample of young women and a graph of height distribution give useful indications of the level of health and physique in a community. This is related to the fact that, even today in Britain, many do not reach their genetic potential for height because of a faulty environment in childhood. It seems probable that this handicap will not be confined to the skeleton but will affect most tissues and organs of the body, and so reproductive efficiency in general will be lowered.

DISCUSSION REFERENCES

Abramowicz, M.; Kass, E.H.: Pathogenesis and Prognosis of Prematurity. New Engl J Med 275(1966)878-885, 938-853, 1001-1007, 1053-1059.

Garn, S.M.; Clark, D.C.: Economics and Fatness. Ecol Food Nutr 3(1974)19-20

Garn, S.M.; Bailey, S.M.; Cole, P.E.; Higgins, I.T.T.: Level of Education, Level of Income and Level of Fatness in Adults. Am J Clin Nutr, in press

Rush, D.M.; Davis, H.; Susser, M.: Antecedent of Low Birth Weight in Harlem. New York City. Int J Epid 4(1972) 375-387

Thomson, A.M.; Billewicz, W. Z.; Hytten, F.E.: The Assessment of Fetal Growth. J Obstet Gynaec Brit Cwlth 75(1968)903

Time Trends in Low Birth Weight in the United States, 1950-1974

Helen C. Chase, Dr. P.H.

During the 1950s, the rate of decline of the infant mortality rate for the United States was decelerating. For several years during the decade there was little change in the rate (Shapiro, Schlesinger and Nesbitt, 1968). National attention was turned to the problem, and low birth weight was among the important correlates of infant mortality which came under scrutiny. Two major reports (Chase and Byrnes, 1972; Chase, 1973) summarized the low birth weight trends of live born infants in the United States through 1968. The purpose of this presentation is to update the trends in low birth weight ratios through 1974.

At the time of the earlier publications, a number of relevant developments were already under way. There were food stamp programs, and the program specifically aimed at women, infants and children (WIC) followed. Under this program, preference was given to areas with the highest infant mortality, low birth weight ratios and low incomes (U.S. Department of Agriculture, 1973). A second significant development was a stated change in the attitude towards the upper limit of desirable weight gain for pregnant women: an average of 24 pounds, with a range of 20–25 pounds, became accepted as a reasonable level of weight gain during pregnancy (National Academy of Sciences, 1970). Newborn intensive care units were also developed, and high risk women became the focus of intensified prenatal care (American Medical Association, 1971).

Since the close of the period covered by earlier reports, other important changes have also occurred. The restraints on abortion have been legally relaxed so that early terminations of unwanted pregnancies are now much more readily available (U.S. Department of Health, Education and Welfare, Center for Disease Control, 1976). In addition, family planning services have become widely available through public as well as private sources (U.S. Department of Health, Education and Welfare, National Center for Health Statistics, various years). Because these developments have some bearing on the birth weight distribution of infants born in the United States, it is appropriate to examine changes in birth weight distributions since 1968.

The data presented here are taken from the annual volumes of *Vital Statistics of the United States* and from unpublished tabulations provided by the National Center for Health Statistics, U.S. Department of Health, Education, and Welfare.

LIVE BIRTHS

The number of live births has undergone marked changes since 1950 (Table 1). In that year, they numbered over 3.5 million: the post-World War II baby boom was underway. In 1961, the number reached its peak of about 4.3 million. Since then, there has been a gradual general decline. In 1974, live births numbered around 3.2 million, which was lower than any year since 1950, with the single exception of 1973. When the trend was converted to relative terms, the number of live births in the peak year (1961) was found to be 20.1% *higher* than in 1950, and the number in 1974 was 26.0% *lower* than in 1961.

Color and Race [1]

Since 1950, the United States has experienced a declining trend in the proportion of live births which are white (86.2% in 1950 to 81.5% in 1974), and a complementary increase (13.8 to 18.5%) in births in the Other category. The increase has occurred among Negro, and All other infants as well.

Negro infants have remained by far the predominant group among Other births, but their relative proportion has declined, while that for races in the All other category has increased:

---

[1] In this presentation, racial designations are White, Negro and "All other." Color designations are White and "Other" (i.e., Negro and "All other").

	Negro	*All other races*
	(As percent of Other)	
1950	95.1	4.9
1955	94.8	5.2
1960	91.7	8.3
1965	91.3	8.7
1970	89.4	10.6
1974	86.8	13.2

Plurality and Sex

There appears to have been a small increase in single births, but no change was suggested in the sex ratio:

	Single Births	*Male Births*
	(As percent of live births)	
1950	97.9	51.3
1955	97.9	51.2
1960	98.0	51.2
1965	98.0	51.2
1970	not available	51.3
1974	98.1	51.3

Gestation

In 1968, a new standard certificate of live birth was introduced and recommended for adoption in the United States. Among other new items, the certificate indicated that the first day of the last normal menstrual period be entered. In 1968, certificates for 36 states and the District of Columbia contained the new item; by 1974, 40 states and the District were using the new form of report. The proportion of certificates for which gestation was not computed because the date of last normal menses was missing remains low and unchanged (0.4% in 1968 and 1974).

Since 1968, there has been a suggested shift in the distribution of live births toward longer gestations:

	1968	*1974*
(As percent of live births)		
Less than 20 weeks	0.03	0.03
20-39 weeks	46.4	41.5
40 weeks	22.7	22.7
41 weeks or more	30.9	35.7

Table 1. Live Births by Race: United States, 1950–1974

Year	Total	White	Negro	All other	Total	White	Negro	All other
	Number				Percentage distribution			
1950	3,554,149	3,063,627	466,718	23,804	100.0	86.2	13.1	0.7
1951	3,750,850	3,237,072	489,282	24,496	100.0	86.3	13.0	0.7
1952	3,846,986	3,322,658	497,880	26,448	100.0	86.4	12.9	0.7
1953	3,902,120	3,356,772	517,576	27,772	100.0	86.0	13.3	0.7
1954	4,017,362	3,443,630	544,288	29,444	100.0	85.7	13.5	0.7
1955	4,047,295	3,458,448	558,251	30,596	100.0	85.5	13.8	0.8
1956	4,163,090	3,545,350	584,572	33,168	100.0	85.2	14.0	0.8
1957	4,254,784	3,621,456	596,050	37,278	100.0	85.1	14.0	0.9
1958	4,203,812	3,572,306	594,500	37,006	100.0	85.0	14.1	0.9
1959	4,244,796	3,597,430	605,962	41,404	100.0	84.7	14.3	1.0
1960	4,257,850	3,600,744	602,264	54,842	100.0	84.6	14.1	1.3
1961	4,268,326	3,600,864	611,072	56,390	100.0	84.4	14.3	1.3
1962	4,167,362	[1]3,394,068	[1]584,610	[1]56,970	100.0	[1]84.1	[1]14.5	[1]1.4
1963	4,098,020	[1]3,326,344	[1]580,658	[1]58,270	100.0	[1]83.9	[1]14.6	[1]1.5
1964	4,027,490	3,369,160	607,556	50,774	100.0	83.7	15.1	1.3
1965	3,760,358	3,123,860	581,126	55,372	100.0	83.1	15.5	1.5
1966	3,606,274	2,993,230	558,244	54,800	100.0	83.0	15.5	1.5
1967	3,520,959	2,922,502	543,976	54,481	100.0	83.0	15.4	1.5
1968	3,501,564	2,912,224	531,152	58,188	100.0	83.2	15.2	1.7
1969	3,600,206	2,993,614	543,132	63,460	100.0	83.2	15.1	1.8
1970	3,731,386	3,091,264	572,362	67,760	100.0	82.8	15.3	1.8
1971	3,555,970	2,919,746	564,960	71,264	100.0	82.1	15.9	2.0
1972	3,258,411	2,655,558	531,329	71,524	100.0	81.5	16.3	2.2
1973	3,136,965	2,551,030	512,597	73,338	100.0	81.3	16.3	2.3
1974	3,159,958	2,575,792	507,162	77,040	100.0	81.5	16.0	2.4

Note: Data for the years 1950 and 1955 are based on 100% of records; for the years 1951–54, 1956–66 and 1968–71, on 50% samples; for the year 1967 on a 20–50% sample; beginning with 1972 on 100% of records in selected states and 50% in the remaining states.
Excludes Alaska for the years 1950–58 and Hawaii for 1950–59; those areas were not states during the specified years.
[1] Excludes New Jersey for the years 1962–63; identification of the race was not required on the vital records in the specified years.

The proportion of infants at less than 20 weeks and those at 40 weeks remained unchanged; the proportion at 20–39 weeks decreased from 46.4 to 41.5%, while those at 41 weeks or more increased from 30.9 to 35.7%. How much of this change is attributable to the new method of reporting this item and how much represents a real shift in gestation periods is unknown at the present time. However, the change is greater than one might expect because of the addition of four states to the 36 states and the District of Columbia which required the first day of the last normal menstrual period in 1968.

LOW BIRTH WEIGHT RATIOS

The low birth weight ratio (percent 2500 gm. or less at birth) in the United States increased from 7.7% in 1960 to a peak of 8.3% in the years 1965 and 1966 (Table 2). Since then, the low birth weight ratio has been declining, and in 1974 it reached a low of 7.4%—a level achieved in only one other year in recorded vital statistics (1954).

Low birth weight infants represent a significant public health problem by virtue of their numbers. Although their absolute numbers have declined due both to the decreasing numbers of births and the decreasing proportions of low birth weight infants, they continue to account for over 200,000 live births each year:

1960	331,420
1965	311,014
1970	294,478
1974	233,750

Color and Race

The differentials in the low birth weight ratio by color are well established (Fig. 1). The differences between White and "Other" infants increased from 1950 until 1965, with a narrowing thereafter. Since 1969, data by race indicate a wide difference in low birth weight ratios between Negro and the remaining other-than-white infants, with the latter more similar to the ratios for White infants. While the low birth weight ratios for all of the groups are declining, a marked differential between Negro and All other infants persists. Negro infants are the prime contributors to the level of the low birth weight ratio for other-than-white infants.

Table 2. Low Birth Weight Ratios Among Live-born Infants for Urban Places and Other Areas in Metropolitan and Nonmetropolitan Counties by Color 1960–74 and by Race 1969–1974: United States (Excludes birth weight not stated)

Area and race	1960	1961	1962	1963	1964	1965	1966	1967	1968	1969	1970	1971	1972	1973	1974
							Percent								
United States	7.7	7.8	8.0	8.2	8.2	8.3	8.3	8.2	8.2	8.1	7.9	7.7	7.7	7.6	7.4
White	6.8	6.9	7.0	¹7.1	7.1	7.2	7.2	7.1	7.1	7.0	6.8	6.6	6.5	6.4	6.3
Negro and all other	12.8	13.0	¹13.1	¹13.6	13.9	13.8	13.9	13.6	13.7	13.5	13.3	12.7	12.9	12.5	12.4
Negro	—	—	—	—	—	—	—	—	—	14.1	13.9	13.4	13.6	13.3	13.1
All other	—	—	—	—	—	—	—	—	—	8.5	8.2	7.6	7.7	7.5	7.3
Urban places	8.1	8.3	8.4	8.6	8.9	8.9	9.0	8.9	8.8	8.8	8.5	8.2	8.3	8.1	8.0
White	7.0	7.1	7.2	¹7.3	7.4	7.4	7.5	7.4	7.3	7.3	7.0	6.7	6.7	6.6	6.5
Negro and all other	13.7	13.9	¹13.9	¹14.4	14.7	14.6	14.7	14.3	14.3	14.1	13.7	13.3	13.3	13.0	12.8
Negro	—	—	—	—	—	—	—	—	—	14.6	14.2	13.8	13.9	13.6	13.4
All other	—	—	—	—	—	—	—	—	—	8.4	8.3	7.8	7.7	7.6	7.4
Balance of area	7.0	7.1	7.3	7.4	7.4	7.5	7.5	7.4	7.5	7.3	7.2	6.9	6.9	6.9	6.7
White	6.5	6.5	¹6.7	¹6.8	6.8	6.9	6.9	6.8	6.8	6.7	6.6	6.4	6.3	6.3	6.1
Negro and all other	10.8	11.0	¹11.3	¹11.8	12.2	12.1	12.0	12.0	12.3	12.2	12.0	11.3	11.7	11.5	11.4
Negro	—	—	—	—	—	—	—	—	—	12.9	12.8	12.1	12.6	12.4	12.4
All other	—	—	—	—	—	—	—	—	—	8.6	8.0	7.2	7.6	7.3	7.3
Metropolitan Counties	8.0	8.1	8.2	8.4	8.5	8.5	8.6	8.4	8.5	8.4	8.1	7.8	7.8	7.7	7.6
White	6.9	7.0	7.1	¹7.2	7.2	7.3	7.3	7.2	7.2	7.1	6.9	6.6	6.5	6.4	6.3
Negro and all other	13.7	13.8	13.9	¹14.4	14.6	14.5	14.6	14.2	14.3	14.0	13.6	13.1	13.2	12.7	12.6
Negro	—	—	—	—	—	—	—	—	—	14.5	14.1	13.6	13.8	13.4	13.3
All other	—	—	—	—	—	—	—	—	—	8.6	8.2	7.7	7.7	7.4	7.3
Urban places	8.3	8.4	8.6	8.8	9.0	9.1	9.2	9.0	9.0	8.9	8.6	8.3	8.4	8.2	8.0
White	7.0	7.1	7.3	¹7.4	7.4	7.5	7.5	7.4	7.4	7.3	7.0	6.7	6.7	6.5	6.4
Negro and all other	13.9	14.1	¹14.1	¹14.6	14.8	14.8	14.8	14.4	14.4	14.2	13.8	13.3	13.4	13.0	12.7
Negro	—	—	—	—	—	—	—	—	—	14.7	14.3	13.8	13.9	13.6	13.4
All other	—	—	—	—	—	—	—	—	—	8.4	8.3	7.8	7.7	7.6	7.3

	(1)	(2)	(3)	(4)	(5)	(6)	(7)	(8)	(9)	(10)	(11)	(12)	(13)	(14)	(15)
Balance of area	6.9	7.0	7.1	7.2	7.2	7.3	7.3	7.1	7.2	7.0	6.9	6.6	6.6	6.4	6.4
White	6.5	6.6	6.7[1]	6.8[1]	6.8	6.8	6.8	6.7	6.8	6.7	6.5	6.3	6.1	6.0	6.0
Negro and all other	12.1	11.9	12.4[1]	12.7[1]	12.9	12.9	13.0	12.4	12.9	12.5	12.0	11.3	11.8	10.9	11.4
Negro	—	—	—	—	—	—	—	—	—	13.4	12.8	12.1	12.8	11.9	12.4
All other	—	—	—	—	—	—	—	—	—	9.2	8.1	7.4	7.6	6.8	7.4
Nonmetropolitan Counties	7.3	7.4	7.6	7.7	7.8	7.8	7.9	7.8	7.7	7.6	7.6	7.3	7.3	7.3	7.2
White	6.7	6.7	6.9[1]	7.0[1]	6.9	7.0	7.1	7.0	6.9	6.8	6.8	6.6	6.5	6.5	6.4
Negro and all other	11.1	11.4	11.6[1]	12.1[1]	12.4	12.2	12.3	12.2	12.4	12.4	12.4	11.7	12.0	11.9	11.8
Negro	—	—	—	—	—	—	—	—	—	13.0	13.1	12.5	12.8	12.8	12.7
All other	—	—	—	—	—	—	—	—	—	8.3	8.0	7.3	7.6	7.6	7.4
Urban places	7.6	7.7	7.9	8.0	8.2	8.3	8.4	8.1	8.0	7.9	7.9	7.7	7.7	7.6	7.7
White	6.9	6.9	7.1[1]	7.2[1]	7.2	7.4	7.4	7.2	6.9	7.0	6.9	6.7	6.7	6.5	6.6
Negro and all other	12.6	12.7	12.9[1]	13.4[1]	14.0	13.4	14.2	13.5	13.4	13.4	13.4	12.8	13.0	12.7	13.0
Negro	—	—	—	—	—	—	—	—	—	13.9	13.9	13.5	13.7	13.2	13.6
All other	—	—	—	—	—	—	—	—	—	8.9	8.4	8.4	7.2	8.1	8.1
Balance of area	7.1	7.2	7.4	7.6	7.6	7.7	7.7	7.5	7.6	7.5	7.5	7.2	7.2	7.2	7.0
White	6.5	5.5	6.7[1]	6.8[1]	6.8	6.9	6.9	6.3	6.5	6.8	6.8	6.5	6.5	6.5	6.3
Negro and all other	10.4	10.7	10.9[1]	11.5[1]	12.0	11.8	11.7	11.8	12.1	12.1	12.1	11.3	11.7	11.7	11.4
Negro	—	—	—	—	—	—	—	—	—	12.8	12.8	12.1	12.5	12.6	12.4
All other	—	—	—	—	—	—	—	—	—	8.2	8.0	7.1	7.6	7.5	7.2

Note: Data for the years 1950 and 1955 are based on 100% of records; for the years 1951–54, 1956–66, and 1968–71 on 50% samples; for the year 1967 on a 20–50% sample; beginning with 1972 on 100% of records in selected states and 50% samples in the remaining states.

[1] Excludes New Jersey for the years 1962–63; identification of race was not required on the vital records in the specific year.

Source: *Vital Statistics of the United States* for the years 1960–72, and unpublished data from the National Center for Health Statistics for the years 1973 and 1974.

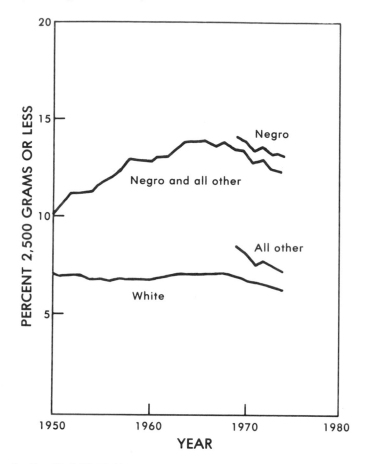

Figure 1. **Low Birth Weight Ratios Among Live Births by Color, 1950–1974, and by Race, 1969–74: United States.**

Geographic Differences

Differences in low birth weight ratios between White and Other infants exist in metropolitan and nonmetropolitan counties (Table 2 and Fig. 2). The geographic difference for white infants which existed in 1960 has apparently been eliminated over this period, and in 1974 the two ratios were virtually identical (6.3 and 6.4%).

For the remaining infants, who were between 85 and 95% Negro over this period, the geographic difference between metropolitan and nonmetropolitan counties also narrowed but was not eliminated. While the low birth weight ratios for Other-than-white infants in metropolitan counties continue to be higher, they are falling more rapidly than in nonmetropolitan counties.

Plurality, Color and Sex

Among the three characteristics of plurality, color and sex, the greatest differential in low birth weight ratios was between single and plural births (Table 3). Among live born infants in plural births, over half weighed 2500 gm. or less at birth. Decreases in the low birth weight ratios between 1968 and 1974 were distributed throughout the plurality, color and sex categories, but the relative change among births in plural deliveries was smaller than for single births.

Maternal Age and Live Birth Order

The proportions of low birth weight infants varied with maternal age, roughly approximating a reverse-J curve (Table 4). The highest propor-

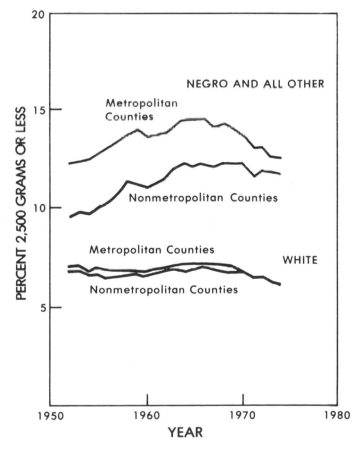

Figure 2. **Low Birth Weight Ratios Among Live Births by Geographic Classification and Color: United States, 1952–74.**

Table 3. Low Birth Weight Ratios for Live Births by Plurality, Color and Sex: United States, 1968 and 1974 (Excludes birth weight not stated)

Race and sex	All births		Single births		Births in plural deliveries	
	1968	1974	1968	1974	1968	1974
	Percent					
Total	8.2	7.4	7.2	6.5	55.8	54.2
Male	7.5	6.8	6.6	6.0	52.3	51.1
Female	8.9	8.1	7.9	7.1	59.4	57.2
White	7.1	6.3	6.2	5.5	54.0	52.1
Male	6.5	5.8	5.7	5.0	50.6	49.2
Female	7.7	6.8	6.7	5.9	57.4	55.1
Negro and all other	13.7	12.4	12.5	11.3	63.4	61.7
Male	12.5	11.3	11.4	10.3	59.5	58.2
Female	14.9	13.5	13.6	12.4	67.0	65.2
Negro	—	13.1	—	12.0	—	62.4
Male	—	12.0	—	10.9	—	59.1
Female	—	14.3	—	13.2	—	65.8
All other	—	7.3	—	6.6	—	55.2
Male	—	6.9	—	6.2	—	50.8
Female	—	7.8	—	7.0	—	59.9

tion of low birth weight infants (15.8%) was among infants born to mothers under 15 years of age. The ratio was at its lowest level for infants born to mothers 25-29 years of age, with steadily increasing ratios up to the oldest group 45-49 years of age (9.9%). Similar patterns were found among White and "Other" infants, although the ratios for the latter were consistently higher.

Variation in the low birth weight ratios by live birth order was less marked than by maternal age. For all births, the range for various maternal age groups was 9.7% (from 6.1 to 15.8); while for births orders, the range was only 2.4% (from 6.7 to 9.1).

There was a slight elevation in the low birth weight ratios for first births. The lowest ratio (6.7%) was for second births, increasing to the highest ratio (around 9%) for sixth or higher births. For both White and "Other" infants, sixth births had the highest low birth weight ratios.

When maternal age and live birth order were considered simultaneously, the lowest proportions of low birth weight infants were for second live born infants with mothers 25-29 years of age—the optimal combination. For White infants, the ratio was 4.7%, and for "Other" infants, 9.0%. Elevated low birth weight ratios were found among higher birth orders.

Detailed Birth Weight

Although the low birth weight ratio is a convenient index, a closer examination of the detailed categories provides additional insight. Changes in the birth weight distributions were spread over a range of birth weight categories, as is illustrated in the comparison between 1968 and 1974 (Table 5).

The proportions of live born infants remained unchanged between 1968 and 1974 for infants who weighed 500 gm. or less. These are very small groups of infants which, because of their extremely low weight, do not contribute to low birth weight survivors.

For each birth weight category less than 3501 gm. for white and 3001 gm. for Negro and All other infants, the proportions of live born infants decreased between 1968 and 1974. Compensating increases were observed between 3501 and 5000 gm. for the remaining infants. Above

Table 4. Low Birth Weight Ratios by Color, Age of Mother, and Infant's Live Birth Order: United States, 1974. (Excludes birth weight not stated.)

Color and age of mother (years)	All birth orders	1	2	3	4	5	6	7	8	Not Stated
					Percent					
Total	7.4	7.7	6.7	7.4	8.1	8.5	9.1	8.9	9.1	8.3
Under 15	15.8	15.5	*	*	*	—	—	—	—	*
15-19	10.0	9.2	12.3	15.9	20.5	*	*	*	*	10.7
20-24	7.1	6.6	6.6	8.9	11.2	12.5	14.7	14.8	*	7.2
25-29	6.1	6.3	5.2	6.3	7.5	8.7	10.0	10.5	13.2	6.8
30-34	6.9	8.3	6.1	6.0	6.9	7.7	8.3	8.4	9.5	8.1
35-39	8.2	11.7	8.0	8.1	7.4	7.4	8.4	7.9	8.1	9.0
40-44	9.5	13.6	10.7	8.8	9.1	8.7	9.0	10.0	8.7	*
45-49	9.9	*	*	*	*	*	*	*	8.8	*
White	6.3	6.5	5.7	6.3	7.0	7.4	7.7	7.4	7.3	6.7
Under 15	12.9	12.6	*	*	*	—	—	—	—	*
15-19	8.1	7.6	9.9	13.1	15.8	*	*	*	*	8.4
20-24	6.0	5.8	5.6	7.4	8.9	10.6	11.6	*	*	5.7
25-29	5.5	5.8	4.7	5.6	6.8	7.6	8.2	8.0	10.1	6.3
30-34	6.2	7.6	5.5	5.4	6.3	7.0	7.2	6.9	7.6	7.3
35-39	7.3	10.6	7.0	7.4	6.8	6.6	7.5	6.7	6.5	7.3
40-44	8.5	12.1	10.0	7.8	8.7	7.9	8.0	9.0	7.5	*
45-49	9.7	*	*	*	*	*	*	*	*	*
Other	12.4	12.6	12.0	12.3	12.4	12.1	12.9	12.4	12.0	13.4
Under 15	17.7	17.5	*	*	*	—	—	—	—	*
15-19	14.4	13.4	16.4	18.6	23.3	*	*	*	*	14.8
20-24	12.0	11.4	11.5	12.7	14.7	14.5	17.2	*	*	13.1
25-29	10.4	10.5	9.0	10.8	10.6	11.5	13.1	13.7	16.4	9.5
30-34	10.9	12.1	10.2	10.1	10.7	11.1	11.5	11.5	12.1	11.6
35-39	12.1	17.7	12.5	11.9	11.0	11.6	12.1	11.4	11.2	*
40-44	13.1	*	*	*	11.2	*	13.8	13.7	11.4	*
45-49	10.8	*	*	*	*	*	*	*	*	*

* Ratio not computed; based on less than 500 live births with birth weight stated.
Source: Unpublished data from the National Center for Health Statistics.

Table 5. Distribution of Live Births by Birth Weight and Color: United States, 1968 and 1974 (Excludes birth weight not stated)

Birth weight (gm.)	Total		White		Negro and all other		Negro	All other
	1968	1974	1968	1974	1968	1974	1974	1974
			Percentage Distribution					
Total	100.0	100.0	100.0	100.0	100.0	100.0	100.0	100.0
2,500 or less	8.2	7.4	7.1	6.3	13.7	12.4	13.1	7.3
2,501 or more	91.8	92.6	92.9	93.7	86.3	87.6	86.9	92.7
500 or less	0.1	0.1	0.1	0.1	0.2	0.2	0.2	0.1
501–1,000	0.5	0.4	0.4	0.3	0.9	0.8	0.9	0.3
1,001–1,500	0.7	0.6	0.6	0.5	1.3	1.1	1.2	0.6
1,501–2,000	1.5	1.4	1.3	1.2	2.7	2.4	2.6	1.4
2,001–2,500	5.4	4.9	4.8	4.2	8.7	7.8	8.3	4.9
2,501–3,000	19.5	18.0	18.1	16.4	26.4	25.1	25.7	21.0
3,001–3,500	38.5	38.1	38.7	37.9	37.6	38.9	38.5	41.1
3,501–4,000	25.6	27.3	27.3	29.2	17.6	18.9	18.2	23.9
4,001–4,500	6.8	7.6	7.4	8.5	3.8	3.9	3.7	5.5
4,501–5,000	1.2	1.4	1.3	1.5	0.7	0.7	0.6	1.0
5,001 or more	0.2	0.2	0.2	0.2	0.1	0.1	0.1	0.1

these weight levels, the proportion of infants remained unchanged between 1968 and 1974.

Maternal Age and Legitimacy

Low birth weight ratios are shown in Table 6 for maternal age groups for 1967 and 1974. The more recent data provide information for some maternal age groups which were not available for 1967. Low birth weight ratios were higher among illegitimate than legitimate births in 1974 for almost every maternal age category of both White and Negro infants; the two exceptions were White and Negro infants whose mothers were 15 years of age. Insofar as the period between 1967 and 1974 was concerned, the low birth weight ratios declined throughout the age groups which are shown.

INFANT AND NEONATAL MORTALITY

The inverse relationship between birth weight and infant or neonatal mortality is established and well known. Both infant and neonatal mortality decrease as birth weight increases, except for an elevation in the birth weight groups of 4001 gm. or more. Mortality data by birth weight are available only for periods when birth and infant death records are linked, and the most recent complete national data are those for 1960. Neonatal mortality among infants who weighed 2500 gm. or less was over 30 times that of other infants in the 1960 national study (Chase, 1972).

Changing Demographic Trends and Mortality

Since 1950, the racial composition of live births has been changing. The racial group with a particularly high proportion of low birth weight infants is the Negro group. As a proportion of all live born infants, Negro babies increased from 13.1 to 16.0% between 1950 and 1974.

The changes according to plurality or sex at birth have been minor and would have had little effect on mortality had these been the only ones which occurred.

The data showed an increasing proportion of live births with gestations of 41 weeks or more, but this observation was difficult to assess. If the shift was real, it should have contributed to the decline in the low birth weight ratio and would have been reflected in lowered infant and neonatal mortality.

Estimates have been made of the reduction in infant mortality associated with the changes in the maternal age/birth order distributions which have been altered markedly by family planning practices (Wright 1972; Morris, Udry and Chase, 1975). For the period 1965–1972, it was estimated that about one-fourth of the decline in infant mortality was associated with the changing maternal age/birth order distribution, and could be attributable to family planning practices. This assessment must be interpreted with caution, however, since maternal age and birth order were the only variables considered in the adjustment.

Table 6. Low Birth Weight Ratios Among Live Births by Race, Age of Mother and Legitimacy Status: Reporting states, 1967 and 1974 (Excludes birth weight not stated)

Race and age of mother (years)	Total		Legitimate		Illegitimate	
	1967	1974	1967	1974	1967	1974
	Percent					
All races	8.2	7.5	7.6	6.7	13.6	12.9
Under 15	18.1	15.6	14.0	12.9	19.0	16.1
15–19	10.5	10.1	9.4	8.5	13.8	13.0
15	—	12.8	—	11.5	—	13.5
16	—	11.8	—	10.1	—	13.3
17	—	10.5	—	9.0	—	12.8
18	—	10.0	—	8.5	—	13.2
19	—	8.7	—	7.6	—	12.5
20–24	7.6	7.1	7.1	6.4	12.5	12.3
25–29	7.1	6.2	6.9	5.8	12.9	12.8
30–34	7.8	6.9	7.5	6.5	14.8	13.9
35 and over	8.9	8.5	8.5	8.1	16.2	14.2
35–39	—	8.2	—	7.7	—	14.5
40–44	—	9.6	—	9.3	—	13.8
45–49	—	10.4	—	10.9	—	*
White	7.0	6.3	6.8	6.1	10.2	10.1
Under 15	13.5	12.9	14.8	12.4	12.6	13.2
15–19	8.5	8.2	8.3	7.8	9.5	9.9
15	—	10.4	—	10.7	—	10.2
16	—	9.7	—	9.5	—	10.0
17	—	8.6	—	8.4	—	9.6
18	—	8.2	—	7.8	—	10.3
19	—	7.2	—	6.8	—	9.4
20–24	6.6	6.0	6.4	5.8	9.9	9.6
25–29	6.4	5.5	6.3	5.4	10.6	10.2
30–34	6.8	6.1	6.7	6.0	12.4	11.8
35 and over	8.0	7.6	7.9	7.4	16.2	12.8
35–39	—	7.3	—	7.1	—	12.9
40–44	—	8.8	—	8.6	—	13.0
45–49	—	9.9	—	9.9	—	*

Table 6. (Continued)

Race, and age (years) of mother	Total		Legitimate		Illegitimate	
	1967	1974	1967	1974	1967	1974
Negro	13.9	13.2	12.8	11.6	16.0	14.9
Under 15	20.2	17.4	*	*	20.7	17.4
15–19	15.9	14.8	15.0	13.9	16.5	15.1
15	—	15.7	—	18.5	—	15.5
16	—	15.6	—	15.2	—	15.6
17	—	14.8	—	14.6	—	14.9
18	—	14.8	—	14.0	—	15.2
19	—	13.9	—	12.9	—	14.6
20–24	13.3	12.6	12.6	11.4	14.9	14.2
25–29	12.4	11.6	11.8	10.5	14.7	14.7
30–34	12.8	12.2	12.1	11.2	16.3	15.4
35 and over	12.9	12.7	12.3	11.0	16.1	15.5
35–39	—	12.6	—	11.6	—	15.9
40–44	—	13.1	—	12.6	—	14.8
45–49	—	11.5	—	*	—	*

* Ratio not computed; based on less than 200 live births with birth weight stated.

Source: U.S. Dept. of Health, Education and Welfare: Trends in Low Birth Weight Ratios, United States and Each State, 1950–68, and unpublished data from the National Center for Health Statistics.

Note: Includes states reporting legitimacy: 34 States and District of Columbia in 1967, and 38 States and District of Columbia in 1974

Changes in the birth weight distribution also have a potential for reducing neonatal and infant mortality. As was noted earlier, during the period 1960 throughout 1974, the low birth weight ratio increased from 7.7 in 1960 to 8.3 in 1965–66 and decreased to 7.4 in 1974 (Fig. 3). Over the same period, infant mortality declined from 26.0 to 16.7 and neonatal mortality declined from 18.7 to 12.3 per 1000 live births. It is obvious that both infant and neonatal mortality have been declining more rapidly than the low birth weight ratio. These relationships, too, must be regarded with caution for they do not include other relevant factors such as gestation, maternal age or birth order.

To estimate the possible effect of the changing color/birth weight distributions, the cohort neonatal mortality rates for 1960 (Chase, 1972) were applied to the basic live birth distributions in 1968 and 1974 by color and weight (in 500 gm. groups):

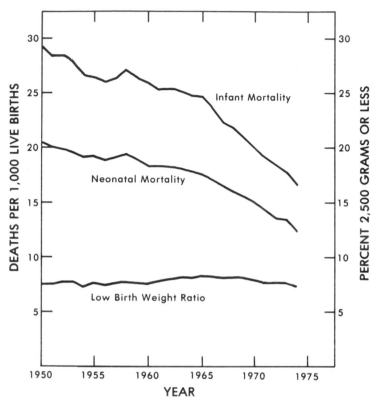

Figure 3. **Infant and Neonatal Mortality, and Low Birth Weight Ratios Among Live Births: United States, 1950–74.**

	Neonatal mortality		
	1960 live birth cohort	*1968*	*1974*
Actual	18.4	16.1	12.3
Estimated	18.4	18.6	16.7

The actual reduction in neonatal mortality was sizable in contrast to the smaller changes suggested in the estimated rates, had weight-specific mortality remained constant and had the color/birth weight distributions changed as they did over the interval between 1960 and 1974. The changes in the color/birth weight distributions, therefore, could account for little of the actual decline in the overall national neonatal mortality rates. These associations must also be regarded with caution since color and birth weight were the only variables considered in the adjustment.

In summary, it seems that, within the limits of the available data, the greatest contribution to the decline in infant mortality in the latter half of the 1960s and the early part of the 1970s was associated with changing maternal age/birth order distributions, but these changes may have accounted for only about one-fourth of the decline. The adjustment procedures have suggested the magnitude of the changes which could have been associated with alterations in some of the basic characteristics. However, the adjustments do not take into account the decreases in mortality in specific subgroups for which data are lacking. Since the most recent comprehensive study of infant mortality at the national level was for 1960, the existing data are now 16-years old. There is a need for more current national data from linked birth and infant death records.

International Standings

Despite the decreases in infant mortality since 1960, the position of the rate of the United States relative to that of other countries remains essentially unchanged. The ranking prepared by the National Center for Health Statistics for 1973 shows the rate for the United States (17.6) as 15th. If the data for the United States were limited to White infants (14.8 per 1000), the country's rank would be 8th. Thus, while the exclusion of Other-than-white births makes a significant difference in the ranking of the United States, one cannot explain away the differences between the US and other lower ranked countries on the basis of racial composition alone. The lowest infant mortality rate in the ranking, that of 9.6 for Sweden, suggests that despite the salutary progress which has been made in reducing infant mortality in the United States, attainable goals still remain to be achieved.

CONCLUSION

Since 1960, there have been a number of important demographic changes with regard to births in the United States. There has been a marked decrease of about one-fourth in the number of live births. The proportion of White infants has fallen; among remaining births, the proportion of Negro infants has also fallen and that of births in the "All others" category has increased. There was a suggested shift toward longer gestation periods and a lesser shift toward heavier birth weight categories. Changes in plurality were relatively minor. There was no discernible trend in the sex distribution at birth.

During the same interval, infant and neonatal mortality declined markedly. Changes in the maternal age/birth order distributions may have been associated with about one-fourth of the decline, and changes in the color/birth weight distributions appeared to have had a lesser effect. This assessment leaves unexplained the major part of the decrease in infant or neonatal mortality between 1960 and the present, and this decline may represent true reductions in mortality within specific subgroups. To evaluate the changes in infant and neonatal mortality since 1960 in a comprehensive fashion, current data from linked live birth and infant death records are needed.

Although the decreases in infant and neonatal mortality since 1960 have been significant, and the present infant mortality in the United States is the lowest it has ever been, data from other advanced countries indicate that attainable goals still remain to be achieved.

TEXT REFERENCES

American Medical Association: Proceedings of the House of Delegates, June 20–24, 1971. Section J, Centralized Community and Regionalized Pertinatal Intensive Care. American Medical Association, Chicago, 1971

Chase, H. C.; Byrnes, M. A.: Trends in "Prematurity," United States, 1950–67. U.S. Department of Health, Education and Welfare, DHEW Publication No. (HSM) 72-1030, Rockville, Md., 1972

Chase, H. C.: Comparison of Neonatal Mortality from Two Cohort Studies. U.S. Department of Health, Education, and Welfare, DHEW Publication No. (HSM) 72-1056, Rockville, Md., 1972

Chase, H. C.: Trends in Low Birth Weight Ratios, Each State and the United States, 1950–68. U.S. Department of Health, Education and Welfare, DHEW Publication No. (HSM) 73-5117, Rockville, Md., 1973

Morris, N. M.; Udry, J. R.; Chase, C. L.: Shifting Age-Parity Distribution of Births and the Decrease in Infant Mortality. Am J Publ Health 65(1975)359–362

National Academy of Sciences: Maternal Nutrition and the Course of Pregnancy. Report of the Committee on Maternal Nutrition, National Research Council, Washington, D.C., 1970

Shapiro, S.; Schlesinger, E. R.; Nesbitt, R. E. L., Jr.: Infant, Perinatal, Maternal, and Childhood Mortality in the United States. Harvard University Press, Cambridge, Mass. 1968 U.S. Department of Agriculture, Food and Nutrition Service: Food and Nutrition, 1973

U.S. Department of Health, Education, and Welfare, Center for Disease Control: Abortion Surveillance, Annual Summary, 1974. DHEW Publication No. (CDC) 76-8276, Atlanta, Ga., 1976

U.S. Department of Health, Education, and Welfare, National Center for Health Statistics: Provisional Data from the National Reporting System for Family Planning Services, Rockville, Md., various years

Wright, N. H.: Some Estimates of the Potential Reductions in the United States Infant Mortality Rate by Family Planning. Am J Publ Health 62(1972)1130–1134

DISCUSSION

Dr. Reed: Your graphs show that the curve for low birth weight was very flat from 1950 to 1968. In 1968 it started to drop dramatically for non-whites and slightly for whites. I wondered if you have any ideas about what happened?

Dr. Chase: There were a number of things that were changing and we don't have data on all of them. Consequently, when we look at low birth weight or infant mortality, which are single-end points reflecting perhaps six or eight or ten different factors which have been changing along the line, we really can't separate the independent factors very well.

Take improved nutrition, for example. We hear about the food stamp programs. We know that there have been programs specifically aimed at women, infants and children. What has the impact been in terms of different states in the United States, and which groups were really affected the most? For example, did they affect the lower-level white group as much as they affected the non-white group? We are just not in a position to answer questions like that.

Dr. Rush: I think that the great tragedy of this is that we don't know and that the nature of our epidemiologic enterprise has been a lot of observational speculation without the sort of expensive and tedious intervention studies that are necessary to formulate this into policy.

Dr. Susser: There may be another approach. Harvey Brenner has related mental hospital admissions and various mortality rates to national economic indices, and this work looks promising. It is obviously a complex statistical enterprise, but it seems to me we have had a number of indices and time-defined interventions over the last 15 years that might be added into analyses of this kind and could give us some leads.

Dr. Stein: Also, I am sure that Dr. Chase has data to show the changes in rates of low birth weight between 1968 and 1974 that take into consideration changes in the child bearing populations arising from family planning and induced abortion, putting these together with demographic factors like race, parity and age, since each of these things predict birth weight. These patterns surely have changed with family planning and induced abortion.

One really wants to see now what the low birth weight rate is inside specific groups, I think.

Dr. Baird: The number of deaths contributed by women having a fourth or later pregnancy has fallen to one-third of that of 10 years ago because families are now much smaller. The death rate in fourth or later pregnancies has risen because a majority of the women have had previous abortions or perinatal deaths and are attempting to complete their families of 2 or 3 children, but they are obviously high risk cases. On the other hand, when families were large a majority of the women had a very good past obstetric history and perinatal death rates were low.

Dr. Terris: I would like to back up what Dave Rush said about the difficulties of observational studies, or rather observational non-studies, because what Brenner does and what we have been talking about is trying to look at it after the fact. One of the difficulties is illustrated by the fact that, as we all know, the US infant mortality rate reached a plateau for a number of years and now it is back down again, for reasons which none of us understand.

Now, we think it might be family planning, it might be abortion, it might be this, or it might be that. But we really have no idea, no way of knowing, and to illustrate that, take a look at Europe. In Europe those rates, as far as I know, just kept going right on down without family planning programs, without sudden abortion programs, and so on. So we are stuck when we do these observational studies, and we have to go to a more intensive experimental approach, perhaps, to try to get at what is causing the change.

Did you get a chance to look at the rates among the American Indians? There was once a very provocative paper presented at APHA indicating that the rates in American Indians were extremely low. If that is so, that leads to a good deal of interesting speculation.

Dr. Chase: The data were surprising. The postneonatal mortality rates were high, and the neonatal rates were very low. As a statistician, I worried about statistical artifacts and incomplete registration of early neonatal deaths. For example, the 1960 national linked infant mortality study showed the highest rates of linkage failure in states with high proportions of Indian births. I asked several people who worked on the Indian reservations about this. When I talked to physicians stationed at Indian hospitals, I was told that all of the births occur in hospitals so the rates have to be valid. When I talked to public health nurses, some of whom still went out on horseback, their story was that the Indian women tended to hide their pregnancies, and the nurses felt that the neonatal deaths which occurred soon after birth and outside hospitals could be underreported. In an area like the Indian desert reservations, one is apt not to get very complete reporting, especially if the women are not close to hospitals. So I have not completely accepted the relationship between the low neonatal mortality and high postneonatal mortality among Indian infants which is suggested by the vital statistics data.

Dr. Rush: There is a coherent explanation for the seeming paradox. The postneonatal mortality rate almost always reflects the level of available public health and medical services. With better nutrition, clean water supply and control and treatment of infection, postneonatal rates will fall, and they are thus a good index of the status of social and health services.

Neonatal mortality rates, on the other hand, are little affected by health services, but rather reflect birth weight and are thus associated with those factors which determine birth weight. There are many independent reports on the high birth weight of American Indians (e.g., Rosa and Resnick, 1965). Since American Indians, compared to other Americans, are economically deprived and of short stature, their high birth weight is almost surely of genetic origin. Similarly, Fijians have higher birth weight than Asiatic Indians living in Fiji and also lower neonatal mortality, while the postneonatal mortality rates of the two groups more accurately reflect their relative economic status (Rosa, 1974).

The disparity is consistent with data on American urban-rural differences: rates of low birth weight and neonatal mortality tend to be lower in rural areas, while postneonatal mortality rates are higher than in urban areas, probably because of less access to preventive and curative health services.

Dr. Kass: We can now identify in carefully studied American populations about seven variables that have been shown to affect significantly the birth weight. Although the variables do not affect mortality in exactly the same order, the same ones tend to appear. Maternal weight, smoking, blood pressure, race and past reproductive history are the recurrent factors, although all together they predict only a minority of early deliveries.

More recently, we have evidence that the presence of two mycoplasmas adds significantly to the previous variables. In those people who have infected urinary tracts, there is now little doubt that clinical pyelonephritis adds significantly both to the lowered birth rate and to infant mortality. Dr. Sever will have more data about this later.

DISCUSSION REFERENCES

Rosa, F. W.: Birth Weight in Fiji and Western Samoa: A Pacific Prescription for Pregnancy? AM J Obstet Gynec 119(1974)1121-1124

Rosa, F.; Resnick, L.: Birth Weight and Perinatal Mortality in the American Indian. Am J Obstet Gynec 91 (1965)972-976

Worldwide Variations in Low Birth Weight

Rosanne Boldman, M.P.H.
Dwayne M. Reed, M.D., Ph.D.

The geographic distribution of disease has exercised a fascination for researchers for many generations, with some considering the *Handbook of Geographical and Historical Pathology,* published in 1850, to be a forerunner of the systematic discipline of epidemiology. Part of our interest in observing how diseases are distributed internationally relates to the belief that the observed patterns contain clues to the nature of the disease process and any adverse environmental factors involved.

The purpose of this investigation was to collect the available information concerning the worldwide frequencies of prematurity, to examine the data for meaningful patterns and to learn if there were any associations with some general indicators of economic and social conditions.

METHODS

For the purposes of this report, we used the low birth weight (LBW) ratio (the percentage of all live births weighing 2500 gm. or less) as the measure of "prematurity." As there is no standard international publication of LBW frequencies, all ratios used here were obtained from a search of the available literature (see appendix).

In selecting some indicator variables of economic and social conditions of the different countries, we followed the guidelines suggested by

Shin (1975) and selected six variables which were available for most of the countries involved. These were:

1. Per capita national income, as a reflection of the standard of living, availability of regular food supplies and level of environmental sanitation.

2. Per capita energy consumption, as an indicator of the level of industrialization.

3. Daily newspaper circulation per 1000 population, as a measure of the level of literacy and the availability of education.

4. Population per physician, as an indicator of the availability of health care services.

5. Percent of the population living in urban places, as an indicator of the development of a society from traditional to modern ways of life.

6. Radio and TV receivers per 1000 population, as an indicator of the level of economic development.

All these data were obtained from the United Nations Demographic series (1974), the United Nations *Statistical Yearbook* (1971), the *World Bank Atlas* (1974), Quinn (1972 and 1974), the National Center for Health Statistics' *Infant Mortality Trends* (1965), and Davis (1969).

Table 1 shows the LBW ratios by geographic area and time period. There was a great range of LBW values, from 4.1% in Sweden to 45% in India; however, the values were between 4 and 10% for 34 (68%) of the 50 countries and territories. Only India, Burma, Singapore and Papua, New Guinea had values over 20%.

The highest LBW ratios were in Asia with the available values generally exceeding 20%, followed by Africa and the Middle East with ratios between 10 and 20% and the Americas with ratios of between 6 and 13%. Europe had consistently low values, nearly all of which were less than 10%. There were no obvious associations with latitude and longitude. Of 21 countries with values available over time, 19 had ratios which were quite steady, while only two (Italy and parts of India) showed any dramatic change.

One question which arose in making these comparisons of different countries was that of whether the LBW ratio was related to racial characteristics. We cannot answer such a question with this type of observation. While searching for reports from different countries, we did come across figures showing that persons of the same racial group can have quite different ratios in different areas. For example, the ratios for Chinese were 16.6% in Malaya (Terris, 1966), 11% in Singapore (Millis, 1958), 7.3% in Hawaii (Terris, 1966) and 4% in New Guinea (Jansen, 1962). For Indians the ratios varied from 8% to 45% in India.

In order to look for associations between LBW ratios and environmental indicators of economic and social conditions, the mean LBW

Table 1. Low Birth Weight Ratios (percentage of live births under 2500 gm.) By Geographical Area and Time.*

Country	Area	before 1940	1940-1949	1950-1959	1960-1969	1970-1976
AFRICA						
Congo (Zaire)	All				10.0-24.4	
Ethiopia	All				16.5	8.8-16.5
Nigeria	Lagos	13.0				
Rhodesia	All			16.6	11.0	
Sudan	All				17.3	
Tanzania	Dar Es Salaam			5-7		
	Tanganyika			15.6		
	Sumve			14.0		
U. of S. Africa	All			11.5	8.2-16.0	
ASIA						
Burma	Rangoon			25.0		
China	All			11.3		
	Canton	14.0				
Fed. of Malaysia	Singapore			21.0	16.8	
India	Andhra (Conoor)			38.4		
	New Delhi			29.0	40.0	
	Maharashtra (Bombay)			37.0		
	Tamilnadu (Madras)		8.1			
	Utter Pradesh (Agra)				26.0	
	Utter Pradesh (Kanpur)				45.0	
	West Bengal (Calcutta)			34.7		
Japan	All			8.0	11.3	5.3
Korea	All				10.0	

Table 1. Low Birth Weight Ratios (percentage of live births under 2500 gm.) By Geographical Area and Time.* (Cont'd)

Country	Area	before 1940	1940–1949	1950–1959	1960–1969	1970–1976
AMERICA						
Canada	All					6.3
U.S.A.	All			7.8		7.5
	Total White			6.9	7.0	6.4
	Total Non-White			11.6	12.5	12.5
	Total Indian				6.0	
Guatemala	All				13.3	
Mexico	Mexico City			11.0		
Jamaica	Kingston				11.0	
Puerto Rico	All			8.9	9.8	9.2–9.4
Virgin Islands	All			8.8	10.5	
Brazil	Ribeirao Preto					
Dutch Guiana (Surinam)	Stoelmanseiland			12.0	8.0	
Venezuela	All				7.9	
EUROPE						
Austria	All				6.0	
Czechoslovakia	All			6–7	6.0	
Denmark	All			4.6	5.6	
East Germany	All			6–7	5.8	
Finland	All	10–12			4.7	
	Helsinki		5.6			
France	All				9.5	
Greece	All				10.2	
Hungary	All				5.1	
Italy	All			17.0	5.9	
Ireland	North					
Netherlands	All				5.5	

Country	Area							
Norway	All							
	Oslo	7.3					5.2	4.9
Poland	All						5.8	
Scotland	Edinburgh				6.7	6.6		
	Aberdeen				6.4–7.6		6.0–7.1	
Sweden	All		5–6	7.6			4.9	4.1
United Kingdom	England and Wales				4.8			
	Great Britain			6.4	6.7		6.2–7.4	6.5
	Middlesex County			5.7			7.5	
	Birmingham			5.4				
Yugoslavia	Bosnia & Herzegovina						7.6	
	Montenegro						5.1	
	Croatia						7.1	
	Macedonia						7.5	
	Slovenia						6.1	

MIDDLE AND NEAR EAST

Country	Area							
Iran	All						14.2	
Israel	All						5.5	
Lebanon	All						7.4–11.9	
Syria	All						19.9	

OCEANIA

Country	Area							
Australia	Queensland						6.4	
	New South Wales (Sydney)					7.5		
Guam	All				8.2			
Hawaii	All						8.8	8.3–9.7
New Zealand	All		5.6					
Papua, New Guinea	New Britain Islands				15.0			
	New Ireland				30.0			
Phillipines							14.2	

*If more than one ratio was available for an area during any given decade, the range is shown.

ratios were calculated for each of the various indicator variables. This information was available for only 39 countries (Fig. 1).

As shown in Figure 1, those countries with high levels of urbanization, per capita income and per capita energy consumption had lower mean LBW ratios. The same inverse relation existed for newspaper circulation and radio and TV receivers per 1000 population, down to a LBW ratio of 7%. The relationship between percent low birth weight and population per physician was direct, that is, the ratios increased as there were more people to share the medical services.

Statistical correlations of LBW ratios with the indicator variables for 21 countries are shown in Table 2. LBW ratios were significantly correlated (coefficient exceeding ± 0.4) with each of the independent variables. An examination of the correlation matrix suggested that the indicator variables were also highly correlated with each other. This was further evident when the partial correlations were computed with the effect of per capita income removed, as shown in the second column of Table 2.

In a stepwise regression, per capita income was selected initially and contributed 70% of the total observed variability. Adding in population per physician increased the multiple correlation to 74%. No remaining variable could further increase the multiple correlation.

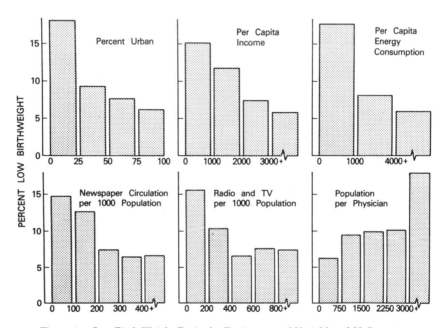

Figure 1.   **Low Birth Weight Ratios by Environmental Variables of 39 Countries.**

Table 2.   Correlation of Low Birth Weight* With Environmental Variables of 21 Countries.

Variables	Zero Order Correlations	Partial Correlations (income)
Percent Urban	− 0.78	− 0.14
Per Capita Income	− 0.84	−
Per Capita Energy Use*	− 0.83	− 0.24
Newspaper Circ./1000 Pop.	− 0.70	− 0.06
Physician/1000 Pop.*	− 0.82	− 0.35
Radio & TV/1000 Pop.*	− 0.77	− 0.25

*Log or Logit transformations were performed to reduce kurtosis (long tail distribution).

CONCLUSION

There are many problems associated with this indirect approach to examining the worldwide variations in LBW ratios. The differences in quality of health facilities influence the reliability and the completeness of the data, and the indicator variables are crude measures which are difficult to relate to biologic phenomena. Despite these problems, patterns of LBW ratios and implications do emerge.

The great variations in LBW ratios among different areas and the variations in ratios among single racial groups living in different areas indicate that, despite genetic variability, the causes of LBW are embedded in the environment. The association of LBW ratios with crude indicators of economic and industrial development and education suggests that the differences have resulted from factors controlling socio-economic development rather than specific efforts aimed at the control of prematurity. Indeed, to a large extent it is difficult to explain how these changes came about.

An ecologist (Stallones, 1971) would say that income, food supplies, sanitation, industrialization, education, urbanization, social customs and medical care systems all interact with each other, and that these interactions determine how much prematurity there will be.

This notion that great changes in the risk of LBW have occurred through the operation of factors which could potentially be influenced by us opens the door to a different approach to prevention. Certainly we cannot ignore the usefulness of specific therapeutic measures. We should, however, also concern ourselves with gaining a deeper appreciation of the clusters and combinations of the environmental experiences which relate to prematurity. An understanding of these factors and their modes of interaction may offer us a new means of disease control.

Acknowledgements

We wish to acknowledge the assistance of Howard Hoffman and Ernest Harley in the analysis of the data.

APPENDIX

AFRICA

Congo (Zaire)	Rosa (1970)
Ethiopia	Tafari and Sterky (1974)
	Höjer (1972)
	Rosa (1970)
Nigeria	Meredith (1970)
Rhodesia	McLaren (1959)
	Houghton and Ross (1953)
	Rosa (1970)
Sudan	Rosa (1970)
Tanzania	Ebrahim and D'sa (1966)
	Oomen and Smulders (1960)
	McLaren (1959)
Union of South Africa	Salber (1955)
	Rosa (1970)

ASIA

Burma	Postmus (1958)
China	Uttley (1940)
	Rosa (1970)
Federation of Malaysia	Millis (1958)
	Rosa (1970)
India	Terris (1966)
	Gosh and Beri (1962)
	Walia et al. (1963)
	Saigal and Srivastava (1969)
	Basavarajappa, Deshpande and Ramachandran (1962)
	Kalra, Kishone and Dayal (1967)
	Verhoestraete and Puffer (1958)
	Chaudhuri (1955)
	Meredith (1970)
Japan	Meredith (1970)
	Pharoah (1976)

	Rosa (1970)
Korea	Kang and Cho (1962)

AMERICA

Canada	Vital Statistics, Canada (1973, 1974)
U.S.A.	Chase and Byrnes (1970)
	Wallace (1970)
	US D.H.E.W. (1970-73)
Guatemala	Rosa (1970)
Mexico	Torregrosa, Nieto and Montemayor (1960)
Jamaica	Grantham, Desai and Back (1972)
Puerto Rico	US D.H.E.W. (1955, 1965, 1970-74)
Virgin Islands	US D.H.E.W. (1955, 1965, 1970-74)
Brazil	Woiski et al. (1965)
Dutch Guiana	Doornbos, Jonxis and Visser (1968)
(Surinam)	
Venezuela	Rosa (1970)

EUROPE

Austria	Czeizel et al. (1970)
Czechoslovakia	Czeizel et al. (1970)
	Fraccaro (1958)
Denmark	Czeizel et al. (1970)
	Verhoestraete and Puffer (1958)
	Dawson (1946)
East Germany	Czeizel et al. (1970)
	Meredith (1970)
Finland	Räihä (1947)
	Pharoah (1976)
	Official Statistics of Finland (1967-1968)
France	Meredith (1970)
Greece	Rosa (1970)
Hungary	Czeizel et al. (1970)
Italy	Czeizel et al. (1970)
	Meredith (1970)
North Ireland	Rosa (1970)
Netherlands	National Center for Health Statistics (1967)
Norway	Medical Birth Registry of Norway (1976)
	Blegen (1953)
Poland	Meredith (1970)
	Czeizel et al. (1970)

Scotland	Drillen and Richmond (1956)
	Baird (1974)
	Terris (1966)
Sweden	Meredith (1970)
	Czeizel et al. (1970)
	Hedberg and Holmdahl (1970)
	Pharoah (1976)
United Kingdom	Czeizel et al. (1970)
	Ashford, Read and Riley (1973)
	National Center for Health Statistics (1965)
	National Center for Health Statistics (1967)
	Meredith (1970)
	Blegen (1953)
	Pharoah (1976)
	United Nations Scientific Committee on Effects of Atomic Radiation (1962)
Yugoslavia	Czeizel et al. (1970)

MIDDLE AND NEAR EAST

Iran	Rosa (1970)
Israel	Grossman, Handlesman and Davies (1974)
Lebanon	Rosa (1970)
Syria	Rosa (1970)

OCEANIA

Australia	Dugdale (1968)
	Stevens and Cope (1965)
Guam	US D.H.E.W. (1970, 1973, 1974)
Hawaii	Chase (1973)
New Zealand	Dawson (1946)
	Rose (1964)
	Verhoestraete and Puffer (1958)
Papua, New Guinea	Meredith (1970)
Phillipines	Rosa (1970)

TEXT REFERENCES

Ashford, J. R.; Read, K. L. Q.; Riley, V. C.: An Analysis of Variations in Perinatal Mortality Amongst Local Authorities in England and Wales. Int J Epid 2 (1973)31–46

Baird, D.: The Epidemiology of Low Birth

Weight: Changes in Incidence in Aberdeen, 1948-72. J Biosoc Sci 6(1974)323-341

Basavarajappa, K. G.; Deshpande, V. A.; Ramachandran,: Effect of Sex, Maternal Age, Birth Order, and Socioeconomic Status on Birth Weight of Live Born Infants. Indian J Public Health 1(1962)18-27

Blegen, S. D.: The Premature Child. Acta Paediat 42(1953)Suppl. 88

Chase, H. C.: Trends in Low Birth Weight Ratios, Each State and the United States, 1950-1968. U.S. Department of Health, Education and Welfare, DHEW Publication No. (HSM)73-5117, Rockville, Md., 1973.

Chase, H. C.; Byrnes, M. E.: Trends in "Prematurity": United States, 1950-1967. Am J Public Health 60(1970)1967-1983

Chaudhuri, A.: Mortality Rate and its Relation to Maturity Weight Level. Indian J Paediatr 22(1955)145-154

Czeizel, A.; Bognar, Z.; Tusnady, G.; Revesz, P.: Changes in Mean Birth Weight and Proportion of Low-Weight Births in Hungary. Br J Prev Soc Med 24(1970)146-153

Davis, K.: World Urbanization 1950-1970, Vol. I: Basic Data for Cities, Countries and Regions, Population Monograph Series No. 4, Institute of International Studies, University of California, Berkeley, 1969.

Dawson, J. B.: Obstetrical Causes of Stillbirths and Neonatal Deaths. N Z MED J 45(1946)389-398

Doornbos, L.; Jonxis, J. H. P.; Visser, H. K. A.: Growth of Bushnegro Children on the Tapanahony River in Dutch Guiana. Human Biol 40(1968)396-415

Drillen, C.M.; Richmond, F.: Prematurity in Edinburgh. Arch Dis Child 81(1956)390-394

Dugdale, A.: Prematurity and its Outcome in Queensland. Med J of Australia 1(1968)1092-1095

Ebrahim, G. J.; D'sa, A.: Prematurity in Dar Es Salaam. J Trop Pediatr 12(1966)55-58

Fraccaro, M.: Data for Quantitative Genetics in Men: Birth Weight in Official Statistics. Human Biol 30(1958)142-149

Gosh, S.; Beri, S.: Standard of Prematurity for North Indian Babies. Indian J Child Hlth 11(1962)210-215

Grantham-McGregor, S. M.; Desai, P.; Back, E. H.: A Longitudinal Study of Infant Growth in Kingston, Jamaica. Human Biol 44(1972)549-561

Grossman, S.; Handlesman, Y.; Davies, A. M.: Birth Weight in Israel, 1968-70: I. Effects of Birth Order and Maternal Origin. J Biosoc Sci 6(1974)43-58

Hedberg, E.; Holmdahl, K.: On Relationship Between Maternal Health and Intrauterine Growth of the Foetus. Acta Obstet Gynec Scand 49(1970)225-229

Höjer, B.: Low Birth Weight Infants in Ethiopia. J Trop Pediatr, 18(1972)192-195

Houghton, J. W.; Rose, W. F.: Birth Weight and Prematurity Rates in Southern Rhodesia. Trans Royal Soc Trop Med and Hyg 47(1953)62-65

Jansen, A. A. J.: Birthweight, Birthlength, Prematurity and Neonatal Mortality in New Guineans. Trop Geogr Med, 14 (1962)341-349

Kalra, K.; Kishone, N.; Dayal, R. S.: Anthropometric Measurements in the Newborn: A Study of 1,000 Consecutive Livebirths. Indian J Pediatr 34(1967)73-82

Kang, Y. S.; Cho, W. K.: The Sex Ratio at Birth and Other Attributes of the Newborn from Maternity Hospitals in Korea. Human Biol 34(1962)38-48

McLaren, D. S.: Records of Birth Weight and Prematurity in the Wasukunia of Lake Province, Tanganyika. Trans Royal Soc Trop Med Hyg, 53(1959)173-178

Medical Birth Registry of Norway, Institute of Hygiene and Social Medicine, University of Bergen, unpublished data, 1976.

Meredith, H. V.: Body Weight at Birth of Viable Human Infants: A Worldwide Comparative Treatise. Human Biol 42 (1970)217-264

Millis, J.: Distribution of Birth Weights of Chinese and Indian Infants Born in Singapore: Birth Weight as an Index of Maturity. Ann Hum Genet 23(1958)164-170

National Center for Health Statistics: Infant Mortality Trends 1930-1964. Government Printing Office, Washington, DC, 1965

National Center for Health Statistics: Vital and Health Statistics, Series 3, No. 6, Government Printing Office, Washington, DC, 1967

Oomen, A. P.; Smulders, F.: Six Hundred African Prematures: A Review of the Conditions and the Results of Simple Treatment. Trop Geogr Med, 12(1960) 15-20

Pharoah, P. O. D.: International Comparisons of Perinatal and Infant Mortality Rates. Proc Royal Soc 69(1976)335-337

Postmus, S.: Beriberi of Mother and Child in Burma. Trop Geogr Med 10(1958) 363-370

Puffer, R. R.; Serrano, C. V.: Patterns of Mortality in Childhood. PAHO, Pan American Sanitary Bureau Regional Office of the World Health Organization, Scientific Publication No. 262, 1973.

Quinn, J. R.: China Medicine as We Saw It. Government Printing Office, Washington, DC, 1974

Quinn, J. R.: Medicine and Public Health in the People's Republic of China. Government Printing Office, Washington, DC, 1972

Räihä, C. E.: Incidence of Premature Births. Ann Med Int Fenniae. 36(1947) 619-629

Ann Med Int Fenniae. 36(1947)619-629

Report of the United Nations Scientific Committee on Effects of Atomic Radiation. Suppl. 16 (A/5216) Official Records of 17th session U.N. General Assembly, 1962.

Rosa, F. W.: International Aspects of Perinatal Mortality. In Clin. Obstet. Gynec., 13:1, 57-78 ed. by E. M. Gold, Harper and Row, New York 1970.

Rose, R. J.: Infant and Foetal Loss in New Zealand. New Zealand Department of Health, Special Report 17, 1964.

Saigal, S.; Srivastava, J. R.: Anthropometric Studies of 1,000 Consecutive Newborns with Special References to Determine Criteria of Prematurity. Indian Pediatr 6(1969)24-33

Salber, E. J.: The Significance of Birth Weight. J Trop Pediatr, 1(1955)54-56

Salber, E. J.; Bradshaw, E. S.: Birth Weight of South African Babies. Brit J Soc Med 5(1951)113-119

Shin, E. H.: Economic and Social Correlates of Infant Mortality: A Cross-sectional and Longitudinal Analysis of 63 Selected Countries. Soc Biol 22(1975) 315-325

Stallones, R. A.: Environment, Ecology and Epidemiology. Fourth PAHO/WHO Lecture on the Biomedical Sciences. Pan American Health Organization, Pan American Sanitary Bureau, Regional Office of the World Health Organization, 1971.

Stevens, L.; Cope, T.: Prematurity: Observations upon its Current Significance and Management. Med J Australia 1(1965) 1165-1172

Tafari, N.; Sterkey, G.: Early Discharge of Low Birth Weight Infants in a Developing Country. J Trop Pediatr 20(1974)73-76

The Official Statistics of Finland, 11. Public Health and Medical Care. 70;71, 1967-1968.

Terris, M.: The Epidemiology of Prematurity: Studies of Specific Etiologic Factors. In: Research Methodology and Needs in Perinatal Studies pp. 207-242, ed. by S. Chipman; A. Lilienfeld; A. Greenberg; J. Donnelly. Charles C. Thomas, Springfield, Ill., 1966.

Torregrosa, L. F.; Nieto, J. V.; Montemayor, F. G.: Somatometria del Recien Nacido. Ann Inst Nae Antrop Hist 11(1960)199-217

United Nations, Department of Economic and Social Affairs: Demographic Yearbook, 26th edition. New York, 1974.

United Nations, Department of Economic and Social Affairs: Statistical Yearbook, 23rd edition. New York, 1971.

U.S., Department of Health, Education and Welfare, P.H.S.: Vital Statistics of the U.S., Vol. II: Mortality, Part A., 1955, 1965, 1970, 1973, 1974.

U.S., Department of Health, Education and Welfare, P.H.S.: Vital Statistics of the U.S., Vol. I: Natality, 1955, 1965, 1970-1974.

Uttley, K. H.: The Birth Weight of Full Term Cantonese Babies. Chinese Med J 58(1940)582-591

Verhoestraete, L. J.; Puffer, R. R.: Challenge of Fetal Loss, Prematurity, and Infant Mortality-World View. JAMA 167 (1958)950-959

Vital Statistics, Canada. Catalog # 84-204, Vol. I-Births, 1973, 1974.

Walia, B. N. S.; Khetarpal, S. K.; Mehta, S.; Ghai, O. P.; Kapoor, P.; Taneja, P. N.: Observations on 1,000 Live-Born Infants. Indian J Child Health 12(1963) 243-249

Wallace, H. M.: Factors Associated with Perinatal Mortality and Morbidity. In: Clin. Obst. Gynec., 13:1, p. 13-43, ed by E. M. Gold, Harper and Row, New York, 1970.

Woiski, J. R.; Romera, J.; Correa, C. E. C.;

Raya, L. C.; Lima-Filho, E. C.: Indices Somaticos Dos Recem Nascidos Normais no Hospital das Clinicas de Ribeirao Preto. Rev Paul Med 66(1965)12–23

World Bank: World Bank Atlas: Population, Per Capita Product and Growth Rates. Washington, D.C., 1974.

DISCUSSION

Dr. Hardy: I was involved in a tangential way in a double blind nutrition study (unpublished work) which was carried out in a rural area in southeast Taiwan. I was amazed to find that the average birth weight in the study population was actually larger than the average birth weight in the Johns Hopkins Hospital in Baltimore.

I simply couldn't believe this and dug into the data and was left with the conclusion that the observation was correct. The prematurity rate in that same population was about 7%. However, when one came to examine the situation around Taipei, which is the big urban center, there was a very marked socioeconomic relationship with birth weight and with the frequency of prematurity. The point that I would make from this is that I am not sure how helpful it is to try to compare the overall results of one country with those of another.

I think that there is much to be learned about the factors which affect birth weight and perinatal mortality, but I think we are at the point where this knowledge must be gained by digging into the interrelationships between many factors, and a simplistic approach is not apt to be very helpful.

Dr. Rush: It is important, given the large amount of variance in birth weight that is contributed by inheritance, to look within ethnic and racial groups. Between-group comparisons that assume that groups differ only by environmental factors may lead to confusion.

Dr. Reed: If we look at another example, perhaps it will clarify our point. Mortality rates for tuberculosis dropped dramatically during the past century, long before we had any knowledge of the disease's etiology, treatment or prevention. We may deduce that the decline of this disease was in response to environmental changes that are even now not completely understood, but are usually considered to be general improvements in the quality of life. The use of this example is to call attention to the idea that a great deal of the burden of problems such as prematurity is part of the environmental situation, and to suggest that if we can gain a better understanding of the interrelatedness of these environmental determinants, we may develop more effective ways of prevention.

Dr. Kass: There is a huge difference between observing what has happened and being concerned about what accounts for it. Before we intervene, it is useful to know what the array of priorities is. There are some fairly strong suspicions that crowding and perhaps nutrition are two large variables, but these aren't worked out as precisely as one would like and intervention studies, too soon, may be doomed to failure.

Dr. Morton: Some of this variation is eliminated in Hawaii, where the Chinese infants weigh about 165 gm. less than the Caucasian infants. The prematurity rate, however, is lower, but I think this is to be anticipated because the Chinese are better educated and more affluent than the Caucasians.

Dr. Garn: I would like to point out that the data you have presented are susceptible to two equally good explanations, simultaneously. One, the degree to which they match the data provided by the National Cancer Institute, showing the relationship between per capita income and cancer, is very dramatic. At the same time, you can explain the data by assuming fairly reasonably that you had two populations: one of European ancestry, with higher birth weight and greater access to the world's "goodies," and the other, with lower birth weight and less access to the world's "goodies."

I think the opportunity here is to see the extent to which both explanations are operational and the extent to which both are separable.

Dr. Terris: I think that the work that Reed and Boldman have done is a further extension of something that we have known for 30 years. I would challenge the people who doubt the implications of this material and say there are different interpretations to be made. You will always get the same result, both within countries and between countries. This is a fact of life about prematurity.

I think the thing that was missed in the discussion is one which I consider very important, namely, the fact that they looked at the same ethnic groups in different situations and different countries. They gave you the data for Chinese living in four different places, with rates that varied from 4–16.6%, an enormous variation. The same is true for Indians in different parts of India, where the variation is even greater. Apparently two things are at work: there are genetic and very powerful environmental factors. This is what we are dealing with.

National Variations in Prematurity (1973 and 1974)

Margaret W. Pratt
Zelda L. Janus
Naresh C. Sayal

Dr. Chase has already presented data to you on trends in prematurity in the US as reflected in low birth weight ratios for various groups from 1950 to 1974. I will discuss with you the current status in the US of the problem of prematurity as reflected in the percentage of low weight births and its variations by geographic areas and by selected categories of characteristics of the mothers or infants.

As one would expect, the data used in this paper are from the Natality Files of the National Center for Health Statistics. Fortuitously in terms of this seminar, the Information Sciences Research Institute has a grant from the Bureau of Community Health Services which includes funds for acquiring and using natality and mortality data from NCHS for various research and program planning studies. Since early this year, the Maternal and Child Health Studies Project at the Institute has been collaborating with the University of California (Berkeley) School of Public Health, Maternal and Child Health Section on an analysis of the relationship of low weight births to other birth characteristics of such infants and their mothers. Most of the materials included in this discussion are preliminary data being analyzed in connection with that research study.

Supported, in part, by Grant No. MC-R-110387-01 from the Bureau of Community Health Services, HSA, Department of Health, Education and Welfare, Rockville, Maryland.

The materials to be presented will largely be information from the 1974 Natality Files on all live births and the 1973 total and single live births in the NCHS sample. The most detailed analyses of the relationship of low weight births to other birth characteristics of the infant and mother which I will present use the 1973 data. One purpose of the study now under way is to enable the low weight ratio for the US (or any area) to be a more meaningful number when examined by persons considering it (and other data) in connection with health problems and the health status of the population of an area.

Before I begin, I want to tell you that there will be different total numbers of low weight births on the various tables. They are the counts of single low weight births in the areas of the US which reported the data covered in the individual tables and, as a result of differences in reporting, these numbers will not be the same in all cases. The first seven tables and five figures will examine variations by selected characteristics of the mother or infant at the national level.

The basic picture of low weight births for all births and single births in the US is shown in Table 1. The staff at the Institute and our associates at BCHS often look at low weight percentages of all births in our materials developed for planning and program review, but for the study with Berkeley it was decided that only single births would be examined in detail. We believe, however, that it is useful to see how the two groups differ or are similar before proceeding with the use of the single-live birth group in our detailed analyses.

The basic distributions show that, as would be expected, the single births group has a slightly smaller proportion of low weight births than the total births group, with 6.6 low weight births per 100 live births in the former group compared with 7.5 low weight births per 100 live births in the latter group. In both groups, as is already known, low weight births among blacks are over twice the proportion of the white race percentage. The all other group (other than white or black) is small, and in both the total and single birth groups, the low weight ratio is virtually the same as the total low weight ratio. This probably would not be true in smaller areas.

Table 2 provides some information on the relationship of low weight births to gestational age. Although the data are limited to areas reporting on the last menstrual period, they include over 75% of all births, and the total percentages of low weight births by race (last 3 lines of the table) are virtually the same as the percentage totals shown in Table 1.

Table 3 shows a further breakdown of the percent of low weight single births by a somewhat more detailed set of low weight categories: under 1001 gm., 1001-1500 gm., 1501-2000 gm., 2001-2500 gm. and over 2501 gm. The major point seems to be that of the 6 to 7 low weight infants per 100 live single births, 4.5 are in the 2001-2500 gm. range

Table 1. 1973 Births: Total Live Births and Single Live Births by Weight Group and Race*

	All Births				Single Births			
		Distribution				Distribution		
Race	Number	<2501 Gms.	≥2501 Gms.	Not Stated	Number	<2501 Gms.	≥2501 Gms.	Not Stated
Total	3,136,965	7.5	92.2	0.3	3,079,244	6.6	93.1	0.3
White	2,551,030	6.4	93.3	0.3	2,505,833	5.6	94.2	0.3
Black	512,597	13.2	86.5	0.3	501,221	12.1	87.6	0.3
Other	73,338	7.5	92.2	0.3	72,190	6.7	93.0	0.3

*For this and subsequent tables in this chapter: Preliminary materials from a collaborative study of natality characteristics under preparation by Information Sciences Research Institute and University of California, Berkeley. Tables prepared by: Maternal and Child Health Studies Project, Information Sciences Research Institute, Washington, D.C., November 1976.

Table 2. 1973 Births: Percent of Live Births by Gestational Age and Birth Weight (All Births and Single Births) and Percent Difference Between Percent of Low Weight Births For All Births and Single Births (Refers only to births to residents occurring within areas reporting the last menstrual period)

Gestational Age (wks) and Race	All Births				Single Births				Percent Difference Between % Low Weight for All Births and % Low Weight for Single Births
	Total Number	Percent Distribution			Total Number	Percent Distribution			
		<2501 Gms.	≥2501 Gms.	Not Stated		<2501 Gms.	≥2501 Gms.	Not Stated	
Total	2,385,917	7.5	92.2	0.3	2,341,382	6.6	93.1	0.3	12.0
20–27	11,203	79.6	18.2	2.2	9,839	77.8	20.4	1.8	2.3
28–31	20,090	69.4	29.4	1.2	17,805	66.3	32.7	1.0	4.5
32–35	85,028	41.4	58.2	0.4	78,223	37.7	62.0	0.3	8.9
36	56,584	21.2	78.6	0.2	53,409	18.7	81.1	0.2	11.8
37–39	671,318	5.9	93.9	0.2	657,407	5.2	94.7	0.1	11.9
40	424,291	2.3	97.6	0.1	420,750	2.1	97.8	0.1	8.7
41–42	463,863	1.9	97.9	0.2	461,199	1.6	98.2	0.2	15.8
43 & over	159,081	2.6	97.2	0.2	157,988	2.5	97.3	0.2	3.8
Not Stated	494,459	9.5	89.7	0.8	484,762	8.5	90.7	0.8	10.5
White	1,919,470	6.3	93.4	0.3	1,884,971	5.5	94.2	0.3	11.1
Black	402,519	13.2	86.5	0.3	393,489	12.1	87.6	0.3	8.3
Other	63,928	7.4	92.3	0.3	62,922	6.7	93.0	0.3	9.5

Table 3.   1973 Single Births: Percent of Live Births by Gestational Age, Weight Group and Race

Race and Gestation	Total Percent[1]	Percent Distribution					
		<1001 Gms.	1001-1500 Gms.	1501-2000 Gms.	2001-2500 Gms.	2501 Gms. & Over	Not Stated
Total							
Total	100.0	0.4	0.5	1.2	4.5	93.1	0.3
20-27 wks.	100.0	50.3	15.5	6.4	5.6	20.4	1.8
28-31 wks.	100.0	5.7	24.5	24.2	11.9	32.7	1.0
32-35 wks.	100.0	0.3	2.1	10.8	24.5	62.0	0.3
36 wks.	100.0	0.1	0.4	2.5	15.7	81.1	0.2
37-39 wks.	100.0	0.0	0.1	0.5	4.6	94.7	0.1
40 wks.	100.0	0.0	0.0	0.2	1.9	97.8	0.1
41-42 wks.	100.0	0.0	0.0	0.1	1.5	98.2	0.2
43 wks. & over	100.0	0.1	0.1	0.3	2.1	97.3	0.2
Not Stated	100.0	0.7	0.8	1.8	5.4	90.7	0.8
White							
Total	100.0	0.4	0.4	1.0	3.8	94.2	0.3
20-27 wks.	100.0	54.4	14.6	5.2	4.7	19.1	2.0
28-31 wks.	100.0	6.0	25.9	26.0	11.0	30.0	1.1
32-35 wks.	100.0	0.3	2.0	10.5	25.6	60.8	0.4
36 wks.	100.0	0.1	0.4	2.4	15.2	81.7	0.2
37-39 wks.	100.0	0.0	0.1	0.5	4.0	95.3	0.2
40 wks.	100.0	0.0	0.0	0.1	1.6	98.1	0.1
41-42 wks.	100.0	0.0	0.0	0.1	1.3	98.4	0.2
43 wks. & over	100.0	0.1	0.0	0.2	1.7	97.8	0.2
Not Stated	100.0	0.5	0.6	1.3	4.4	92.4	0.8
Other-Than-White							
Total	100.0	0.8	1.0	2.1	7.4	88.4	0.3
20-27 wks.	100.0	43.5	17.0	8.5	7.2	22.2	1.5
28-31 wks.	100.0	5.2	21.9	20.8	13.3	38.0	0.7
32-35 wks.	100.0	0.5	2.3	10.6	22.1	64.2	0.3
36 wks.	100.0	0.1	0.4	2.9	17.0	79.4	0.2
37-39 wks.	100.0	0.1	0.1	0.8	6.7	92.1	0.1
40 wks.	100.0	0.1	0.1	0.4	3.6	95.8	0.1
41-42 wks.	100.0	0.1	0.0	0.4	3.2	96.1	0.2
43 wks. & over	100.0	0.1	0.1	0.6	4.1	95.0	0.1
Not Stated	100.0	1.2	1.3	2.6	8.4	85.9	0.7

[1] Percents were rounded independently and may not add to total.

(not always viewed as truly premature) but slightly over 2 per 100 live single births are in the under 2001 gm. group. This is still a significant number of infants born at high risk of death or health problems associated with low weight.

Figure 1 depicts the black/white ratios of percents of low weight single births in 1973. In the early gestational ages, blacks have a slight advantage over whites, but beginning with the 36th week of gestation, the disadvantage of blacks becomes marked and approaches 3:1 during the 41-42 week gestational age group. For the all other group (not shown on the figure), the percent of low weight births is slightly higher than for whites, but they do not have nearly as high a relative disadvantage to whites as blacks do.

Table 4 presents data for 1973 single live births on the percent of low weight births by onset of prenatal care by race. These data present a striking picture of the differences in low weight proportions of births in all groups receiving prenatal care versus those with no prenatal care. However, it is not easy to interpret the meaning. Do the percentages of low weight births reflect the results of care? When we compare the black/white ratios, even in categories receiving care, it would seem better to hope not. When one looks at the percent of low weight births in the no-care group versus the group receiving care starting in the first trimester, one would like to think that the care helps. The actual number of births reported as having no prenatal care was about 37,500: white, 22,000; black, 14,000; and other, 1,500. These figures are probably low since many hospitals will show prenatal care in the third trimester on the birth record if the birth occurs in the hospital. Also, there has been no correction applied to the figures for births occurring before the third trimester. Births for which the mother had no prenatal care represent 1.5% of all single births for which there was reporting of prenatal care.

Figure 1. **1973 Single Live Births: Ratio of Percent Black Low Weight Births to Percent White Low Weight Births.**

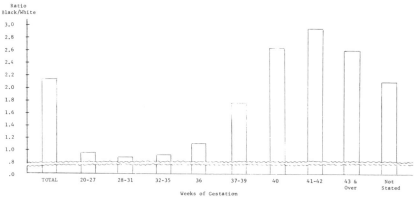

Table 4. 1973 Single Live Births: Percent of Low Weight Births By Race and Trimester of Onset of Prenatal Care (Refers only to births occurring within areas reporting month of pregnancy prenatal care began)

Onset of Care	Number of Births	Percent of Births <2501 Gms.					Ratios	
		Total	White	Black	Other	Black and Other	Black and Other/White	Black/White
Total	2,656,590	6.5	5.6	12.1	6.7	11.4	2.04	2.16
1st Trimester	1,798,463	5.7	5.1	11.0	6.1	10.3	2.02	2.16
2nd Trimester	573,322	7.7	6.3	12.1	6.8	11.6	1.84	1.92
3rd Trimester	131,698	7.8	6.3	11.7	6.0	10.9	1.73	1.86
None	37,520	19.8	16.2	25.6	15.8	24.6	1.52	1.58
Not Stated	115,587	8.8	7.1	14.2	8.7	13.8	1.94	2.00
Ratio:								
None								
1st Trimester	N/A	3.47	3.18	2.33	2.59	2.39	N/A	N/A

N/A = Not applicable.

Figure 2.   1973 Single Live Births: Percent of Low Weight Births in Each Race by Onset of Prenatal Care Category.

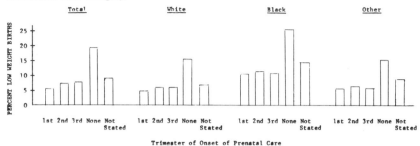

Figure 2 graphically depicts the percent of low weight babies in each category of onset of prenatal care. The picture is similar for all racial groups, although the levels of low weight percentages vary by race in the now familiar pattern of blacks having substantially higher low weight ratios than whites or "others."

Figure 3 shows the percent of low weight babies by mother's race and educational level. The black race shows a substantially higher proportion of low weight births in each educational category. Even black college graduates have a higher percentage of low weight births than those in any white or "other" educational category. There appears to be little difference in the percent of low weight babies by educational level through 11 years of schooling, after which the levels reduce substantially. This is different from a recent study of NYC data (Kessner et al., 1973), which showed fairly substantial differences between the groups with 0–8 years of schooling and 9–11 years of schooling. There is much less variation in the "other" race percentages of low weight births by mother's educational level than in the white and black races.

Figure 4 presents the relationship of wedlock status by race to percent of low weight births. The differences are clear for all race groups. The "in wedlock" results are better, ranging from somewhat over 5 low

Figure 3.   1973 Single Live Births: Percent of Low Weight Births Within Each Category of Mothers Race and Education (Refers only to births occurring within areas reporting educational attainment).

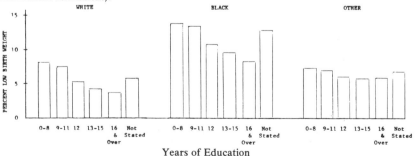

Figure 4. 1973 Single Live Births: Percent of Low Weight Births by Wedlock Status by Race (Refers only to births occurring within areas reporting wedlock status).

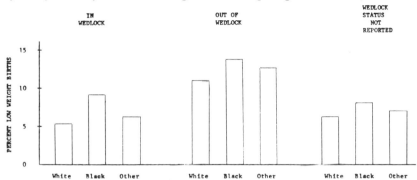

weight births per 100 single live births to whites to almost 10 for blacks. The "out of wedlock" group ranges from well over 10 low weight births for whites in each 100 single live births to almost 15 low weight black births.

Table 5 shows another characteristic which is often of concern in defining pregnancy risk: mother's age. The results of the analysis, which are found in the lower-right quarter of the table, reflect the current knowledge and expectations that, in all racial groups, young mothers and older mothers have a much higher proportion of low weight babies than those in between.

Table 6 confirms the expected relationship of total birth order to the risk of a low weight birth, and Figure 5 shows this information graphically.

These materials, examining prematurity from a representative national sample, emphasize not only that there are clearly defined variations in percentages of low weight births based on such characteristics as

Figure 5. 1973 Single Births: Percent of Low Weight Births by Race and Total Birth Order.

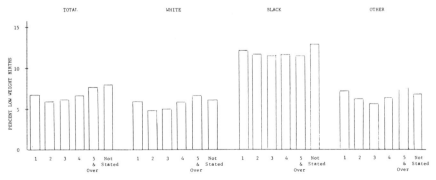

Table 5. 1973 Single Live Births: Number of Births and Percent of Low Weight Births by Age of Mother and Race

Mother's Age (yrs.)	Numbers				Percent[1]			
	Total	White	Black	Other	Total	White	Black	Other
Total Live Births								
Total	3,079,244	2,505,833	501,221	72,190	100.0	100.0	100.0	100.0
<15	12,735	4,859	7,702	174	0.4	0.2	1.5	0.2
15–17	235,838	151,900	80,143	3,795	7.7	6.1	16.0	5.3
18–19	360,957	268,200	86,150	6,607	11.7	10.7	17.2	9.2
20–24	1,082,607	889,652	170,751	22,204	35.2	35.5	34.1	30.8
25–29	869,647	758,632	88,427	22,588	28.2	30.3	17.6	31.3
30–34	360,907	305,993	43,138	11,776	11.7	12.2	8.6	16.3
35–39	123,468	100,369	19,007	4,092	4.0	4.0	3.8	5.7
40–44	31,167	24,753	5,512	902	1.0	1.0	1.1	1.2
45 & over	1,918	1,475	391	52	0.1	0.1	0.1	0.1
Low Weight Births								
Total	204,912	139,535	60,524	4,853	6.6	5.6	12.1	6.7
<15	1,918	562	1,336	20	15.1	11.6	17.3	11.5
15–17	24,345	12,536	11,526	283	10.3	8.2	14.4	7.5
18–19	30,685	18,662	11,460	563	8.5	7.0	13.3	8.5
20–24	68,509	47,314	19,750	1,445	6.3	5.3	11.6	6.5
25–29	46,490	35,977	9,136	1,377	5.4	4.7	10.3	6.1
30–34	21,301	16,082	4,478	741	5.9	5.3	10.4	6.3
35–39	8,975	6,444	2,172	359	7.3	6.4	11.4	8.8
40–44	2,522	1,843	616	63	8.1	7.4	11.2	7.0
45 & over	167	115	50	2	8.7	7.8	12.8	3.8

[1] For total live births, this is a percent distribution by age of mother in each race category. For the low weight births, the percent is that of low weight births in each mother's age-race category.

Table 6. **1973 Single Live Births: Number of Births and Percent of Low Weight Births in Each Race-Total Birth Order Category**

Total Birth Order[1]	Total	Race		
		White	Black	Other
Number of Births				
Total	3,079,244	2,505,833	501,221	72,190
1st Child	1,160,254	950,988	181,948	27,318
2nd Child	863,364	727,270	115,512	20,582
3rd Child	436,403	360,010	65,984	10,409
4th Child	217,604	175,401	37,077	5,126
5th Child	113,455	88,875	21,877	2,703
6th Child	61,738	46,690	13,521	1,527
7th Child	35,316	25,823	8,512	981
8th Child & more	55,370	36,837	16,750	1,783
Not Stated	135,740	93,939	40,040	1,761
Percent Low Weight Births[2]				
Total	6.6	5.6	12.1	6.7
1st Child	6.9	6.0	12.3	7.2
2nd Child	5.9	4.9	11.9	6.4
3rd Child	6.2	5.2	11.7	5.7
4th Child	6.8	5.8	11.9	6.5
5th Child & more	7.8	6.6	11.7	7.5
Not Stated	8.1	6.2	12.8	6.9

[1] Includes fetal deaths.
[2] Percent low weight births are for each race-total birth order category.

race, length of gestation, onset of prenatal care, mother's education, wedlock status and total birth order, but they give specific national baseline information about the actual low weight ratios in terms of these characteristics. Further analysis, not yet completed, in our collaboration with the Berkeley group will attempt to define the significance of the contributions of these categories to the percent of low weight births.

At this time, I would like to examine national variations in prematurity in terms of geographic areas.

Map 1 shows the US with states defined into quartiles by numbers of births in 1974. This map is intended to give a quick reference on where the births are occurring. Again, there are few surprises.

Map 2 shows the states defined by quartiles of low weight percentage for total births. There is no apparent relationship between numbers of births and the percent of low weight births. There is, however, some relationship between the percent of births to other-than-white persons and the percent of low weight births, as Maps 3 and 4 will show. It is hoped

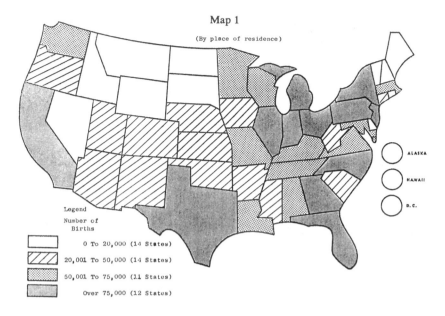

Map 1

(By place of residence)

ALASKA

HAWAII

D. C.

Legend
Number of
Births

0 To 20,000 (14 States)

20,001 To 50,000 (14 States)

50,001 To 75,000 (11 States)

Over 75,000 (12 States)

that our completed study will be helpful in assessing the relationships of the characteristics already discussed to geographic areas at the state level. And certainly, as has been said at this meeting already, other studies will be needed to show low birth weight ratio relationships to mortality, morbidity, socioeconomic characteristics of populations and to geographic areas.

Map 3 shows the states defined by quartiles of low weight birth percentages for the white race. A quick check of the previous map will show that while many states are defined as being in the same quartile as for the total, there are many others which are in different quartiles.

Map 4 shows the states grouped by quartiles of low weight percentages for other-than-white races. This map and the two previous ones suggest the importance of considering the size of a group's contribution to the ratios for an area. Race-adjusted rates would have presented the picture, taking into account the effect of the size of the different groups. I ask you to look at Mississippi as a case in point. Neither the white nor black group has a "bad" rate; in fact each is defined in the "good" or second quartile. However, the proportion of "other-than-white" births puts the total low weight ratio of Mississippi into the lowest quartile. Table 7 provides the back up numbers for the maps for reference.

Another way the studies prepared at the Institute examine information is in terms of groups of counties defined by characteristics which are believed to measure to some extent the population's access to health

Map 2.

(By place of residence)

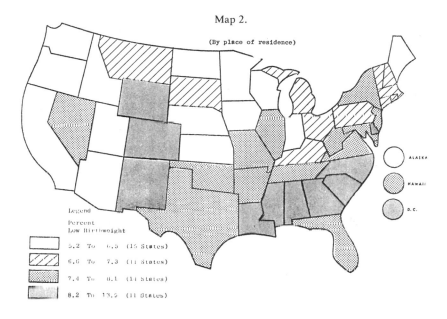

Legend

Percent
Low Birthweight

5.2 To 6.5 (15 States)
6.6 To 7.3 (11 States)
7.4 To 8.1 (11 States)
8.2 To 13.9 (11 States)

ALASKA

HAWAII

D.C.

Map 3.

(By place of residence)

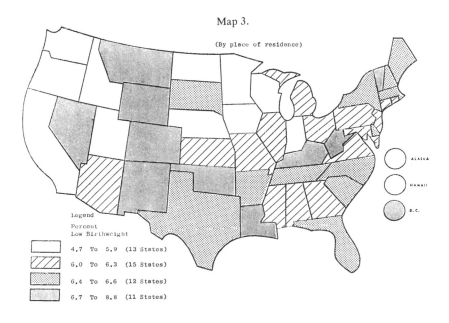

Legend

Percent
Low Birthweight

4.7 To 5.9 (13 States)
6.0 To 6.3 (15 States)
6.4 To 6.6 (12 States)
6.7 To 8.8 (11 States)

ALASKA

HAWAII

D.C.

Map 4.

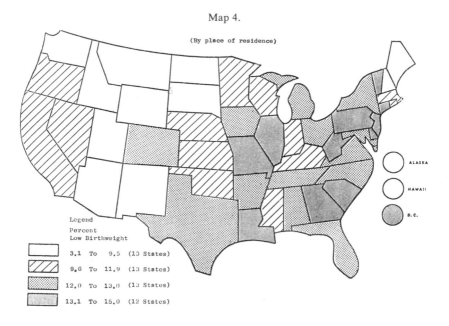

(By place of residence)

ALASKA

HAWAII

D.C.

Legend

Percent
Low Birthweight

	3.1 To 9.5 (13 States)
	9.6 To 11.9 (13 States)
	12.0 To 13.0 (13 States)
	13.1 To 15.0 (12 States)

care and health care facilities. The counties are grouped into five categories as follows:

Greater metropolitan counties: Counties in 1970 Standard Metropolitan Statistical Areas (SMSA) with population of one million or more.

Lesser metropolitan counties: Counties in 1970 Standard Metropolitan Statistical Areas (SMSA) with population less than one million.

Adjacent counties: Counties adjacent to the metropolitan counties and having easy access to the central city in the metropolitan area.

Isolated semirural counties: Counties other than those in the first three groups and having an incorporated place of population of 2500 or more.

Isolated rural counties: Counties other than those in the first four groups.

The findings regarding these county groups are of interest. There are, for example, significant variations in infant mortality levels in the different groups. There are also significantly different rates of improvement in infant mortality levels (Pratt et al., 1976). Tables 8, 9 and 10 illustrate these differences.

Table 7.   Race Specific Ratios According to Birthweight and Quartile of Low Birthweight Ratio, U.S., 1974 (by place of residence).

State/race	Total Births	Total	Race Specific Ratio							Quartile of low birthweight ratio
			Less than 2501 Gms.	Less than 1001 Gms.	1001–1500 Gms.	1501–2000 Gms.	2001–2500 Gms.	2501 Gms. & over	Not stated	
Alabama	59,451	100.0	8.4	0.5	0.7	1.6	5.5	91.2	0.3	4
White	38,775	100.0	6.2	0.3	0.5	1.2	4.1	93.4	0.2	2
Other	20,676	100.0	12.5	0.8	1.1	2.5	7.9	87.0	0.4	3
Alaska	7,053	100.0	5.2	0.3	0.4	0.9	3.4	94.3	0.3	1
White	4,984	100.0	4.7	0.3	0.4	0.8	3.1	94.9	0.3	1
Other	2,069	100.0	6.4	0.3	0.6	1.3	4.0	92.9	0.5	1
Arizona	39,841	100.0	6.5	0.3	0.5	1.2	4.3	93.2	0.1	1
White	33,658	100.0	6.3	0.3	0.5	1.2	4.2	93.5	0.1	2
Other	6,183	100.0	7.8	0.3	0.7	1.6	5.0	91.7	0.4	1
Arkansas	34,548	100.0	8.1	0.4	0.7	1.5	5.4	91.6	0.2	3
White	25,908	100.0	6.6	0.2	0.5	1.3	4.4	93.1	0.1	3
Other	8,640	100.0	12.5	0.8	1.1	2.1	8.4	86.9	0.4	3
California	311,820	100.0	6.2	0.4	0.5	1.1	4.1	93.3	0.4	1
White	263,710	100.0	5.5	0.3	0.4	1.0	3.6	94.0	0.4	1
Other	48,110	100.0	10.0	0.6	0.9	1.9	6.5	89.5	0.3	2
Colorado	39,042	100.0	8.9	0.4	0.5	1.6	6.2	90.7	0.3	4
White	36,663	100.0	8.6	0.4	0.5	1.5	6.1	90.9	0.3	4
Other	2,379	100.0	12.9	0.6	1.0	2.3	8.9	86.5	0.5	3
Connecticut	36,753	100.0	7.1	0.5	0.6	1.1	4.8	92.6	0.1	2
White	32,203	100.0	6.2	0.4	0.5	0.9	4.2	93.6	0.1	2
Other	4,550	100.0	13.6	1.3	1.1	2.1	8.9	86.1	0.2	4
Delaware	8,276	100.0	8.2	0.6	0.8	1.5	5.1	91.3	0.3	4
White	6,412	100.0	6.5	0.4	0.5	1.1	4.3	93.1	0.3	3
Other	1,864	100.0	13.9	1.1	1.9	2.8	7.9	85.5	0.5	4

Table 7. Race Specific Ratios According to Birthweights and Quartile of Low Birthweight Ratio U.S., 1974 (by place of residence)—Continued

State/race	Total Births	Total	Less than 2501 Gms.	Less than 1001 Gms.	1001–1500 Gms.	1501–2000 Gms.	2001–2500 Gms.	2501 Gms. & over	Not stated	Quartile of low birthweight ratio
District of Columbia	10,034	100.0	13.5	1.1	1.0	2.6	8.7	86.1	0.2	4
White	1,314	100.0	7.7	0.6	0.6	1.3	5.1	91.4	0.7	4
Other	8,720	100.0	14.4	1.2	1.1	2.7	9.2	85.3	0.2	4
Florida	110,350	100.0	8.0	0.5	0.6	1.4	5.3	91.7	0.1	3
White	81,720	100.0	6.4	0.3	0.5	1.1	4.3	93.4	0.1	3
Other	28,630	100.0	12.7	1.0	1.1	2.4	8.1	87.0	0.1	3
Georgia	83,291	100.0	8.6	0.5	0.7	1.8	5.5	87.1	4.2	4
White	54,167	100.0	6.2	0.3	0.4	1.2	4.1	88.4	5.3	2
Other	29,124	100.0	13.1	1.0	1.2	2.7	8.1	84.7	2.1	4
Hawaii	15,503	100.0	7.8	0.6	0.6	1.4	5.0	92.1	0.0	3
White	4,211	100.0	5.3	0.5	0.6	1.0	3.0	94.6	0.0	1
Other	11,292	100.0	8.7	0.6	0.6	1.5	5.8	91.2	0.0	1
Idaho	15,617	100.0	5.8	0.3	0.3	1.0	4.0	93.5	0.6	1
White	15,256	100.0	5.8	0.3	0.4	0.9	4.0	93.6	0.5	1
Other	361	100.0	6.3	0.0	0.0	1.6	4.7	91.4	2.2	1
Illinois	169,215	100.0	7.8	0.6	0.7	1.5	4.9	92.1	0.0	3
White	131,243	100.0	6.1	0.4	0.5	1.1	3.9	93.7	0.0	2
Other	37,972	100.0	13.4	1.1	1.3	2.6	8.3	86.4	0.0	4
Indiana	83,254	100.0	6.5	0.5	0.5	1.2	4.2	93.0	0.4	1
White	74,014	100.0	5.9	0.4	0.5	1.0	3.8	93.6	0.3	1
Other	9,240	100.0	11.3	1.2	1.0	2.0	7.0	88.1	0.4	2
Iowa	40,220	100.0	5.8	0.4	0.5	1.1	3.6	94.0	0.0	1
White	39,136	100.0	5.6	0.4	0.4	1.1	3.5	94.2	0.1	1
Other	1,084	100.0	12.0	1.1	1.3	2.1	7.4	87.9	0.0	3

Kansas	32,919	100.0	6.4	0.4	0.5	1.2	4.2	93.5	0.0	1
White	29,957	100.0	6.0	0.4	0.4	1.1	3.9	93.9	0.0	2
Other	2,962	100.0	10.8	0.8	1.0	2.5	6.4	89.1	0.0	2
Kentucky	53,443	100.0	7.1	0.4	0.5	1.4	4.7	92.6	0.1	2
White	48,655	100.0	6.7	0.3	0.4	1.3	4.5	93.0	0.2	4
Other	4,788	100.0	11.5	0.7	1.0	2.4	7.2	88.4	0.0	2
Louisiana	65,819	100.0	9.2	0.5	0.7	1.9	6.1	90.4	0.2	4
White	39,926	100.0	6.7	0.3	0.4	1.3	4.5	93.0	0.1	4
Other	25,893	100.0	13.2	0.8	1.1	2.7	8.4	86.5	0.2	4
Maine	15,120	100.0	6.5	0.5	0.4	1.1	4.3	93.1	0.3	1
White	14,962	100.0	6.5	0.5	0.4	1.1	4.4	93.1	0.3	3
Other	158	100.0	3.1	0.0	0.6	0.0	2.5	96.2	0.6	1
Maryland	53,470	100.0	7.9	0.5	0.5	1.4	5.3	91.7	0.2	3
White	39,047	100.0	6.3	0.4	0.4	1.1	4.3	93.4	0.2	2
Other	14,423	100.0	12.4	1.0	0.9	2.5	7.9	87.2	0.3	3
Massachusetts	70,083	100.0	6.7	0.5	0.4	1.2	4.4	93.1	0.1	2
White	64,834	100.0	6.4	0.4	0.4	1.1	4.2	93.4	0.1	3
Other	5,249	100.0	10.1	0.8	0.8	1.9	6.6	89.8	0.0	2
Michigan	137,636	100.0	7.3	0.5	0.6	1.3	4.7	92.0	0.6	2
White	113,151	100.0	6.1	0.4	0.5	1.1	4.0	93.1	0.6	2
Other	24,485	100.0	12.8	1.2	1.2	2.3	8.0	86.8	0.2	3
Minnesota	55,789	100.0	5.5	0.3	0.5	1.0	3.6	93.3	1.1	1
White	53,621	100.0	5.3	0.3	0.5	1.0	3.4	93.4	1.1	1
Other	2,168	100.0	9.9	0.7	0.1	1.4	7.5	89.6	0.3	2
Mississippi	44,122	100.0	8.9	0.5	0.7	1.7	5.8	90.8	0.2	4
White	22,985	100.0	6.1	0.3	0.4	1.2	4.1	93.7	0.1	2
Other	21,137	100.0	11.9	0.7	1.0	2.3	7.7	87.7	0.2	2
Missouri	69,624	100.0	7.4	0.4	0.6	1.4	4.8	92.3	0.1	3
White	58,239	100.0	6.2	0.3	0.5	1.2	4.1	93.5	0.1	2
Other	11,385	100.0	13.4	1.1	1.2	2.7	8.2	86.3	0.1	4

Table 7. Race Specific Ratios According to Birthweights and Quartile of Low Birthweight Ratio U.S., 1974 (by place of residence)—Continued

State/race	Total Births	Total	Less than 2501 Gms.	Less than 1001 Gms.	1001-1500 Gms.	1501-2000 Gms.	2001-2500 Gms.	2501 Gms. & over	Not stated	Quartile of low birthweight ratio
					Race Specific Ratio					
Montana	12,266	100.0	6.8	0.3	0.5	1.6	4.3	93.0	0.0	2
White	11,069	100.0	6.8	0.3	0.5	1.6	4.3	93.0	0.0	4
Other	1,197	100.0	7.1	0.4	0.7	1.5	4.5	92.7	0.0	1
Nebraska	23,711	100.0	6.0	0.4	0.5	1.1	4.0	93.8	0.0	1
White	22,336	100.0	5.8	0.3	0.4	1.0	3.8	94.0	0.0	1
Other	1,375	100.0	10.4	0.7	1.3	1.7	6.5	89.3	0.1	2
Nevada	8,966	100.0	8.1	0.6	0.6	1.4	5.4	91.7	0.1	3
White	7,618	100.0	7.4	0.4	0.3	1.2	5.2	92.4	0.0	4
Other	1,348	100.0	11.9	1.6	1.8	2.2	6.2	87.7	0.2	2
New Hampshire	11,642	100.0	6.6	0.4	0.6	1.2	4.3	93.2	0.0	2
White	11,524	100.0	6.6	0.4	0.6	1.2	4.2	93.2	0.0	3
Other	118	100.0	7.6	0.0	1.6	0.8	5.0	92.3	0.0	1
New Jersey	94,950	100.0	7.8	0.5	0.6	1.5	5.1	91.9	0.1	3
White	76,411	100.0	6.3	0.3	0.4	1.2	4.2	93.4	0.1	2
Other	18,539	100.0	13.8	1.1	1.2	2.6	8.8	85.9	0.1	4
New Mexico	21,319	100.0	8.8	0.4	0.5	1.4	6.5	90.9	0.2	4
White	17,881	100.0	8.8	0.4	0.5	1.3	6.5	90.9	0.2	4
Other	3,438	100.0	8.9	0.3	0.4	1.6	6.3	90.6	0.4	1
New York	239,504	100.0	7.9	0.5	0.6	1.4	5.2	91.8	0.2	3
White	189,142	100.0	6.5	0.4	0.5	1.2	4.4	93.1	0.2	3
Other	50,362	100.0	12.9	1.0	1.2	2.4	8.2	86.8	0.1	3
North Carolina	84,244	100.0	8.5	0.5	0.7	1.6	5.5	91.3	0.0	4
White	57,803	100.0	6.6	0.4	0.5	1.2	4.4	93.2	0.0	3
Other	26,441	100.0	12.7	0.8	1.1	2.6	8.1	87.1	0.0	3

North Dakota	9,972	100.0	5.2	0.5	0.4	0.9	3.3	94.1	0.5	1
White	9,157	100.0	5.2	0.4	0.3	0.9	3.4	94.1	0.5	1
Other	815	100.0	5.8	0.9	0.7	1.7	2.4	93.6	0.4	1
Ohio	160,609	100.0	7.2	0.4	0.5	1.4	4.7	92.6	0.1	2
White	139,000	100.0	6.3	0.4	0.4	1.2	4.2	93.5	0.1	2
Other	21,609	100.0	12.7	1.0	1.1	2.6	7.9	87.1	0.1	3
Oklahoma	42,450	100.0	7.7	0.5	0.5	1.5	5.1	92.0	0.1	3
White	34,727	100.0	7.1	0.4	0.4	1.4	4.7	92.6	0.2	4
Other	7,723	100.0	10.6	0.7	0.9	2.0	6.7	89.2	0.1	2
Oregon	32,519	100.0	5.6	0.3	0.4	1.0	3.7	94.3	0.0	1
White	30,829	100.0	5.3	0.3	0.4	0.9	3.6	94.5	0.0	1
Other	1,690	100.0	9.9	0.5	1.0	2.0	6.3	89.9	0.1	2
Pennsylvania	151,439	100.0	7.3	0.6	0.6	1.3	4.7	92.5	0.1	2
White	132,267	100.0	6.3	0.5	0.5	1.1	4.1	93.4	0.1	2
Other	19,172	100.0	13.8	1.3	1.2	2.6	8.6	85.9	0.2	4
Rhode Island	11,388	100.0	6.6	0.6	0.5	1.2	4.2	93.1	0.2	2
White	10,640	100.0	6.3	0.6	0.4	1.2	4.0	93.4	0.2	2
Other	748	100.0	11.3	1.3	1.2	1.7	7.0	88.3	0.2	2
South Carolina	48,554	100.0	9.0	0.6	0.7	1.8	5.8	90.6	0.2	4
White	29,551	100.0	6.4	0.4	0.4	1.3	4.2	93.3	0.1	3
Other	19,003	100.0	13.1	1.0	1.0	2.6	8.4	86.5	0.2	4
South Dakota	11,193	100.0	7.0	0.6	0.6	1.2	4.4	92.8	0.0	2
White	9,712	100.0	6.6	0.6	0.6	1.2	4.1	93.2	0.0	3
Other	1,481	100.0	9.5	0.6	0.8	1.3	6.6	90.3	0.1	1
Tennessee	64,265	100.0	7.9	0.5	0.6	1.5	5.1	91.6	0.4	3
White	50,275	100.0	6.5	0.3	0.5	1.2	4.2	93.1	0.3	3
Other	13,990	100.0	12.9	1.2	1.0	2.4	8.3	86.2	0.7	3
Texas	211,063	100.0	7.5	0.4	0.6	1.4	5.0	92.3	0.0	3
White	178,089	100.0	6.6	0.3	0.5	1.2	4.4	93.2	0.0	3
Other	32,974	100.0	12.7	1.0	1.0	2.5	8.0	87.1	0.0	3

Table 7. Race Specific Ratios According to Birthweights and Quartile of Low Birthweight Ratio U.S., 1974 (by place of residence)—Continued

State/race	Total Births	Total	Less than 2501 Gms.	Less than 1001 Gms.	1001–1500 Gms.	1501–2000 Gms.	2001–2500 Gms.	2501 Gms. & over	Not stated	Quartile of low birthweight ratio
					Race Specific Ratio					
Utah	29,966	100.0	5.3	0.3	0.3	0.9	3.8	93.8	0.7	1
White	29,036	100.0	5.3	0.3	0.3	0.8	3.7	93.9	0.7	1
Other	930	100.0	7.5	0.2	0.0	1.5	5.8	91.1	1.2	1
Vermont	6,887	100.0	6.7	0.4	0.5	1.2	4.5	93.0	0.1	2
White	6,847	100.0	6.7	0.4	0.5	1.2	4.4	93.1	0.1	4
Other	40	100.0	15.0	0.0	0.0	2.5	12.5	85.0	0.0	4
Virginia	71,091	100.0	7.5	0.5	0.6	1.4	4.8	92.3	0.0	3
White	54,316	100.0	6.1	0.4	0.4	1.1	4.0	93.7	0.0	2
Other	16,775	100.0	12.0	1.0	1.3	2.3	7.2	87.8	0.1	3
Washington	50,045	100.0	6.0	0.4	0.5	1.1	3.9	93.8	0.1	1
White	45,548	100.0	5.7	0.3	0.4	1.0	3.8	94.1	0.1	1
Other	4,497	100.0	9.2	1.2	0.8	2.3	4.8	90.4	0.2	1
West Virginia	27,878	100.0	7.5	0.4	0.5	1.5	4.9	92.2	0.2	3
White	26,609	100.0	7.2	0.4	0.5	1.5	4.7	92.5	0.1	4
Other	1,269	100.0	13.5	1.5	1.2	2.5	8.1	86.1	0.3	4
Wisconsin	65,203	100.0	6.0	0.4	0.5	1.1	3.8	93.9	0.0	1
White	60,360	100.0	5.6	0.4	0.5	1.0	3.6	94.3	0.0	1
Other	4,843	100.0	10.9	0.9	0.7	1.9	7.3	89.0	0.0	2
Wyoming	6,541	100.0	8.5	0.2	0.5	1.3	6.3	91.2	0.1	4
White	6,294	100.0	8.5	0.3	0.5	1.3	6.3	91.2	0.1	4
Other	247	100.0	8.0	0.0	0.8	0.0	7.2	91.9	0.0	1

Table 8. Infant Mortality Rate (per 1000 live births, by place of residence): 1961–1965 and 1969–1973

Degree of Urbanization	Total		White		Other	
	Rate	Ratio[1]	Rate	Ratio[1]	Rate	Ratio[1]
1961–1965						
United States	25.1	100.0	21.9	100.0	41.0	100.0
Greater Metropolitan	24.0	95.6	20.9	95.4	37.7	92.0
Lesser Metropolitan	24.2	96.4	21.7	99.1	38.8	94.6
Adjacent	25.4	101.2	22.6	103.2	44.9	109.5
Isolated Semi Rural	27.9	111.2	23.6	107.8	47.8	116.6
Isolated Rural	29.1	115.9	24.1	110.0	49.4	120.5
1969–1973						
United States	19.3	100.0	17.1	100.0	29.3	100.0
Greater Metropolitan	18.8	97.4	16.2	94.7	28.3	96.6
Lesser Metropolitan	18.7	96.9	16.9	98.8	28.2	96.2
Adjacent	19.7	102.1	17.9	104.7	31.4	107.2
Isolated Semi Rural	21.2	109.8	18.9	110.5	33.0	112.6
Isolated Rural	21.2	109.8	19.0	111.1	31.9	108.9

[1] Ratio in this column is the rate for the degree of urbanization divided by the United States rate for the column times 100.

Source: Pratt (1976)

Table 9.   Percent Decrease of Infant Mortality Rate 1969-1973 Over 1961-1965

Degree of Urbanization	Percent Decrease		
	Total	White	Other
United States	23.1	21.9	28.5
Greater Metropolitan	21.7	22.5	24.9
Lesser Metropolitan	22.7	22.1	27.3
Adjacent	22.4	20.8	30.1
Isolated Semirural	24.0	19.9	31.0
Isolated Rural	27.2	21.1	35.4

Source: Pratt (1976)

Table 11 presents material on number and percent of low weight births by race in each county group. There are variations, but these are relatively minor and seem to follow the US picture in each county group, with the races following the pattern we have seen before.

We used the county level computer mapping techniques developed by the National Cancer Institute (Mason, et al., 1975).

Map 5 presents low weight percentages of all births, showing quartile definitions of the over 3000 counties of the US. Clearly, the "best" counties with respect to this variable are located primarily in the northeast, north central, northwest and west. This roughly parallels Map 2.

The group of counties with highest ratios are concentrated in the south and in the high altitude areas of New Mexico, Colorado and Wyoming. The relationship of low weight ratios to higher altitude has been noted in other studies (Grahn and Kratchman, 1963; Lichty et al., 1957), and it is portrayed quite clearly on this map. Interestingly, alti-

Table 10.   Differentials [1] of Other-than-white to White Infant Mortality Rates (per 1000 live births, by place of residence and age-at-death):1969-1973

Degree of Urbanization	Age-At-Death				
	<1 Year	<1 Day	1-6 Days	7-27 Days	28-364 Days
United States	1.71	1.59	1.37	1.77	2.30
Greater Metropolitan	1.75	1.72	1.48	1.69	2.11
Lesser Metropolitan	1.67	1.64	1.38	1.62	2.05
Adjacent	1.75	1.39	1.32	2.08	2.77
Isolated Semirural	1.75	1.38	1.28	2.23	2.82
Isolated Rural	1.68	1.20	1.10	2.29	2.96

[1] Differential is calculated by dividing the rate for other-than-white infants by rate for white infants.
Source: Pratt (1976)

Table 11.   1973 Single Births: Numbers of Births and Percent of Low Weight Births by County Group and Race (By place of residence)

County Group[1]		Race		
	Total	White	Black	Other
Number of Births				
Total	3,079,244	2,505,833	501,221	72,190
Greater Metropolitan	1,139,747	876,316	237,451	25,980
Lesser Metropolitan	936,414	778,617	136,681	21,116
Adjacent	499,761	432,826	59,911	7,024
Isolated Semirural	423,231	351,377	58,663	13,191
Isolated Rural	80,091	66,697	8,515	4,879
Percent Low Weight				
Total	6.6	5.6	12.1	6.7
Greater Metropolitan	7.0	5.5	12.4	6.3
Lesser Metropolitan	6.5	5.6	11.9	7.1
Adjacent	6.3	5.6	11.5	6.8
Isolated Semirural	6.6	5.7	12.0	6.6
Isolated Rural	6.3	5.8	10.3	7.3

[1] See text for definitions.

tude apparently is not so great a factor in Arizona, Utah and Idaho, where the populated areas are at lower altitudes.

The county level map of the white race distribution of low weight percentages by quartile (Map 6) shows a picture roughly similar to the total.

The map of "other-than-white" low weight percentages (Map 7) shows that the "bad" and "worst" counties are mainly in the south. We had thought the Indians might be reflected in the higher altitude counties, but there are more of these counties shown in the total and white population maps as having "bad" and "worst" low weight ratios.

As is always the case, the Institute is concerned not only with fascinating statistical variations, but with the size of a problem. Thus, it should be noted that the quartile arrays presented on the "total births" map have the following numbers of low weight births: quartile 1-11,497; quartile 2-64,628; quartile 3-82,149; and quartile 4-75,476.

I would like to make a few final comments—not as a summary or conclusion, but to emphasize some of the points which seem significant to us at this time.

1. By the definition of prematurity as infants weighing under 2501 gm. at birth, this problem is a significant one with 6.6 such births out of every 100 single births. Even in the gestational age with the best low

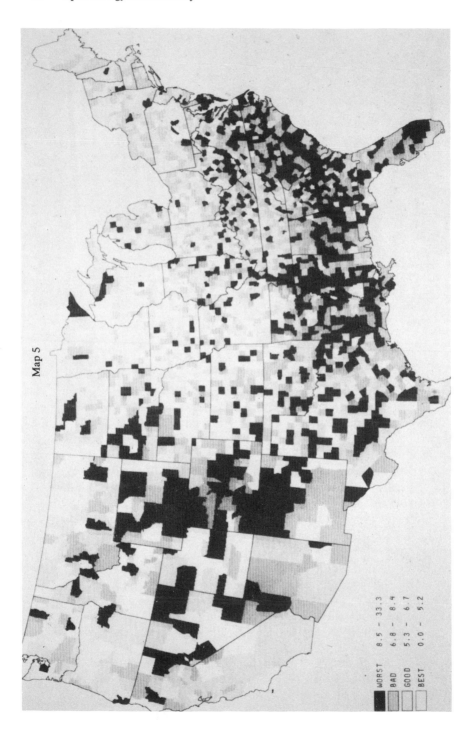

Map 5

WORST   8.5 - 33.3
BAD   6.8 - 8.4
GOOD   5.3 - 6.7
BEST   0.0 - 5.2

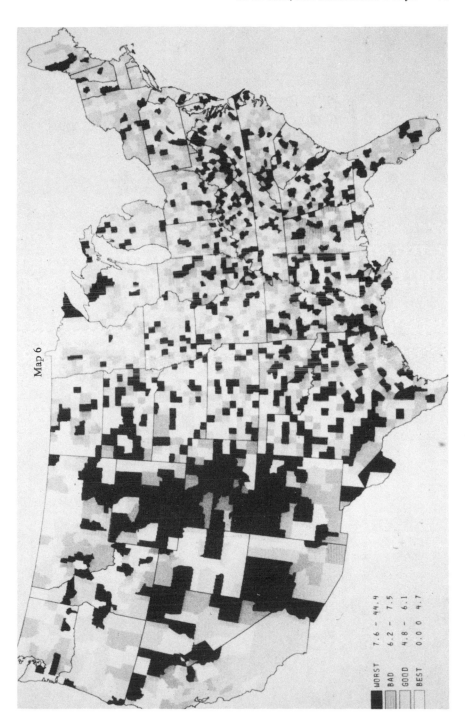

Map 6

WORST	7.6 − 44.4
BAD	6.2 − 7.5
GOOD	4.8 − 6.1
BEST	0.0 0 4.7

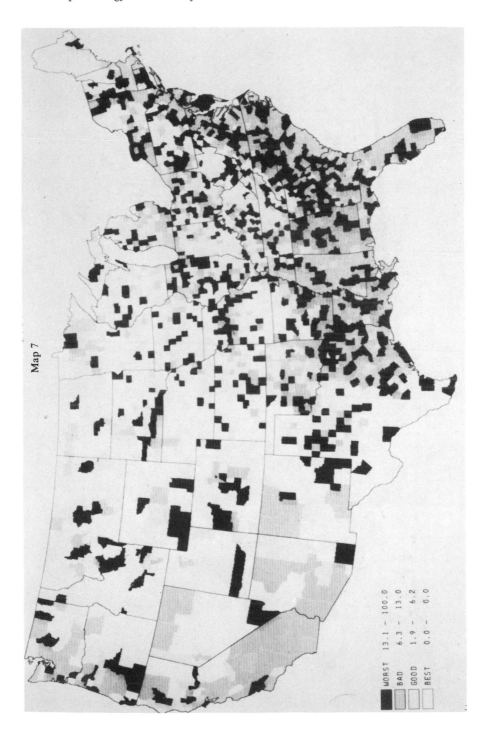

Map 7

WORST 13.1 — 100.0
BAD   6.3 — 13.0
GOOD   1.9 —   6.2
BEST   0.0 —   0.0

weight ratio (41–42 weeks), there are 1.5 low weight births per 100 single births. Most groups have substantial percentages of low weight births, even when they are not in the dramatically high categories.

2. There are those who would question whether a baby weighing between 2001 and 2500 gm. should be classified as a truly premature baby, particularly in the gestational ages over 36 weeks. If this weight group is omitted, there are still slightly more than 2% of babies (single births) that are clearly premature and who are at risk of suffering the problems often related to prematurity, which are the reasons for our concern at this seminar.

3. These national baseline data support the BCHS program's concern for the risk of a poor pregnancy outcome for the young, unwed, poorly educated mother whose problems are further compounded if she is black and does not seek prenatal care. If the mother is older and is having the fifth or higher order birth, she is at the highest risk of all of bearing a low weight infant, especially if she also has some of the other characteristics already mentioned.

4. The maps show that the largest ratios of low weight births tend to occur in the states with large black populations and in the very high altitude states. Two-thirds of the low weight births occur in the counties in the "bad" and "worst" quartiles for low weight ratios.

5. The severe relative disadvantage between blacks on the one hand and the "other" races and whites on the other in terms of the percents of low weight births suggest again the need for a very careful look at the low weight black infant.

Source of Data

National Center for Health Statistics, Vital Statistics Data on Computer Tapes 1973, 1974. National Vital Statistics Division, Public Health Service, US Department of Health, Education and Welfare.

TEXT REFERENCES

Grahn, D.; Kratchman, J.: Variation in Neonatal Death Rate and Birth Weight in United States and Possible Relations to Environmental Radiation, Geology and Altitude. Am J Human Genetics 15(1963)329–52

Kessner, D. M.; Singer, J.; Kalk, C. E.; Schlesinger, E. R.: Infant Death. An Analysis by Maternal Risk and Health Care. Institute of Medicine, National Academy of Sciences, Washington, D.C., 1973

Lichty, J. A.; Ting, R. Y.; Burns, P. D.; Dyar, E.: Studies of Babies Born at High Altitudes. AMA J Diseases of Children 93(1957)666–669

Mason, T. J.; McKay, F. W.; Hoover, R.; Robert, B.; William, J.; Fraumeni, J. F., Jr.: Atlas of Cancer for U.S. Counties, 1950–1969. DHEW Pub. #(NIH) 75-780, USDHEW, PHS, NIH, 1975

Pratt, M. W.; Hutchins, V. L.; Janus, Z. L.; Sayal, N. C.: Infant and Perinatal Mortality Rates by Age and Race, United States, Each State and County: 1961–1965, 1966–1970, 1969–1973. Maternal and Child Health Studies Project, MSRI, Washington, D.C., 1976

DISCUSSION

Mr. Hoffman: I have one comment on Figure 1. I think this figure could be misinterpreted by the unaware. The definition of below 2500 gm. is consistent with most black and white babies born before 36 weeks weighing under 2500 gm. This particular figure is conditional upon weeks, so it is not saying anything at all to the effect that more black babies are, in fact, born prematurely than whites. So this is a rather misleading figure.

Ms. Pratt: The overall ratio of black premature or low weight births to whites is well over 2 to 1, as shown on the chart. We considered that it was a significant point that in the earlier weeks of gestation (after 20 weeks), the blacks actually had an advantage over the whites in the ratio of low weight births. In later periods of gestation, the ratio of black low weight births to white is almost 3 to 1. In terms of total numbers of low weight births, in 1973 there were over 163,000 white low weight infants and somewhat under 68,000 black low weight infants.

Dr. Rush: When relating prenatal care to outcome, did you control for gestation? Have you accounted for the effect of those women who had no prenatal care because they delivered prior to the point where they might have sought care?

Ms. Pratt: No. This study is in its very early design stages, and the results presented here are a pre-analysis to make some determinations on the quality of the data.

Dr. Stanley: It really would be quite interesting to look at the maps again by birth weight and gestational age, and at the differences between low birth weight babies at different altitudes, for example.

Effects of Maternal Smoking and Altitude on Birth Weight and Gestation

Mary B. Meyer, Sc.M.

Maternal smoking and high altitude appear to have very similar effects on pregnancy. In both of these situations, the supply of oxygen available to the fetus is reduced, either by reduced oxygen tension at high altitudes or by the presence of carboxyhemoglobin in maternal and fetal blood when the mother smokes. Because oxygen is critical for maintaining life, a variety of adaptive mechanisms are available to insure an adequate supply for mother and fetus.

In this paper I shall present data showing the effects of high altitude and of maternal smoking on birth weight and on gestation separately, conforming as much as possible to the new ICD definitions (World Health Organization, 1975). I shall try to put these findings in perspective as either physiological or pathological responses in order to direct our attention to the areas most in need of future study.

To clarify the interrelationship between birth weight and gestation, Figure 1 shows the components of maternal weight gain by gestation (Hytten and Leitch, 1964). As fetal weight increases with time, the products of conception account for an increasing proportion of maternal weight gain, from roughly 20% at 20 weeks to 30% at 30 weeks and 40% at term. As this happens, the implications of delivery change drastically. Before 20 weeks, survival of a delivered baby is said to be impossible. The probability of survival if delivered increases gradually between 20 and 32 weeks, rapidly from 32 weeks to term, and decreases somewhat again after term. Any factor that increases the risk of early delivery will therefore increase neonatal mortality. The high mortality of these preterm babies, if otherwise normal, is largely due to their gestational immaturity, and their low weights are due to the fact that they have had too little time to grow.

During gestation many factors reduce the rate of fetal growth, some of which also jeopardize fetal survival, others of which have no effect on survival, and some of which are benign or even beneficial. As birth weight is an outcome indicator of a complex variety of forces acting during pregnancy, we need to evaluate whether a factor that reduces birth weight also has other detrimental consequences. Does it increase perinatal or later mortality? Does it affect physical or mental development in measurable ways? If so, are these changes directly related to reduced birth weight or are they parallel, independent effects of the factor?

Figure 2 (Hytten and Leitch, 1964) shows the components of increased oxygen consumption during pregnancy, and suggests especially that fetal weight and fetal oxygen consumption are correlated.

I shall present data from studies of smoking and pregnancy, most of which are epidemiologic, and from studies of altitude and pregnancy, where the main interest has been in physiological responses to reduced oxygen tension. I shall try to relate findings from both areas and to draw a logical picture of what happens in these pregnancies. We should bear in mind that some measurable changes may represent successful physio-

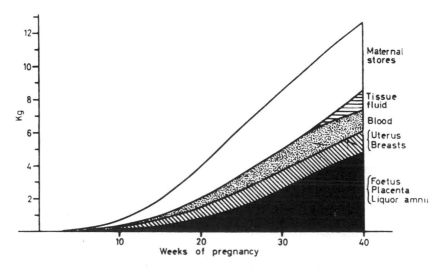

Figure 1.   **The Components of Maternal Weight Gain in Normal Pregnancy.**   Source: Hytten and Leitch (1964). Reproduced by permission of Blackwell Scientific Publications Ltd. Oxford.

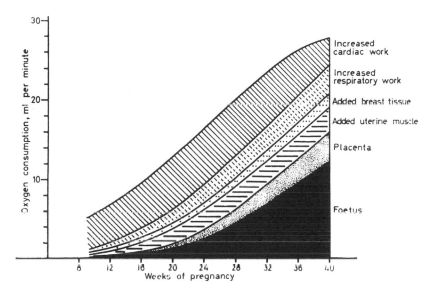

Figure 2. **The Components of Increased Oxygen Consumption in Normal Pregnancy.**
Source: Hytten and Leitch (1964).

logical responses to hypoxic stress, whereas others may represent either failures of these responses to do enough or pathological consequences related or unrelated to hypoxia.

BIRTH WEIGHT

Smoking in pregnancy has been a popular subject for epidemiologic studies since Simpson's paper was published in 1957. Since then more than half a million births have been analyzed by over 45 studies from all over the world—some large, some small, some of whole populations and some highly selective, some well controlled and others not. Since the beginning the relationship between maternal smoking and reduced birth weight has been shown clearly and consistently under all conditions. Typical patterns from published studies by others and from our analysis of the Ontario Perinatal Mortality Study data will illustrate the strength of this association.

Figure 3 shows the most important feature, namely, that for smoking mothers the whole distribution of birth weights is shifted downwards (MacMahon, Alpert and Salber, 1965). In most studies the mean shift is 150-250 gm., and the proportion of births under 2500 gm. usually doubles for smoking mothers. The birth weight reduction is not due to a

INFANT WEIGHT AND PARENTAL SMOKING HABITS

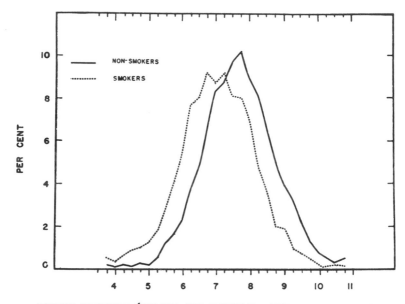

BIRTH WEIGHT (SCALE IN POUNDS; INTERVALS OF 4 OZ.)

Figure 3. **Percentage Distribution by Birth Weight of Infants of Mothers Who Smoked 1 Pack or More of Cigarettes per Day.**   Source: MacMahon, Alpert and Salber (1965). Infant weight and parental smoking habits. Reproduced by permission of the American Journal of Epidemiology.

similar shift in mean gestation, as illustrated by the lower mean weights for smokers at each gestational age in Figure 4 (Butler and Alberman, 1969).

The weight reduction is directly proportional to the number of ciga-rettes smoked, and is independent of other factors such as maternal weight, height, age, parity, number of prenatal visits, previous pregnancy history and all others examined.

To illustrate this point, Figure 5 shows that within classes of maternal weight, the mean birth weight is inversely correlated with smoking level (Underwood, Kesler and O'Lane, 1967). Figure 6 shows that the effect of maternal smoking on birth weight is also independent of maternal weight gain, a strongly gestation-dependent measurement. Within each maternal weight gain class, the more the mothers smoke, the higher the proportion of low birth weight babies. The direct correlation of birth weight with maternal weight gain shown in some recent studies is at least partly due to the fact that the same products of conception are weighed as they grow *in utero* and again at the time of birth.

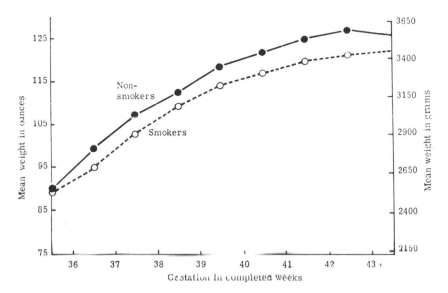

Figure 4. **Mean Birth Weight for Week of Gestation According to Maternal Smoking Habit.** Control week singletons. Source: Butler and Alberman (1969). Reproduced by permission of Churchill Livingstone.

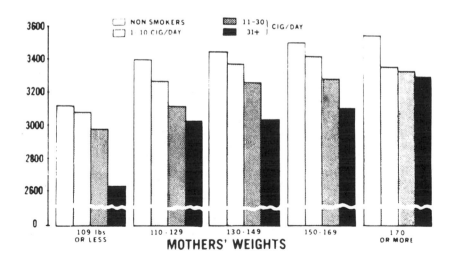

Figure 5. **Mean Birth Weights by Maternal Weight Group and Number of Cigarettes Smoked per Day During Pregnancy.** Source: Underwood et al. (1967) Reproduced by permission of Obstetrics and Gynecology, 29:1–8, 1967.

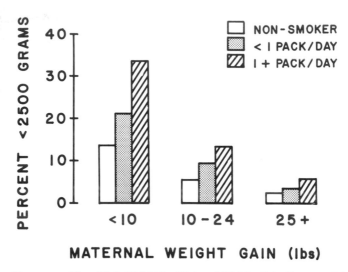

Figure 6.   **Frequency of Low Birth Weight by Maternal Weight Gain Group and Amount Smoked During Pregnancy. (Ontario data.)**

Table 1 summarizes the birth weight findings from five studies, showing the proportion of the low birth weight problem attributable to smoking for smoking mothers and for the whole population (Andrews and McGarry, 1972; Niswander and Gordon, 1972; Yerushalmy, 1971; Fabia, 1973; and Meyer, Jonas and Tonascia, 1976). The figures can be used to calculate the impact on the incidence of low birth weight in the population if pregnant women did not smoke.

A multiple regression analysis of risk factors for low birth weight, using Ontario data, measures the independent effect of maternal smoking. Table 2 shows rates of low weight births by smoking level, simultaneously adjusted for the effects of hospital pay status, mother's birthplace, height, prepregnant weight, previous pregnancy history, age-parity and sex of child. With the effects of the other factors held constant, smokers of less than a pack per day had a 53% increase and smokers of a pack or more per day a 130% increase in the incidence of births under 2500 gm., compared with nonsmokers. Maternal smoking had a more significant effect on birth weight than any other factor in the regression (Meyer et al., 1976). $(F = 182.8, df = 2, \infty)$. It is clearly essential to include maternal smoking information in all studies of birth weight if the results are to be interpretable.

Although there are few real epidemiologic studies of altitude and birth weight, all existing data show that the picture is the same as for smoking. Mean birth weights are inversely proportional to elevation, as shown in Figure 7 (Grahn and Kratchman, 1963). Again it appears that all births are

Table 1. Maternal Smoking and Low Birth Weight (Data from five studies)

Study	Total Births	Percent Smokers	Percent Weight < 2500 g		Percent Attrib. Risk	
			Nonsmokers	Smokers	Smokers	Total
Cardiff (Andrews & McGarry 1972)	13,414	46	4.1	8.1	49	31
U.S. Collaborative (Niswander & Gordon 1972)	18,247	54	4.3	9.5	55	39
Kaiser-Permanente *(Yerushalmy 1971)	5,334	40	3.5	6.4	45	25
Montreal (Fabia 1973)	6,958	43	5.2	11.4	54	34
Ontario	48,378	44	4.5	9.0	50	31

*White births only

Table 2. Birth Weight < 2500 Grams by Maternal Smoking and Other Significant Factors. Adjusted Rates* per 1000 Births. Ontario Data.

	< 2500 per 1000 births	F ratio
Maternal smoking		
None	49	182.8
<1 pack	76	
1 + packs	114	
Prepregnant weight		
<120 lb	85	87.5
120–134 lb	58	
135 + lb	46	
Previous pregnancy history		
No previous pregnancy	70	123.5
Previous preg., no loss	58	
Previous preg., loss	135	

*Each rate adjusted for the effects of the others listed, and also for those of hospital status, mother's birthplace, height, age-parity and sex of child.
Source: Meyer, Jonas and Tonascia, 1976.

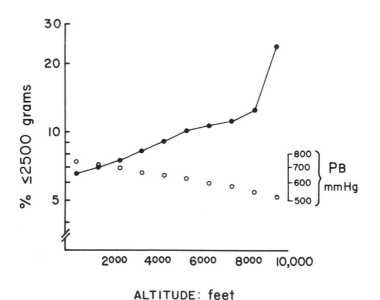

ALTITUDE: feet

Figure 7. **Frequency of Low Birth Weight by Elevation and Barometric Pressure: U.S. Mountain States, 1952–1957, White Population.**   Adapted from Grahn and Kratchman (1965).

affected, the whole distribution of weights shifting downwards with increasing altitudes as seen in Figure 8 and 8a (Lichty et al., 1957, Grahn et al., 1963). In general these babies are not born preterm, so again the weight reduction is independent of gestational age.

PLACENTA

Characteristics of the placenta are vital in the transfer of oxygen to the fetus, and we might expect the placenta to play an important part in adaptation to varying levels of oxygen availability. As both uterine and umbilical blood flows are generally high, the limiting factor for oxygen transfer is the resistance of the villous membrane. The diffusing capacity of the placenta can be increased by an increase in the surface area of villi and fetal capillaries and by a decrease in the distance between maternal and fetal blood. Fetal growth and increased oxygen consumption in the last third of pregnancy are maintained by a large increase in the number of terminal villi, with a decrease in size of the individual villus. This maintains fetal oxygen supply at a time when the fetus is growing faster than the placenta and the ratio of placental weight to baby weight is declining (Bartels, 1970; Laga, Driscoll and Munro, 1973).

The possible role of the placenta in adaptation to hypoxic conditions can be measured by comparisons of placental ratios, dimensions, shapes, gross and microscopic examination and morphometry. Some of this has

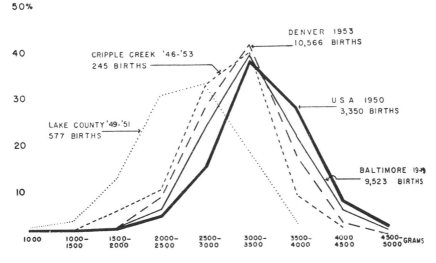

Figure 8. **Percentage Distribution by Birth Weight of Infants Born at Different Elevations in the U.S.**   Source: Lichty et al. (1957) Reproduced by permission of the AMA Journal of Diseases of Children, 93:666, 1957. Copyright 1957, American Medical Association.

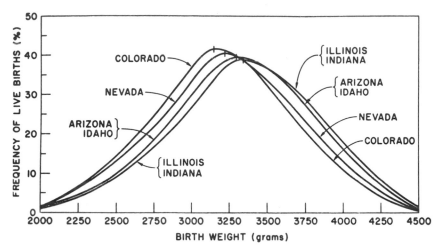

Figure 8a.   **Percentage Distribution by Birth Weight of Infants Born in Indicated States, 1956–57, White Population.**   Source: Grahn (1965).

been done, and again the findings from studies of altitude and of smoking effects are similar. A number of studies of placentas at different altitudes have shown that the placental ratio increases with altitude. Table 3 summarizes findings from the carefully controlled study by McClung (1968) of births in Lima and Cuzco, showing significantly lower birth weights, a higher placental ratio, increased diameter to thickness ratio and a much higher incidence of placenta previa in Cuzco at 3400 m. than in Lima at 200 m. Significantly, more high altitude than sea level placentas have irregular shapes (Chabes et al., 1968). Morphometric studies indicate that the high altitude placenta has a higher ratio of parenchyma to stroma, a greatly increased villous surface area with diminution of intervillous space, increased vascularity and a larger area of attachment than its sea level counterpart (Kadar and Saldana, 1971).

A few previous studies in which placentas were weighed indicated that while birth weights decreased with maternal smoking, placenta weights were similar for smokers and nonsmokers, with a consequent increase in the placental ratio for smokers. This has been confirmed by the carefully controlled, large study by Wingerd et al., (1976), the results of which are reported in Figure 9, giving placental ratios by smoking level and gestation. Although the ratio declines towards term, the direct increase with smoking level is clearly seen at each gestational age. As for the birth weight, this change in the placental ratio seems to occur in all pregnancies. A recent histological study (Spira et al., personal communication) of placentas from births to smoking and nonsmoking mothers shows that

Table 3.   Birth Weight and Placental Data by Altitude.

Mean values	CUZCO (3416 m) N = 60	LIMA (203 m) N = 80
Birth weight	3093	3312
Placental ratio	0.17	0.15
Placental diameter: depth	7.4	6.3
Placenta previa (%)	27	1

Source: McClung (1969)
p < 0.01 for all differences.

the smokers have significantly more placentas with diminished intervillous space relative to the space occupied by villi and fetal capillaries. We and others have found significant increases in the incidence of placenta previa and other placental complications among smoking mothers, to be discussed in detail later.

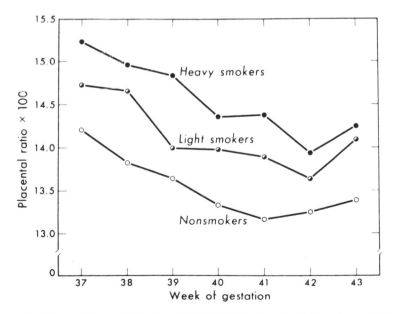

Figure 9.   **Ratio of Placental Weight to Birth Weight by Length of Gestation and Maternal Smoking Category.**   Source: Wingerd et al. (1976). Reproduced by permission of the American Journal of Obstetrics and Gynecology, 124:671–675, 1976.

GESTATION

In many studies the finding of reduced birth weight with maternal smoking has raised the obvious question of whether it is due to a shorter gestation. The negative answer to this question comes from the fact that the downward shift of mean gestation is minimal—perhaps three days—if the mother smokes. However, the different question of whether the incidence of preterm delivery increases with smoking does show a significant relationship, as illustrated in Table 4. The distribution of gestation times from the Ontario study shown in Figure 10 indicates the reason for this apparent discrepancy. Because the vast majority of births occur around term, the mean is an insensitive measure unless all births are affected

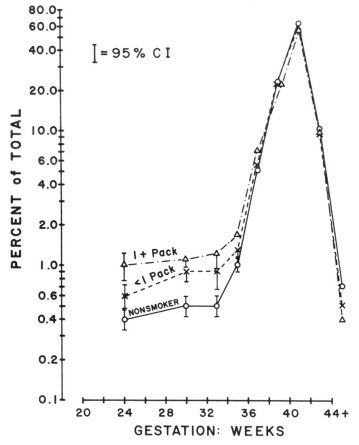

Figure 10.   **Percentage Distribution by Weeks of Gestation of Births to Non-Smokers, Smokers of Less than a Pack per Day, and Smokers of One Pack per Day or More. (Ontario Data.)**

Table 4. Preterm * Births by Maternal Smoking Habit: Relative and Attributable Risks Derived from Published Studies.

Study	Smokers (proportion)	Preterm births per 100 total births		Relative risk, smoker: non-smoker	Attributable risk (%)
		Nonsmoker	Smoker		
Cardiff	.465	6.7	9.2	1.36	14
Great Britain (Butler & Alberman, 1969)	.274	4.7	6.9	1.47	11
Montreal	.432	7.7	10.6	1.38	14
Ontario‡	.435	7.4	10.1	1.36	14
California					
White	.402	5.9	6.5	1.10	4
Black	.338	13.4	16.7	1.25	8

*Cardiff and Ontario data are for < 38 weeks. All others are for < 37 weeks.
‡Unpublished, derived from original data.
Source: Meyer, Jonas and Tonascia (1976). Reproduced with permission.

similarly, as is the case for birth weight. The picture here is that there is a significant increase in the risk of preterm delivery with maternal smoking level, but that only a small proportion of births are affected. The increased rate of perinatal mortality with maternal smoking is closely related to this increase in preterm delivery, whereas it appears to be unrelated to birth weight reduction. In fact, the case fatality rate for low weight babies is higher for nonsmokers than for smokers.

Although there are no real epidemiologic studies showing gestation by altitude, the clinical impression is quoted that high altitude babies are small but gestationally mature (Lichty et al., 1957). Grahn's analysis (1965) of gestation by altitude shows a slight decline in mean gestation by altitude, with a difference of 2.7 days between Illinois-Indiana and Colorado. Between these two areas, the proportion of births occurring before 36 weeks increases by 41%, similar to the increase observed with smoking (Grahn, personal communication, 1976).

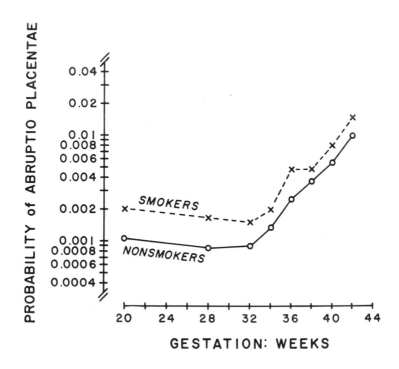

Figure 11.   **Risk of Abruptio Placentae by Gestational Age for Smoking and Nonsmoking Mothers.**   Risks calculated per total pregnancies *in utero* at beginning of each interval. (Ontario Data.)

PREGNANCY COMPLICATIONS AND PERINATAL MORTALITY BY GESTATION

So far, most of our studies have been concerned with smoking-related increases in perinatal mortality. Although this is not the primary concern of the workshop, I would like to show the interrelationships we have found between maternal smoking, certain pregnancy complications, gestation and perinatal mortality. We and others have found that the incidence of bleeding during pregnancy, abruptio placentae, placenta previa and premature and prolonged rupture of membranes increases directly with the level of maternal smoking, as shown in Table 5. To relate these complications to time of delivery, we have calculated risks among the population *in utero* at each period of gestational age for smoking and non-smoking mothers. The risks of abruptio placentae (Fig. 11), placenta previa (Fig. 12) and premature rupture of membranes (Fig. 13) are all significantly increased for smoking mothers who deliver in the earlier weeks observed in the Ontario study, which included all births of at least 20-weeks duration. The excess of perinatal mortality risk associated with maternal

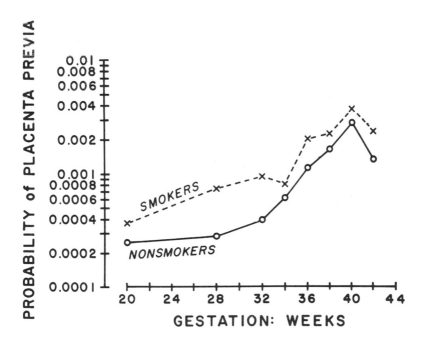

Figure 12.   **Risk of Placenta Previa by Gestational Age for Smoking and Nonsmoking Mothers. (Ontario Data.)**

Table 5. Perinatal Mortality and Selected Pregnancy Complications by Maternal Smoking Level (Ontario Data).

Outcome	Smoking Level (Packs per day)			X^2†
	0	<1	1+	
	(Rates per 1000 total births)			
Perinatal mortality	23.3	28.0	33.4	27.8*
Abruptio placentae	16.1	20.6	28.9	47.3*
Placenta previa	6.4	8.2	13.1	28.6*
Bleeding during pregnancy	116.5	141.6	180.1	201.9*
Rupture of membranes>48 hours	15.8	23.3	35.8	109.9*
Rupture of membranes only at admission	30.3	39.3	45.0	45.7*

*$p < 0.00001$.
†Cochran's chi square for trends.

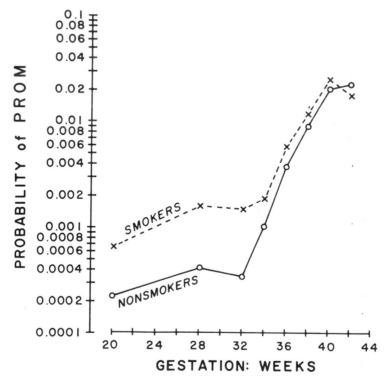

Figure 13.   **Risk of Premature Rupture of Membranes (Admission Diagnosis: Rupture of Membranes Only) by Gestational Age for Smoking and Nonsmoking Mothers. (Ontario Data.)**

smoking is concentrated in these weeks, as shown in Figure 14. This is true for fetal deaths, for which the smoker's excess is concentrated in deaths coded as due to anoxia or to unknown cause, as well as for neonatal deaths where the coded cause is prematurity alone and the closely related code of respiratory difficulty. In other words, excess deaths associated with maternal smoking seem to involve babies without obvious pathology who die *in utero* in association with maternal bleeding and placental complications, or who die neonatally because of premature delivery, especially if the mother has a history of early bleeding (Meyer and Tonascia, 1977, in press).

Neonatal mortality has been shown to increase with altitude in the United States and Peru (Lichty et al., 1957; Mazzess, 1965). Aside from the report of an increased incidence of placenta previa at high altitude in McClung's study (1968), we have not been able to ascertain whether there are also differences at different altitudes in the incidence of bleeding, abruptio placentae or premature rupture of membranes.

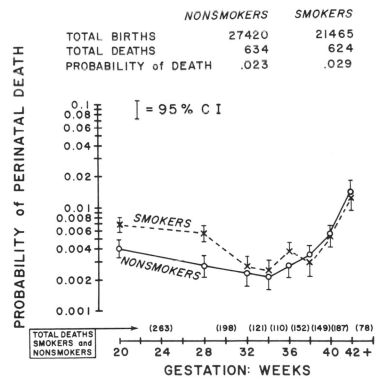

Figure 14. **Probability of Perinatal Death by Gestational Age for Smoking and Non-smoking Mothers. (Ontario Data.)**

DISCUSSION

We have reviewed the changes observed in pregnancies exposed to two forms of hypoxia and have found striking similarities in the results. The most obvious change we have seen is that, as altitude or number of cigarettes increases, birth weight is reduced and the ratio of placental weight to birth weight increases. This change occurs in all births, and for the most part these infants are delivered around term in reasonable shape.

A steady supply of oxygen is crucial for fetal survival and growth, and the supply is protected by a variety of mechanisms which may work to maintain the supply, to redistribute it to the most vital parts or to reduce the demand. A relatively larger placenta with increased villous and capillary surface areas delivers more oxygen, and a smaller fetus demands less. If we think in terms of an optimum birth weight for each baby, depending upon many factors in its makeup and intrauterine environment, perhaps it is an advantage for the high altitude or smoker's baby to be small.

I think our task in future studies of birth weight is to find out whether there is a price paid for this survival at a lower weight. In these pregnancies the fetus grows and develops with a lower driving force of oxygen delivery. Figure 15 illustrates this relationship for carbon monoxide (Longo, 1976). The normally low oxygen tension in the fetal circulation is reduced further by the presence of carboxyhemoglobin in maternal and fetal blood if the mother smokes. There is experimental evidence that exposure to cigarette smoke during pregnancy results in a reduced number of cells in the hindbrain of rats, contrasted with pair-fed unexposed rats and with unrestricted controls (Haworth and Ford, 1972). The British seven- and eleven-year follow-up studies suggest that there are slight deficiencies in physical and mental development associated with maternal smoking during pregnancy (Davie, Butler and Goldstein, 1969). More such studies are needed, and an attempt should be made to determine whether detrimental effects are due to low oxygen tension at the level of fetal tissues during gestation or directly to the smaller size of the baby, or to both.

The increased probability of early fetal death and of preterm delivery (which produces a smoking-related increase in perinatal mortality from approximately 2% to approximately 3%) seems to be quite a separate problem and needs to be studied differently. These occurrences seem to represent cases in which the mechanism for increasing oxygen delivery and reducing oxygen demand have failed, or have led to secondary pathology. Our observation of a strong association between maternal smoking, bleeding during pregnancy, abruptio placentae and fetal death, and similarly, between maternal smoking, early bleeding, premature rupture of membranes, preterm delivery and neonatal death suggests that in some mothers smoking may contribute to pathological conditions of the placental

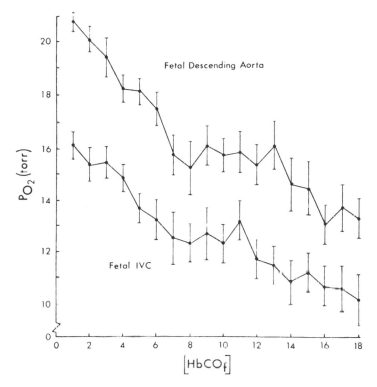

Figure 15.   **Oxygen Partial Pressure in Blood of Fetal Descending Aorta and Fetal In-ferior Vena Cava as a Function of Fetal Carboxyhemoglobin Concentrations (Sheep).** Source: Longo (1976). Reproduced by permission of Science 194:523-525, 1976. Copyright 1976 by the American Association for the Advancement of Science.

bed and spiral arterioles, aggravated by the need for an increased area of attachment (Meyer and Tonascia, 1977).

Studies are needed to determine what risk factors interact with smoking to produce these complications and the consequent increases in perinatal loss in a small proportion of mothers. These should be prospective studies of the characteristics of women with pregnancy complications such as early or late bleeding, placenta previa, abruptio placentae and premature rupture of membranes. These women should be extensively studied using standard personal and historical variables; smoking habits confirmed by analysis of blood or expired air; alcohol use; drug use, including aspirin; blood studies, including clotting factors; levels of certain vitamins, enzymes and hormones; detailed studies of placentas at delivery; and detailed studies of living and dead babies. A sample of total births studied in the same way would be a good control. From these studies it would be pos-sible to identify mothers at highest risk of these complications and to intervene in the case of risk factors where modification is possible, such as vitamin supplementation, stopping smoking and others to be determined. In this connection, we have examined the risk of placental complications for smokers and nonsmokers by maternal age and parity, as shown in Figure 16.

The same approach can be applied to existing data sets, as we have done and are doing with the Ontario data and as Fedrick and Anderson (1976) have done with British data. Outcome variables should include a number of gestational ages (e.g., before 20 weeks, 20–28 weeks, etc.) as the risk factors may differ for these outcomes. The various pregnancy complications should also be analyzed as outcome variables to determine risk factors for their incidence. Multiple regression analyses, with great care taken to avoid inclusion of other outcome variables such as birth weight and gestation in the regression, should also help to identify the relative importance of different risk factors. Studies with follow-up data, such as the British studies and the Collaborative Perinatal Study, should be especially valuable for this approach.

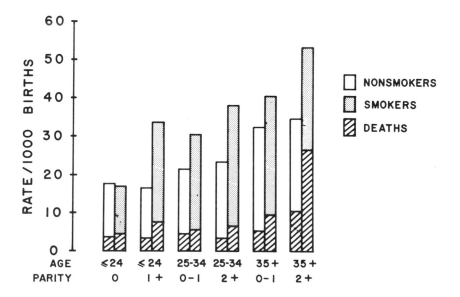

Figure 16.   **Placenta Previa and Abruptio Placentae by Maternal Age and Parity. Incidence and associated perinatal mortality for smoking and nonsmoking mothers. (Ontario Data.)**

TEXT REFERENCES

Andrews, J.; McGarry, J. M.: A Community Study of Smoking in Pregnancy. J Obstet Gynecol Br Commonw 79(1972)1057–1073

Bartels, H.: Prenatal Respiration. North Holland, Amsterdam and London, 1970

Butler, N. R.; Alberman, E. D.: Perinatal Problems. The Second Report of the 1958 British Perinatal Mortality Survey, pp. 72–84. Livingstone, Edinburgh and London, 1969

Chabes, A.; Pereda, J.; Hyams, I.; et al.: Comparative Morphometry of the Human Placenta at High Altitude and at Sea Level. Obstet Gynec 31(1968)178–184

Davie, R.; Butler, N.; Goldstein, H.: From Birth to Seven. Longman, London, 1972

Fabia, J.: Cigarettes Pendant la Grossesse, Poids de Naissance et Mortalité Perinatale. Can Med Assoc H 109(1973) 1104–1108.

Fedrick, J.; Anderson, A. B. M.: Factors Associated with Spontaneous Pre-term Birth. Brit J Obstet Gynaecol 83(1976) 342–350

Grahn, D.: Methodological Problems in the Use of Standard Vital Statistical Data in the Study of Neonatal Mortality and Birth Weight. *In*: Genetics and the Epidemiology of Chronic Diseases. U.S. Dept. Health, Education and Welfare Pub. No. 1163, 1965

Grahn, D.; Kratchman, J.: Variation in Neonatal Death Rate and Birth Weight in the U.S. and Possible Relations to Environmental Radiation, Geology and Altitude. Am J Hum Genetics 15(1963) 329–352

Haworth, J. C.; Ford, J. D.: Comparison of the Effects of Maternal Undernutrition and Exposure to Cigarette Smoke on the Cellular Growth of the Rat Fetus. Am J Obstet Gynec 112(1972)653–656

Hytten, F. E.; Leitch, I.: The Physiology of Human Pregnancy. Blackwell Scientific Publications, Oxford, 1964

Kadar, K.; Saldana, M.: La Placenta en la Altura. Characteristicas Macroscopicas y Morfometrica. *In*: Hurtado, A., ed. Estudios sobre la Gestacion y el Recien Nacido en la Altura. Universidad Peruana Cayetano Heredia, 1971

Laga, E.; Driscoll, S. G.; Munro, H. N.: Quantitative Studies of the Human Placenta. I. Morphometry. Biol Neonate 23(1973)231–259

Lichty, J. A.; Ting, R. Y.; Bruns, P. D.;

Dyar, E.: Studies of Babies Born at High Altitudes. AMA J Dis Children 93(1957) 666–678

Longo, L.: Carbon Monoxide: Effects on Oxygenation of the Fetus in Utero. Science 194(1976)523–525

MacMahon, B.; Alpert, M.; Salber, E. J.: Infant Weight and Parental Smoking Habits. Am J Epidemiol 82(1965)247–261

Mazzess, R. B.: Neonatal Mortality and Altitudes in Peru. Am J Phys Anthropol 23(1965)209

McClung, J.: Effects of High Altitude on Human Birth. Observation on Mothers, Placentas, and the Newborn in Two Peruvian Populations. Harvard University Press, Cambridge, Mass., 1968

Meyer, M. B.; Jonas, B. S.; Tonascia, J. A.: Perinatal Events Associated with Maternal Smoking during Pregnancy. Am J Epidemiol 103(1976)464–476

Meyer M. B.; Tonascia J. A.: Maternal Smoking, Pregnancy Complications, and Perinatal Mortality. Am J Obstet Gynecol 128(1977)494–502

Niswander, K. R.; Gordon, M.: The Women and Their Pregnancies. The Collaborative Perinatal Study of the National Institute of Neurological Disease and Stroke. Saunders, Philadelphia, 1972

Simpson, W. J.: A Preliminary Report of Cigarette Smoking and the Incidence of Prematurity. Am J Obstet Gynec 73(1957) 808–815

Spira, A.; Philippe, E.; Spira, N.; Dreyfus, J.: Smoking during Pregnancy and Placental Histopathology. Personal Communication, 1976

Underwood, P.; Kesler, K. F.; O'Lane, J. M.; Callagan, D. A.: Parental Smoking Empirically Related to Pregnancy Outcome. Obstet Gynecol 29(1967)1–8

Wingerd, J.; Christianson, R.; Lovitt, W. V.; Schoen, E. J.: Placental Ratio in White and Black Women: Relation to Smoking and Anemia. Am J Obstet Gynecol 124(1976)671–675

World Health Organization. Recommendations Regarding Statistics of Perinatal and Maternal Deaths. WHO/ICD9/Rev. Conf./75.24, Rev. 1, 1975 Annex II.

Yerushalmy, J.: The Relationship of Parents' Cigarette Smoking to Outcome of Pregnancy—Implications as to the Problem of Inferring Causation from Observed Associations. Am J Epidemiol 93(1971)443–445

DISCUSSION

Dr. Rush: I want to congratulate Prof. Meyer on a provocative paper, which has suggested an interesting hypothesis linking maternal smoking and low birth weight.

She alluded to our observation of depressed pregnancy weight gain in smokers (Rush, 1974), an observation which was recently confirmed in Wales by Davies et al. (1976). The depressed gain in smokers was far greater than that accounted for by the products of conception. As Prof. Meyer mentioned, the placentae of smokers are the same weight as non-smokers, and the birth weights of infants of smokers are depressed about 150 gm., while the pregnancy weight gain of heavy smokers is two to three kilos lower. Only a small part of the depressed weight gain can therefore be accounted for by lighter products of conception. While this depressed weight gain, presumably of nutritional origin, may not be the only cause of the lowered birth weights of smokers, it is fascinating that a letter to the *Lancet* (Spira and Servent, 1976), following Davies' publication and supposedly contradicting its observation, actually lent further credence to it. For while the correspondents' heaviest smokers did not have depressed weight gain, their infants were also heavier than those of the lighter smokers. This implies a causal relationship, and parallels our own experimental findings.

Prof. Meyer: I think there is considerable evidence for a negative correlation between smoking and body weight. There is also evidence (Pelkonen, Joutpila and Karki, 1972) that smoking alters metabolism and increases the activity of liver enzymes. So it would not be surprising to find some differences in weight gain between smokers and nonsmokers, more probably due to differences in metabolism than in food intake. However, I think that the effect of smoking on birth weight is over and above any effect it may have on weight gain. We plan to look at birth weight by smoking level in five-pound weight gain categories, and expect to observe the smoking-related effect in each subgroup.

As for the relative differences between maternal weight gains and between birth weights for smokers and nonsmokers, I would say that although the ratio of placental weight to fetal weight is higher for smokers, there is nevertheless a correlation between them, so that, in general, the other products of conception would tend to be heavier if the baby is heavy. Hytten and Leitch (1964) estimate that, at term, the products of conception constitute 40% of the maternal weight gain. In Davies' paper, the mean birth weight for male births was reduced by 160 gm. for light to moderate smokers, and by 240 gm. for heavy smokers. Differences in mean maternal weight gain between 20 and 36 weeks were 160 gm. and

2080 gm. for light and heavy smokers compared with nonsmokers. For female babies the birth weight differences were 240 and 330 gm., and the maternal weight gain differences were 640 and 1120 gm. In these studies the babies are weighed inside the mother as they become an increasingly important component of her weight gain and they are weighed again after birth. A slower growing smokers' baby will cause the mother to gain less weight (Davies et al., 1976).

Dr. Hardy: Mary, what was your definition of a smoker?

Prof. Meyer: In the Ontario study mothers were interviewed soon after birth. The question that was asked was: "What is the greatest amount that you smoked at any time during pregnancy?" and it seemed to work out pretty well.

Dr. Hardy: I was very pleased to hear Prof. Meyer's paper because I think that smoking is a very important variable that relates very strongly to birth weight and to immediate pregnancy outcome.

Dr. Mellits and I looked at this in a small, tightly controlled, matched study of 88 pairs some years ago. We took women in the Johns Hopkins part of the Collaborative Perinatal Study who had been followed prospectively through pregnancy, so they were asked about smoking at each visit. We included in the study women who smoked 10 or more cigarettes a day all through pregnancy. We matched these women on a number of variables with women who did not smoke at all. Then we compared immediate and long-range pregnancy outcomes.

As expected, the immediate pregnancy outcome was less successful among those women who smoked through pregnancy. There was a 225 gm. difference in birth weight, and the perinatal mortality was higher for the women who smoked. There was not a significant difference in gestational age. It was about two or three days. So the effect could not be attributed to gestational age.

We expected to find the weight gain of the mothers to be significantly different in the two groups. Interestingly, both the prepregnancy weight and the weight gain were not significantly different. When we came to long-term outcome, there was still a significant difference in body length at age four. But this had disappeared by the time the children were seven. And there was not a significant difference in educational performance at age seven.

It is rather interesting. We found during the neonatal period a significant difference in bilirubin concentration between the babies of smokers and nonsmokers, with the former babies having a lower average bilirubin. We simply couldn't understand this because they were lighter in weight. However, about a year afterward we came across a publication indicating that maternal smoking stimulated the enzyme systems of infants, and perhaps this explains the lower bilirubin.

Dr. Morton: Do women who discontinue smoking before or during pregnancy return to the nonsmoking risk group?

Prof. Meyer: They do. The British data suggest that the smoking effect is not apparent if smoking ceases before the fourth month, but the data aren't clear on this question yet.

Dr. Hardy: There are some preliminary data from the Collaborative Perinatal Study which indicate that babies with the highest average birth weight are those of women who stopped smoking during pregnancy.

Dr. Baird: The primigravidae who continue to smoke during pregnancy tend to be in the high risk category, e.g., under the age of 20, short in stature and from social class V. In such circumstances perinatal deaths are usually associated with "unexplained" low birth weight, malformations of the central nervous system or with antepartum hemorrhage. In such cases in the city of Aberdeen it was found that the women who had deaths of this kind smoked no more than women with the same characteristics who had live births. There is little doubt that smoking should be discontinued in pregnancy, yet in estimating the additional risk of a perinatal death, great care has to be taken to ensure very strict controls.

DISCUSSION REFERENCES

Davies, D.P.; Gray, O.P.; Ellwood, P.C.; Abernethy, M.: Cigarette Smoking in Pregnancy: Associations with Maternal Weight Gain and Fetal Growth. Lancet 1(1976)385-387

Hytten, F.E.; Leitch, I.: The Physiology of Human Pregnancy. Blackwell Scientific Publications, Oxford, 1964

Pelkonen, O.; Joutpila, P.; Karki, N.T.: Effects of Maternal Cigarette Smoking on 3,4-Benzpyrene, N-Methylalanine Metabolism in Human Fetal Liver and Placenta, Toxicology and Applied Pharmacology 23(1972)399-407

Rush, D.: Examination of the Relationship Between Birthweight, Cigarette Smoking during Pregnancy and Maternal Weight Gain. J Obstet Gynaecol Brit Comm 81 (1974)764-752

Spira, A.; Servent, B.: Letter to the Editor. Lancet 1(1976)1146-7

Relationship of Low Birth Weight to Maternal Characteristics of Age, Parity, Education and Body Size

Janet B. Hardy, M.D., C.M.
E. David Mellits, Sc.D.

The data to be presented are from two sources: The National Collaborative Perinatal Study (CPS) of the National Institute of Neurological and Communicative Disorders and Stroke, and the Johns Hopkins Child Development Study (JHCDS). The CPS included a total of some 59,000 pregnancies. The women were followed prospectively from the first prenatal visit through labor and delivery and the postpartum period. Surviving children were followed to age seven or eight years. The families represented a broad spectrum of socioeconomic levels followed in 12 medical centers across the United States. Approximately 20,000 black and 19,000 white women, registering for the first time in the study, formed the core group described by Niswander and Gordon (1972). The JHCDS, which was a part of the CPS, included about 4800 black and white women living in the East Baltimore. They were of lower-middle and lower socioeconomic status (Hardy, 1971).

GESTATIONAL AGE

Figure 1, from the CPS core study, shows the relationship between birth weight and gestational age for white and black infants. Mean birth weight is displayed for each week of gestation, from 28 through 50 weeks. The mean birth weight steadily increases with each week until term, after which fetal growth slows down and the curves flatten out.

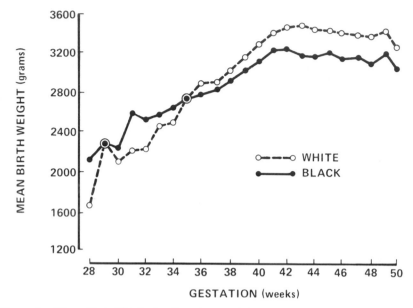

Figure 1. **Mean Birth Weight by Gestation at Delivery by Race.**   Source: updated from Niswander and Gordon, 1972.

The difference between whites and blacks in average birth weight for a given week of gestation is clearly discernible. Black babies are, on the average, larger than white below 35 weeks gestation, but after this point, white infants grow more rapidly than black. This, in conjunction with an average duration of gestation which is nine days longer for white women, results in the mean birth weight of white infants being approximately 200 gm. greater than that of blacks.

LONG RANGE OUTCOMES

While in general the thrust of this conference is directed toward determinants of low birth weight, it is important to remember that birth weight is an intervening variable with important implications for later development. Furthermore, the consequences are modified by interactions between birth weight and gestational age at delivery. The next three figures, which are based on CPS data,[1] provide information suggesting the implications of birth weight for child development and the need for the development of effective intervention strategies to prevent low birth weight.

Figure 2 displays the distribution of mean IQ scores (Weschler In-

[1] The data are from approximately 12,000 white and 12,000 black children with known neonatal bilirubin levels examined at seven years. Unknown bilirubin levels were randomly distributed by weight in surviving children.

telligence Scale for Children) at age seven years for CPS children, by birth weight and gestational age. All infants of 1500 gm. and below were grouped, regardless of gestational age. Above 1500 gm., birth weight was subdivided by 500 gm. increments and gestational age was subdvided into two categories (37 weeks and above, and 36 weeks and below). Among the more mature infants, i.e., those of 37 weeks gestation or more, the relationship between birth weight and IQ score is almost linear: the higher the birth weight, the greater the average IQ. For the less mature infants (below 37 weeks), there is a different pattern, with a decreasing average IQ score above 2500 gm. birth weight. The crossing of the lines in the graphs suggests some disadvantage for both the "small-for-dates" babies above 36 weeks, where more mature infants of 2001–2500 gm. have lower scores than those below 37 weeks, and the "large-for-dates" infants above 2500 gm. (36 weeks and less) whose average IQ scores are below those whose birth weight is appropriate for gestational age. It should be noted that, in spite of the overall average difference in IQ scores between black and white children (which may reflect cultural differences), the children of both races show the same basic relationships between birth weight, gestational age and later IQ scores.

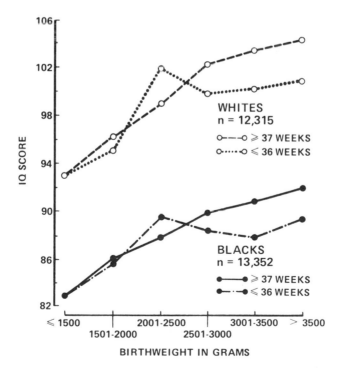

Figure 2.   **Mean WISC IQ (Full Scale) by Birth Weight and Gestation at Delivery.**

Figure 3, which is largely a reciprocal of the proceeding figure, shows the distribution of error scores obtained on the Bender Gestalt Test administered at age seven. A high score is undesirable. This is a test of visual perception which is thought to be indicative of organic neurological impairment. As birth weight increases, the average error score decreases. Again, gestational age is related to performance.

Examination of the physical measures of height and head circumference at seven years revealed similar findings, i.e., a strong relationship with birth weight and a similar effect of gestational age. Examination of body weight yielded less clear-cut results.

Figure 4 shows the relationships between birth weight, gestational age and neurological abnormalities (definite and suspect) identified at seven years of age. The high frequency of such abnormalities in low weight babies is clear.

With these long-range consequences of low birth weight and the interactions with gestational age clearly in mind, some of the factors other than gestational age which are antecedents to birth weight are now discussed.

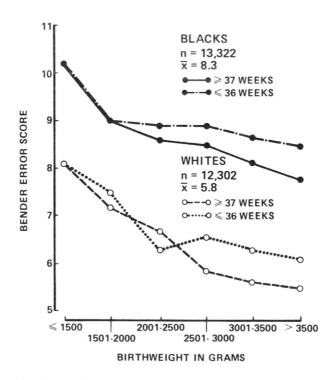

Figure 3.   **Mean Bender Gestalt Performance at 7 Years by Birth Weight and Gestation at Delivery.**

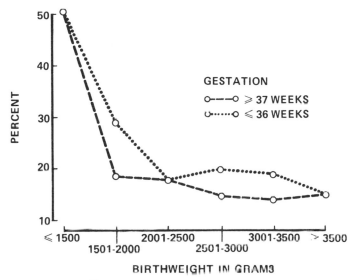

Figure 4. Neurological Abnormalities (Definite and Suspect) at 7 Years by Birth Weight and Gestation at Delivery in 10,825 White Children.

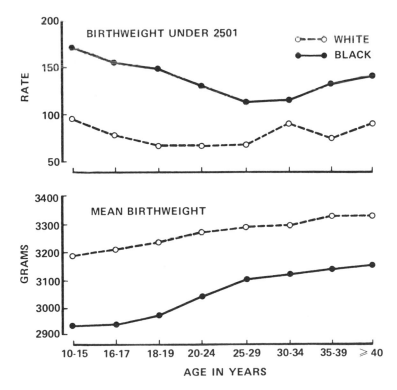

Figure 5. Maternal Age and Race.

MATERNAL AGE AND RACE

Figure 5, from the CPS data, shows the rate of low birth weight per 1000 live births for infants of black and white women by maternal age. The higher frequency of low birth weight for both young and older black women is quite striking. The rate of low birth weight is substantially greater among blacks of all ages. The mean birth weight for infants of women in each age group rises progressively with increasing maternal age.

PARITY

Figure 6, from the CPS, shows the relationships between birth weight, parity and race. The curves are similar to those in Figure 5 for maternal age. The average birth weight increases with increasing parity and the rate of low birth weight falls as parity rises.

Figure 7, from the JHCDS, indicates interactions between maternal age and parity in relation to birth weight. Infants born to multiparous

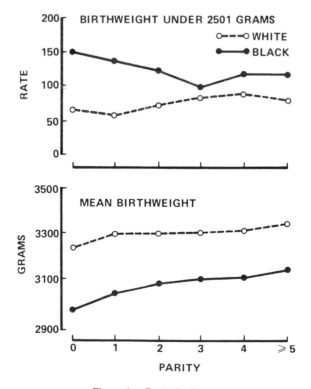

Figure 6.   **Parity by Race.**

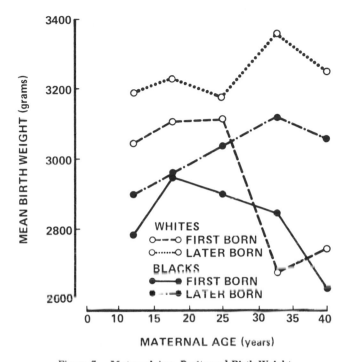

Figure 7.   Maternal Age, Parity and Birth Weight.

women are larger than first born at each maternal age. Below 35 years, there is an increase in birth weight with age. First born infants, on the other hand, decrease in weight with increasing maternal age.

MATERNAL EDUCATION

Figure 8 demonstrates the relationship between maternal education (as a "proxy" for socioeconomic level) and birth weight. Low levels of maternal education, as measured by years of schooling completed, are related to higher rates of low birth weight and to lower mean birth weight. However, women with education beyond the high school level have some increase in frequency of low birth weight and some decrease in mean birth weight, perhaps related to older age.

MATERNAL HEIGHT

Figure 9 shows the distribution of maternal height by race. There is essentially no difference in the distribution for black and white women.

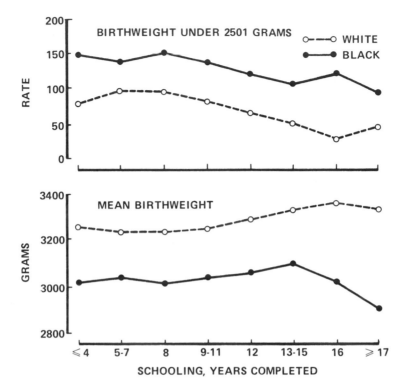

Figure 8. **Maternal Education and Race.**

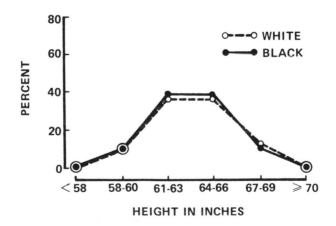

Figure 9. **Maternal Height by Race.**

Figure 10 shows the rate of low birth weight and the mean birth weight as a function of maternal height by race. Substantial differences by race are observed, with black women having higher rates of low birth weight and lower mean birth weight at each height interval than whites. This finding suggests that height may not be an important discriminator of birth weight.

Figure 11 shows that maternal height has little effect on perinatal death rates (per 1000 births) when the infant weighs over 2500 gm. at birth, but when the infant weighs less than 2501 gm. the rate is higher and increases dramatically with increasing maternal height. The findings for black women were similar.

PREPREGNANT WEIGHT

Figure 12 illustrates the distributions of prepregnant weight for black and white women. Again, there is little difference between the two races, white women weighing on the average very slightly less than blacks.

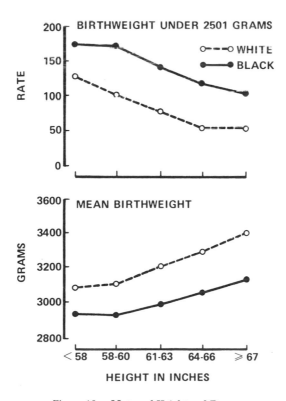

Figure 10. **Maternal Height and Race.**

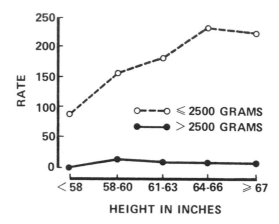

Figure 11.   **Perinatal Deaths in Whites by Maternal Height by Birth Weight.**

Figure 13 provides rates of low birth weight and mean birth weight by prepregnant weight and race. This variable relates strongly to low birth weight, with the largest women having the lowest rate. The heaviest women also have the highest mean birth weight.

Figure 14 shows the distribution of perinatal deaths by prepregnant weight and birth weight for whites. While prepregnant weight seems to have little effect on the rate of perinatal death for babies over 2500 gm. birth weight, with increasing prepregnant weight there is a sharply increasing risk of perinatal mortality for low birth weight infants. The findings for blacks were similar.

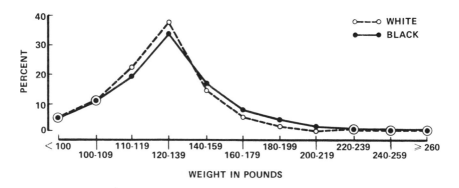

Figure 12.   **Prepregnant Weight by Race.**

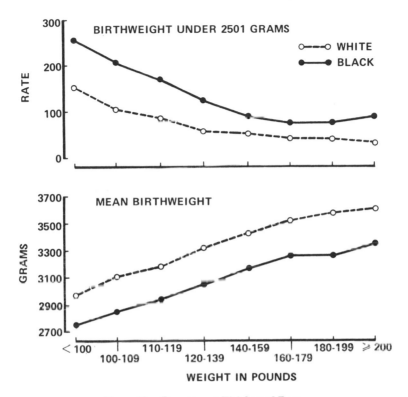

Figure 13.   **Prepregnant Weight and Race.**

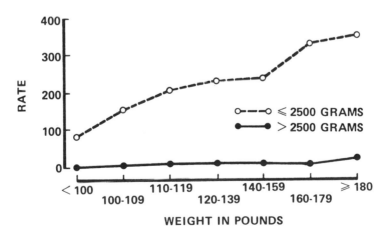

Figure 14.   **Perinatal Deaths in Whites by Prepregnant Weight by Birth Weight.**

WEIGHT GAIN IN PREGNANCY

Figure 15 shows the distribution of mean weight gain by prepregnant weight for black and white women. White women in the lower prepregnant weight ranges (i.e., ≤ 110 lbs) gain slightly more weight during pregnancy than blacks, but over most of the range there is no difference.

Niswander and Jackson (1974), using CPS data, have shown that a maternal weight gain during pregnancy of about 30 pounds is optimal in terms of both birth weight and neonatal mortality.

SUMMARY: MATERNAL FACTORS AFFECTING BIRTH WEIGHT[2]

Weiss and Jackson (1969), using data from large cohorts of white and black multiparous women of 37 weeks or more gestation in the CPS, carried out multiple regression analyses to isolate the relationships with birth weight of 32 individual factors and to rank the individual factors in order of their importance as determinants of birth weight.

Figure 16, which is from their work, shows the 32 antecedent variables studied in the order of the strength of their association with birth weight and the index of association for each. Weight gain during pregnancy is the strongest determinant, but prepregnant weight and birth weight of last prior child are almost as strong. Cigarette smoking during pregnancy also has a significant effect. Interestingly, maternal age and height are near the bottom of the list, with little residual effect after other interacting or confounding variables are accounted for.

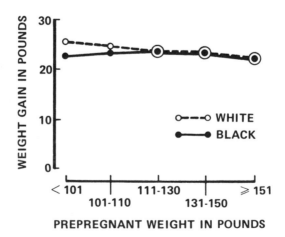

Figure 15.   **Mean Weight Gain in Pregnancy by Race for Gestation 37 Weeks or More.**

[2] Discussion at the end of Chapter 8.

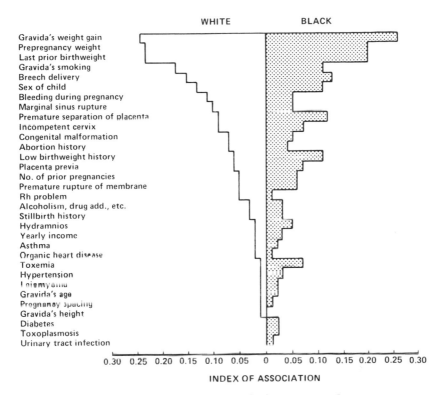

WHITE   BLACK

Gravida's weight gain
Prepregnancy weight
Last prior birthweight
Gravida's smoking
Breech delivery
Sex of child
Bleeding during pregnancy
Marginal sinus rupture
Premature separation of placenta
Incompetent cervix
Congenital malformation
Abortion history
Low birthweight history
Placenta previa
No. of prior pregnancies
Premature rupture of membrane
Rh problem
Alcoholism, drug add., etc.
Stillbirth history
Hydramnios
Yearly income
Asthma
Organic heart disease
Toxemia
Hypertension
Leiomyoma
Gravida's age
Pregnancy spacing
Gravida's height
Diabetes
Toxoplasmosis
Urinary tract infection

0.30 0.25 0.20 0.15 0.10 0.05   0   0.05 0.10 0.15 0.20 0.25 0.30

INDEX OF ASSOCIATION

Figure 16. **Factors Associated with Birth Weight by Race for Multiparous Women.**
Source: Weiss and Jackson, 1969.

Analyses of this kind, based on large cohorts of subjects, are essential to the identification of variables to be considered in the design of intervention programs.

TEXT REFERENCES

Hardy, J. B.: The Johns Hopkins Collaborative Perinatal Project. Descriptive Background. Johns Hopkins Med J 128(1971)5

Niswander, K. R.; Gordon, M.: The Women and Their Pregnancies. W. B. Saunders, Philadelphia, 1972

Niswander, K.; Jackson, E. C.: Physical Characteristics of the Gravida and Their Association with Birthweight and Perinatal Death. AM J Obstet Gynec 119 (1974)306-313

Weiss, W.; Jackson, E. C.: Maternal Factors Affecting Birth Weight. In: Perinatal Factors Affecting Human Development, Pan American Health Organization, pp. 54-59, Washington, DC., 1969

Information Pertaining to Birth Weight, Gestational Age, Placental Weight and Mortality

E. David Mellits, Sc.D.
Janet B. Hardy, M.D., C.M.

We would like to present new results which demonstrate relationships between birth weight, gestational age, placental weight and mortality. This discussion revolves about the four figures herewith presented.

By first describing the relationship between gestational age and birth weight and then adding in stepwise fashion other variables and examining the overall relationships for both prematurity and death rates, we, in our study at the National Institute of Neurological and Communicative Disorders and Stroke, have been trying to separate out many of the variables that are being discussed in this conference. One variable that appears to have emerged as important, over and above the effects of birth weight and gestation, is placental weight.

A simple dichotomization of placental weight at 300 gm. has been employed in the examination of relationships with the variables of birth weight, gestational age and perinatal mortality, stratified by this dichotomization. Interesting results can be seen.

Figure 1 shows low birth weight (live births ≤ 2500 gm.) by gestational age. We repeated this analysis for black children, using a different weight definition (2200 gm.). This, we believe, may be a more proper definition of prematurity for black infants. The results from this alternate definition were approximately the same as those demonstrated by Figure 1.

Figure 1 indicates the proportion of infants born equal to or below 2500 gm. as a function of gestational age. The relationship is what one

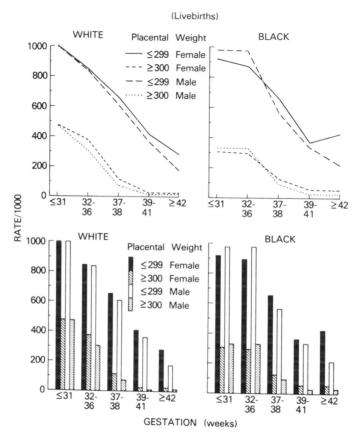

Figure 1. **Prematurity by Weight (≤ 2500 gm) by Gestational Age.**

would expect and has been shown in other papers presented at this conference: a declining prematurity rate with respect to gestational age. There is also a difference between races, which should be emphasized before examining the separate placental weight groups. It has not always been recognized that, on the average, black babies weigh more than whites in the early gestations. The general assumption that everything is less favorable for black children is not always true. It is certainly not the case for the mortality rates in early gestation.

As demonstrated by Figure 2, black infants do better than white infants for preterm gestational age categories. The mortality rates for white children are higher in early gestation than they are for blacks for both placental weight groups. Referring back to Figure 1, it is important to observe that within the races we have somewhat of a sex difference. However, the major difference that one finds when controlled for race and gestation is due to the placental weight dichotomization.

This large, well-defined difference exists over and above the effects of gestation, race and sex. It is much larger than the relationship with either race or sex, and seems to be consistent with respect to gestational age.

Figures 2-4 examine perinatal deaths, defined as stillbirths (20 weeks and above) plus neonatal deaths. Separate analyses for neonatal deaths and stillbirths are also available, but results are similar. The combination provides numbers large enough to permit one to draw conclusions.

Figure 2 examines the perinatal death rate as a function of gestational age, controlled within race, and then illustrated for the different sexes and placental weight dichotomies. There is again a well-defined difference due to placental weight. Note that this difference is demonstrated by simply dichotomizing placental weight at 300 gm. A multiple regression analysis, in which placental weight was utilized as a continuous variable rather than a dichotomy, would be even more enlightening. The top two graphs in Figure 2 demonstrate, for all births, the definite difference between the two placental weight groups, which is not to be unexpected. Again, the shape of the curves is what has been shown before.

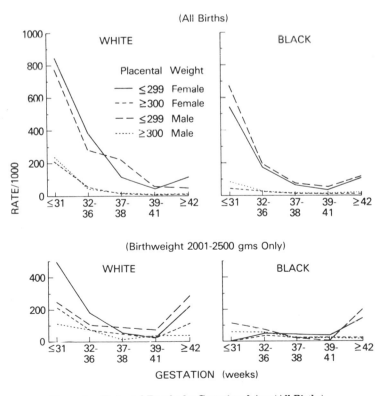

Figure 2.   **Perinatal Deaths by Gestational Age (All Births).**

The perinatal mortality is high for the early gestations, low between 37 and 42 weeks, and then increases again at 42 weeks gestation and above. That pattern exists for both races.

Comparing races across the graphs, the perinatal mortality rate in the early gestations is greater in whites than blacks. If one is to be born early, it is better to be black.

It was reported earlier, in a preliminary analysis on a portion of this same data (Sedlis, 1967), that the differences in mortality by placental weights are entirely explained by birth weight. We find, however, in the larger sample, that the relationship with placental weight is not entirely explained by birth weight. When this analysis was repeated, controlled within birth weight categories, similar results were obtained.

At the bottom of Figure 2, the 2000–2500 gm. birth weight group has been singled out to illustrate this point. Comparing the placental group lines within race and sex, a consistent difference exists, even within this 500 gm. birth weight category, between the high and low placental

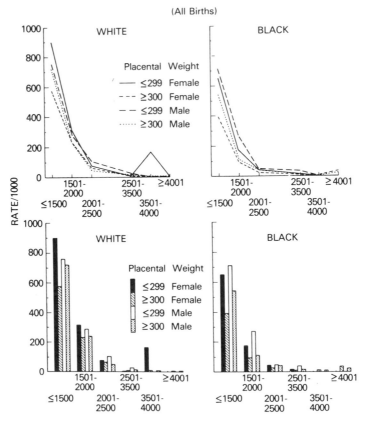

Figure 3.   **Perinatal Deaths by Birth Weight (All Births).**

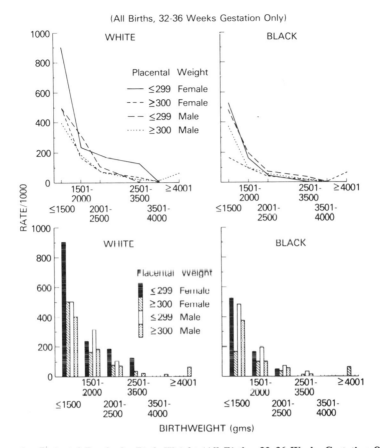

Figure 4.   **Perinatal Deaths by Birth Weight (All Births, 32–36 Weeks Gestation Only).**

weight groups. This difference is pronounced in early gestations. It becomes much less of a factor at term, and then increases again postterm. The differential effect of placental weight, though present in blacks, is much more pronounced in the white population.

Figure 3 presents perinatal mortality as a function of birth weight rather than gestational age. Mortality is shown to be definitely related to birth weight, as expected. Also, the race and sex differences remain consistent and, when controlled for race and sex, the two placental weight groups separate.

Whereas Figure 3 is calculated on all births, Figure 4 demonstrates that the relationships hold for the gestation period 32–36 weeks. This figure is calculated on those infants delivered between 32 and 36 weeks of gestation. Controlling within other gestational age groupings yielded similar results, although as earlier gestation groups and also lower birth weight groups are examined, the basic relationships are more pronounced but the other variables are not as discriminatory. That is, for earlier gestation or lower birth weight, race, sex and placental weight cease to be as important as birth weight or gestational age.

When the relationships are examined for gestation groups above 36 weeks, the effect of birth weight is still apparent but the discrimination due to the other variables extends to higher birth weights.

As placental weight differences are still discernible when controlled within birth weight and gestational age groups, placental weight does indeed appear to have a differential effect on the perinatal death rate and on the prematurity rate, over and above race, sex, birth weight and gestational age.

TEXT REFERENCE

Sedlis, A.; Berendes, H.; Kim, H. S.; et al.: The Placental Weight-Birth Weight   Relationships. Dev Med Child Neuro 9(1967)160-171

DISCUSSION

Prof. Meyer: It seems to me that your data suggest that the births with a higher placental to birth weight ratio have lower mortality, and it might be less confusing if looked at in terms of placental ratio as well. Have you taken smoking into account?

Dr. Mellits: Smoking will be taken into consideration as an independent variable. The placental/birth weight ratio makes an assumption of linearity and of intersecting the origin which I am not willing to make on this data. I don't think the relationship between placental weight and birth weight is linear, and then the ratio is a little misleading.

Dr. Susser: When we analyzed the relationship of fetal age, birth weight and placental weight in 6000 births in the Netherlands, 1934–46, birth weight accounted for virtually the entire relationship between length of gestation and placental weight.

Dr. Mellits: Yes, but contrary to our expectations, in small birth weight categories we found four to ten fold differences between groups, dichotomizing as crudely as placental weight of greater or less than 300 gm. This is based on about 50,000 pregnancies total. I wonder if the reason that this has not been appreciated in the past is because of small numbers, because the effect is only seen when cross classified into these small cells. Although we don't have the data yet, it may be part of the reason why we get the dichotomy in birth weight distributions for early gestations that we do in this country.

I am not suggesting that the mechanism is through the placental weight, but it might be a marker. With the development of sonography, preliminary estimates of birth weight and placental weight might determine obstetric practice on such matters as whether to induce labor or not in the early gestations. You might have a much better idea of which mode of the bimodality they are in in early gestation.

Dr. Morton: I can't see how to interpret these data, except on the assumption that those unfavorable factors which act on black birth weight are mediated through placental weight.

Dr. Mellits: In the early gestations the black infant has an advantage independent of placental weight. This is in the early gestations. I think part of the reason that we get these differential race effects is because of what I call a trunctation problem in the distributions of these studies. We have a selectivity difficulty in the data that we have. The black populations that get into these samples may not be the same in their risk as are the white populations for some reasons, whether having to do with medical care, socioeconomic factors or cultural practices.

Effects of Socioeconomic Status and Race on Weight-Defined and Gestational Prematurity in the United States

Stanley M. Garn, Ph.D.
Helen A. Shaw, B.A.
Kinne D. McCabe, M.D.

INTRODUCTION

As shown in a large number of studies, both race and socioeconomic status (SES) bear on the prevalence of prematurity, as variously defined. In the United States, prematurity is far more common in Blacks than in Whites, and more common in those of low socioeconomic status than in those of higher income, education and occupation. Moreover, race and socioeconomic status are far from independent.

As with the definition of prematurity itself, there are problems with the simple labels White and Black. The census category White properly includes individuals of European, Middle Eastern and North African ancestry, but who lack the characteristic African marker genes. The current census category Black refers to individuals of largely African ancestry (primarily from the Gold Coast, the Ivory Coast and the Slave Coast), but with some 20% accretion of European genes, primarily from northwestern Europe (Garn, 1970). And Puerto Ricans in the mainland US are of largely African ancestry, but with European genes derived from Spain instead of northwestern Europe, and with some Amerindian (Carib) genes.

The research described in this paper was partially supported by Grant No. NO1-NS-5-2308 with the NINCDS.

Socioeconomic categories commonly used include income, education and occupation, or classes or rankings that include combinations of these, and others such as housing. The component SES variables are not only inter-correlated, but they are also age dependent. Thus a low income grouping may include more younger women, as will the lower educational categories, while high education women will of necessity be somewhat older, and because of their backgrounds, somewhat more affluent and more often in managerial and professional positions.

In the United States, moreover, Black women (like Blacks in general) are of lower income, the majority being at or below the poverty level, and of lower status occupations, though more often employed. And there is a further complication we cannot ignore. Poor and uneducated women (both Black and White) tend to be fatter, and more affluent women tend to be leaner, as we have demonstrated in great detail (Garn and Clark, 1974, 1976a; Garn, 1976; Garn et al., 1977a). Fatness and leanness bear on the weight of the conceptus (Frisancho, Klayman and Matos, 1977), but if this were the sole determinant, the affluent newborn would actually weigh less than the poverty level neonate!

In the present analysis, therefore, we will compare the proportion of "premature" births (using various criteria of prematurity) in different income levels, educational levels and occupational groupings, and in relation to smoking for Whites, Puerto Ricans and Blacks. In this way we may make racial comparisons by socioeconomic groupings, so as to separate geographic ancestry from the variables of income, education and occupation. The key question, of pertinence to this country, is the extent to which the larger proportion of premature births in Blacks and Puerto Ricans reflects a biological predisposition and the extent to which it is a reflection of lower income, lesser education and more menial and physically demanding occupations well into pregnancy.

METHOD OF INVESTIGATION

Using data on approximately 45,000 live singling births from the Collaborative Perinatal Project of the National Institute of Neurological and Communicative Disorders and Stroke (NINCDS), we made use of three population groups (Black, Puerto Rican and White) and birth weight and gestation length data. Both "eyeball" and program cleaning were used to eliminate coding and transcription errors and improbable single and combination values, against printouts covering the entire sample.

We employed a set of per-capita-income categories (in $400 per annum groupings), a set of educational level categories and a set of occupational groupings (following the Bureau of Census categories) from "never worked" through "managerial" and "professional." In education, the range was from little or no schooling through to college level and beyond.

Naturally, we took a cursory look at a large number of variables (including maternal height, prepregnancy weight, weight gain, age at menarche, etc.). We also employed a variety of definitions of prematurity at various points in the data analysis. (After all, the conventional weight definition of prematurity encompasses a far smaller percentage of live born singlings than does the conventional gestation length definition.) And we explored the extent of maternal smoking during pregnancy. However, even though we employed, at various points in our data analysis, five different prematurity definitions for three population groups and three socioeconomic variables, what we report here is both limited and intentionally conventional. We report here our findings based on the ≤ 37-week gestation length definition. We do mention specific test restrictions, e.g., the 20–35 year age grouping, a parity-restricted grouping, etc., but our reported analyses are otherwise quite traditional, including the ≤ 2500 gm. weight definition.

The major question was the extent to which the greater prevalence of prematurity in Blacks may have a genetic basis, and the extent to which it may result from the combination of poverty and limited education. To answer this question, we made use of comparisons by income, educational level and occupational grouping. As a further test, we compared not just Blacks and Whites, but Blacks, Puerto Ricans and Whites, thus making use of two groups of largely African ancestry but differing cultural backgrounds.

FINDINGS

With the three-population design (Whites, Puerto Ricans and Blacks) and the three socioeconomic variables (income, education and occupation), what we found is best exemplified and also best illustrated in purely graphic form. Moreover, for presentation, we have grouped the analyses of prematurity first by weight, and then by gestation length, leaving the analyses by parity and with reference to smoking until last. It may be helpful, therefore, to introduce the graphic analyses as follows:

1. Prematurity by birth weight and income group.
2. Prematurity by birth weight and maternal occupation.
3. Prematurity by birth weight and maternal education.
4. Prematurity by gestation length and income.
5. Prematurity by gestation length and occupation.
6. Prematurity by birth weight and education (age-restricted).
7. Prematurity by birth weight, education and parity.
8. Prematurity by birth weight, education and smoking.

Taking the conventional birth weight definition of prematurity first, the results in relation to per capita income are dramatically displayed in Figure 1. For all three racial groups, there is a statistically significant income effect, though the actual magnitude of the effect is small. Far more important is the fact that the prevalence of low birth weight ($\leq$ 2500 gm.) is generally far higher in Blacks than in Whites, and in Puerto Ricans than in Whites, in each per-capita-income group considered.

Taking maternal occupation into account next (Fig. 2), from "never worked" (A) through managerial and professional (I and J), the prevalence of low birth weight singling neonates is clearly higher in Blacks at each occupational grouping compared. (As in Figure 1, absent or empty bars denote a paucity of birth weight data for that category.)

When we turn to maternal education (Fig. 3), socioeconomic and population effects are both highly visible. The higher the level of mater-

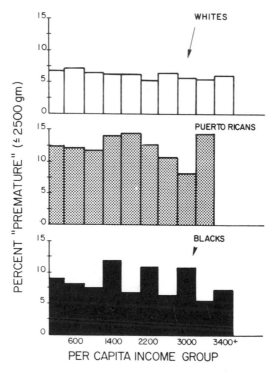

Figure 1. **Interaction of Per Capita Income and Race on Gestational Prematurity.**   As shown, for a total of 21,483 live singling births, prematurity (weight-defined) is least frequent in Whites as compared with Puerto Ricans and Blacks. There is, moreover, a slight income effect as shown by two-way analysis of variance. Yet, income group by income group, Puerto Ricans and Blacks show a higher prevalence of weight-defined prematurity, whereas the income effect itself is relatively small.

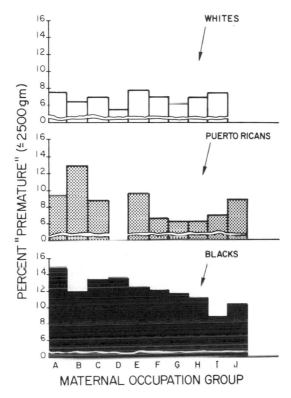

Figure 2. **Interaction of Race and Occupation Level in Whites, Puerto Ricans and Blacks.**   As shown, the prevalence of prematurity (weight-defined) is systematically lower in Whites than in Puerto Ricans or Blacks in each occupational category. Particularly in Blacks, there is a smaller proportion of live neonates with birth weights of 2500 gm. or less in the managerial and professional groupings.

nal education, the lower the prevalence of low birth weights in all three groups. Yet for constant educational level, the prevalence of birth weight prematurity (≤2500 gm.) is far higher in Puerto Ricans and Blacks than in Whites. Education, or years of schooling, however, has such obvious bearing on the prevalence of prematurity as to provide a target minimum for a program of national action.

Repeating the income analysis, but this time in reference to gestational prematurity (≤ 37 weeks), we again see a small though statistically significant income effect in all three groups. However, the prevalence of gestational prematurity in Puerto Ricans and Blacks surely commands attention. As shown in Figure 4, short gestation lengths are approximately twice as prevalent in Puerto Ricans and Blacks than in Whites, however income matched.

Arranged next by maternal occupation (Fig. 5), there is a declining prevalence of prematurity through to the managerial and professional

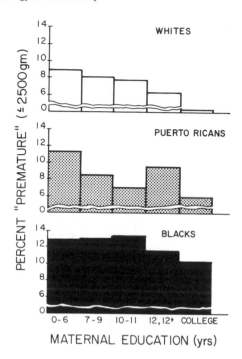

Figure 3. **Interactive Effects of Education and Racial Origin on Prematurity in Whites, Puerto Ricans and Blacks.**   As shown, weight-defined prematurity is systematically less common in Whites than in Puerto Ricans and Blacks and there is a marked inverse relationship between maternal education and the prevalence of prematurity. For all 3 groups, the percent of live born singlings with birth weights of 2500 gm. and less is lowest in the highest educational category.

ranks, but with the same population differences as previously described in Figures 1-4. Matching by occupational level scarcely reduces total sample comparisons of gestational prematurity in Whites, Puerto Ricans and Blacks.

In Figure 6, age restricted maternal education appears as the most relevant socioeconomic variable, so much so as to provide a target minimum when gestational prematurity is considered. Yet the data so clearly show the population differences (despite educational matching) as to suggest that short gestation lengths always must be considered in population context.

Since these comparisons for birth weight (Figs. 1-3) and gestation length (Figs. 4-6) are for live born singlings uncorrected for parity, and since parity bears on both birth size and gestation length, parity correction was next order. And, as shown in Figure 7, parity correction does not alter the general results presented so far. Corrected for parity, and again using the birth weight definition ($\leq$ 2500 gm), there is a major effect of maternal education. There is also a major population effect, with low birth weights still far more prevalent in Puerto Ricans and Blacks.

Further correction for smoking, as shown in Figure 8, reveals the effect of tobacco usage on birth weights, at each level of maternal education, with low birth weights obviously far more common in the smoking mothers. Yet the two-way corrections (smoking and maternal education) once again reiterate the population differences demonstrated in the seven graphs previously presented. So per capita income, maternal occupation and maternal education all bear on the prevalence of prematurity in live born singlings, increasingly in that approximate order. With 12

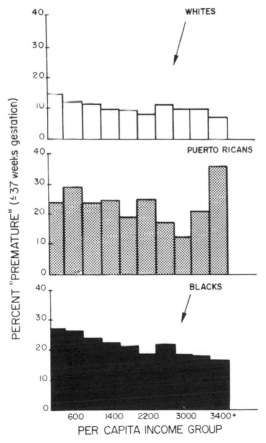

Figure 4. **Interaction of Race and Income on Prematurity (Gestation Length-Defined) in Whites, Puerto Ricans and Blacks.**   As shown, Blacks and Puerto Ricans evidence a higher frequency of short gestation lengths, as compared with Whites, in each per-capita-income grouping. At the same time, there is an inverse relationship between per capita income and gestation length in all 3 groups. In general, the highest income groupings are associated with the lowest frequency of short gestation lengths.

years of education or more, both birth-weight-defined prematurity and gestational prematurity are at their lowest levels. Education thus appears to be the best "prevention" for prematurity, whether weight-defined or defined in terms of gestation length. Yet across income, occupational or educational levels, Blacks and Puerto Ricans have a far higher prevalence of prematurity, whether defined by weight or by gestation length. There are other findings we would like to cite, among them the far lower weight for gestation lengths in Puerto Ricans and Blacks. As presented in another study (Garn and Bailey, 1977), we have shown that, for constant gestation length, Black male neonates have birth weights comparable to those in the White female (singling) newborn. Radiographic measures of skeletal (osseous) maturity separately show that there are Black/White differences in the maturity status of the newborn, holding birth weight or gestation length constant.

But to summarize, as socioeconomic status increases, the prevalence of gravimetric and gestational prematurity markedly decreases, espe-

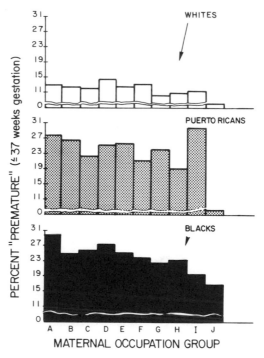

Figure 5. **Interaction Between Race and Occupational Level in the Prevalence of Short Gestation Lengths in Whites, Puerto Ricans and Blacks.**   Arranged by occupational grouping from "never worked" (A) through to managerial (I) and professional (J), short gestation lengths are less common in Whites than in Puerto Ricans or Blacks.

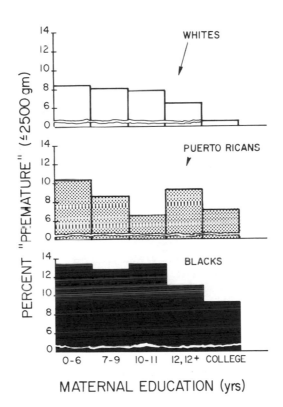

Figure 6. **Interaction Between Race and Education on the Prevalence of Birth Weight-Defined Prematurity in the 20–35 Maternal Age Group.**   As shown, low birth weights are far more common in Puerto Ricans and Blacks than in Whites (with ratios of 1.66 and 2.10 respectively for this comparison). At the same time, there is a marked decrease in the prevalence of short gestation lengths with increasing educational level. These age restricted comparisons reflect the higher prevalence of prematurity (however defined) in Puerto Ricans and Blacks than in Whites grouped by income or maternal or educational level.

cially so when maternal education is the primary variable. However, at each income level, each occupational level and each educational level, whether corrected for parity or not, or smoking or not, Puerto Rican and Black neonates are twice as often premature (using either conventional definition of prematurity) as White neonates.

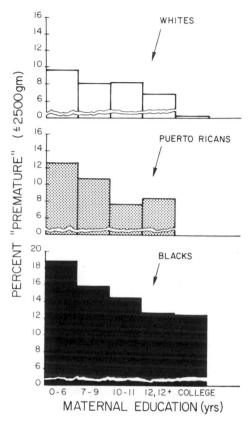

Figure 7. **Interaction Between Race and Maternal Education as They Affect Prematurity.** Here, eliminating neonates of later parity, weight defined-prematurity is still far more common in Puerto Ricans and Blacks than in Whites, but even parity-restricted, the educational factor is clearly involved.

DISCUSSION

What we have shown here in both tabular and graphic form reiterates what we said at the onset, namely, that both African ancestry and low socioeconomic status bear on the prevalence of prematurity, both separately and together. However, the low birth weights and the apparently shorter gestation lengths in Blacks and Puerto Ricans are far from being explained (in the statistical sense) by income, education or occupation. And the socioeconomic variables do not automatically yield a simple nutritional explanation, given what we know about socioeconomic status and nutrition.

These and other data suggest a smaller birth size for term infants of African ancestry, yet one associated with developmental maturity, as judged from radiographic and other indicators. It is impressive that the

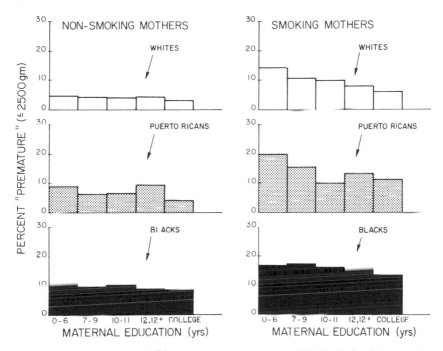

Figure 8.   **Effect of Maternal Education on the Prevalence of Weight-Defined Prematurity after Correction for Smoking.**   Even for non-smoking mothers (left), the prevalence of "premature" progeny is higher in Black and Puerto Rican women at all educational levels. The effect of education is especially apparent in the progeny of smokers (right).

infant of largely African ancestry, though generally smaller at birth and more often premature by conventional standards, is at the same time advanced in postnatal ossification timing, as we have shown in the Ten-State and Pre-School Survey data (Garn et al., 1972; Garn and Clark, 1976b) and as Roche et al. (1974, 1975, 1976) have shown in the National Health Examination data. In fact, Black boys and girls tend to be larger than White boys and girls from ages 2 through 14, as variously shown in the NINCDS, Pre-School, Ten-State and National Health Examination data (Garn et al., 1973a, 1973b; Owen and Lubin, 1973; Garn et al., 1974a). So the lower birth weights and yet higher proportions of statistical prematurity in Blacks and Puerto Ricans, though socioeconomic in part (and therefore preventable), also appear to be genetic in part and therefore to be considered. It is not racism to suggest race specific standards and definitions of prematurity, anymore than it is racism to advocate race specific standards for skeletal mass or for hemoglobins and hematocrits (Garn, et al., 1974b; Garn and Clark, 1976b; and Garn et al., 1977b).

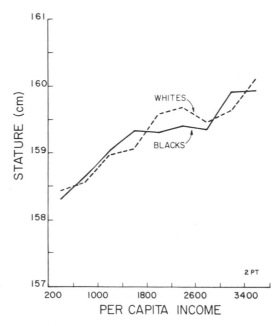

Figure 9. **Systematic Relationship Between Per Capita Income and Stature in Black Mothers (solid line) and White Mothers (dashed line).** The higher the income, the greater the stature and the fat-free weight but the lower the fat weight.

The socioeconomic correlates of prematurity, which cross racial and ethnic boundaries, are complicated and raise questions of national concern both as to the income groupings and the educational groupings or levels at special risk. One can argue that it is educational level and not income that is the primary variable or determinant, and the generic prescription may be educational enrichment rather than just financial advancement. One can also argue that the key determinant of low birth weight within a genetic population is actually nutritional level during pregnancy, and since the poor are more likely to be at nutritional risk, that education (or nutrition education) should be administered forthwith.

But let us again note that the poor woman, regardless of ancestry, tends to be far fatter than the more affluent woman (Garn and Clark, 1974; Garn et al., 1977a). To the extent that stored fat is a factor in prenatal growth, the progeny of the poor should actually be heavier at birth. At the same time, the fatter and heavier poor woman actually has a smaller fat-free weight than her leaner but richer peer (Garn and Clark, 1976a). And to the extent that the fat-free weight is a determinant of fetal growth and uterine continuation (Frisancho, Klayman and Matos, 1977), we might expect the conceptus of the rich woman to be less often premature than the fetus of the poor women who is larger on the outside but a smaller source of nutrients, given her smaller fat-free weight.

Let us not forget the fact that the poor in the US do have a larger proportion of women consuming less than optimal levels of protein intake, and with lower serum and urinary vitamins and lower hemoglobins and hematocrits, too. Prematurity in the poor may be related to these quantitative and qualitative differences in nutritional status. At the same time, poor women (and those of lesser education status) are smaller (i.e., shorter), as neatly shown in Figure 9, and they have smaller fat-free weights as well (Garn and Clark, 1976a). So the higher prevalence of gravimetric and gestational prematurity in their newborn may relate to their smaller cellular mass, and possibly their smaller uterine sizes and reduced reproductive efficiency.

CONCLUSIONS

The facts that we have come out with do not contradict the studies we started with, but we have been able to clarify the interactions between socioeconomic status and geographic race as they bear on 1) low birth weights and 2) short gestation lengths in live born singlings.

Socioeconomic status has an obvious bearing on the prevalence of prematurity in Whites, Puerto Ricans and Blacks, with prematurity (as variously defined) least common in the best educated women, both before and after corrections for parity and smoking. Consideration must be given to nutritional knowledge (which increases with educational level), to interest in health care and to the prepregnancy health status of women of higher educational attainment.

Geographic race also has a major bearing on the prevalence of prematurity at each income, occupational and educational level considered. Both in Black women (comparable in body size to White women) and in Puerto Rican women (of slightly shorter stature), the proportion of low-birth-weight neonates and short-gestation-length newborns is approximately twice that in SES-matched White women. Taking these two factors into account, as well as the smaller birth weights at each week of gestation (and evidences of greater developmental maturity of the newborn), the course of prenatal development appears to be different in those of largely African ancestry.

From the standpoint of national policy, there are two conclusions to reach. First, within each population considered, the far lower prevalence of prematurity in the progeny of women of higher educational and occupational attainment gives us target percentages to strive for. Second, the far higher prevalence of smaller, lower birth weight Black and Puerto Rican neonates suggests the need for race specific standards or definitions, as we move from descriptive findings to action programs designed to reduce the proportion of the premature.

ACKNOWLEDGMENTS

The research described in this paper was partially supported by Grant No. NO1-NS-5-2308 with the National Institutes of Neurological and Communicative Disorders and Stroke and incorporates the statistical and computer assistance of Kenneth E. Guire, Richard L. Miller and Robert L. Wainright. The illustrations were completed by Elizabeth M. Nofs and the manuscript was completed by Linda J. Kelly.

TEXT REFERENCES

Frisancho, A. R.; Klayman, J.; Matos, J.: Influence of Maternal Nutritional Status on Prenatal Growth in a Peruvian Urban Population. Am J Phys Anthrop 46(1977) 265–274

Garn, S. M.: Human Races, 3rd ed. Thomas, Springfield, Ill., 1970

Garn, S. M.: The Origins of Obesity. Am J Dis Child 130(1976)465–467

Garn, S. M.; Bailey, S. M.: Genetics of Maturational Processes. In: Human Growth, F. Falkner and J. M. Tanner, eds. Plenum Publishing Corp., New York, 30(1977b)000–000.

Garn, S. M.; Bailey, S. M.; Cole, P. E.; Higgins, I. T. T.: Level of Education, Level of Income and Level of Fatness in Adults. Am J Clin Nutr 30(1977a)721–725

Garn, S. M.; Clark, D. C.: Economics and Fatness. Ecol Food Nutr 3:(1974)19–20

Garn, S. M.; Clark, D. C.: Trends in Fatness and the Origins of Obesity. Pediatrics 57(1976a)443–456

Garn, S. M.; Clark, D. C.: Problems in the Nutritional Assessment of Black Individuals. Am J Pub Health 66(1976b)262–267

Garn, S.M.; Clark, D. C.; Trowbridge, F. L.: Tendency Toward Greater Stature in American Black Children. Am J Dis Child 126(1973a)164–166

Garn, S. M.; Owen, G. M.; Clark, D. C.: The Question of Race Differences in Stature Norms. Ecol Food Nutr 3(1974a) 319–320

Garn, S. M.; Sandusky, S. T.; Nagy, J. M.; McCann, M. B.: Advanced Skeletal Development in Low-Income Negro Children. J Pediat 80(1972)965–969

Garn, S. M.; Sandusky, S. T.; Nagy, J. M.; Trowbridge, F. L.: Negro-White Differences in Permanent Tooth Emergence at a Constant Income Level. Arch Oral Biol 18(1973b)609–615

Garn, S. M.; Shaw, H. A.; Guire, K. E.; McCabe, K.: Apportioning Black-White Hemoglobin and Hematocrit Differences During Pregnancy. Am J Clin Nutr 30 (1977b)461–462

Garn, S. M.; Smith, N. J.; Clark, D. C.: Race Differences in Hemoglobin Levels. Ecol Food Nutr 3(1974b)299–301

Owen, G. M.; Lubin, A. H.: Anthropometric Differences Between Black and White Pre-School Children. Am J Dis Child 126(1973)168–169

Roche, A. F.; Roberto, J.; Hamill, P. V. V.: Skeletal Maturity of Children 6–11 Years (United States). DHEW Publ. No. (HRA) 75-1622. Series 11, No. 140. 1974

Roche, A. F.; Roberto J.; Hamill, P. V. V.: Skeleton Maturity of Children 6–11 Years: Racial, Geographic Area, and Socioeconomic Differentials (United States). DHEW Publ. No. (HRA) 76-1631. Series 11, No. 149. 1975.

Roche, A. F.; Roberto, J.; Hamill, P. V. V.: Skeletal Maturity of Youths 12–17 Years (United States). DHEW Publ. No. (HRA) 76-0000. Series 11, No. 160. 1976.

DISCUSSION

Dr. Emanuel: Can fat-free weight be influenced very much after adulthood is reached?

Dr. Garn: The fat-free weight can obviously be increased in the adult male by muscle building courses! Whether the tendency towards fitness in the female is doing a similar thing I think is worthwhile observing. There is indirect evidence that people who have moved to the US in adulthood have attained a higher weight, if not a higher fat-free weight.

Dr. Kass: The regression correlation between maternal weight at the twentieth week and total blood volume is around 0.8, and this in turn has a significant relation to outcome. However, all of the red cell mass and blood data get lost in birth weight, and this argues that the amount of fat in these young women, at least in our population (a rather sparc population at the city hospital), may not be important as has been thought.

Dr. Rush: For the record, I think I need to disagree. Weiss et al.'s study (1969) of the women delivering twice in the collaborative study showed that change in prepregnant weight, which was almost surely not lean tissue, as well as changed pregnancy weight gain, were both associated with changes in birth weight. It has also been well argued that in the human the predominant change (aside from blood volume) in the body composition during pregnancy is in fat deposition, especially during the second trimester, and that this fat deposition if the major energy source for the special metabolic needs of pregnancy (Hytten and Leitch, 1971).

Dr. Garn: As long as you only look at weight in the child and weight in the mother, the problem cannot be well resolved. In those cases where we have had the opportunity in other studies to separate maternal weight into fat-free weight and fat weight categories, it becomes clear that the fat-free weight of the mother influences the fat-free weight of the child, and that the fat weight of the mother has particular bearing on the fatness of the off-spring (Garn et al., 1956; Frisancho et al., 1977a,b.).
So I think it is possible to separate these body components, but only when the data are there; whereas weight alone conceals, as we all know, a multitude of skins.

Dr. Morton: I think that terms like "black" and "white" are reasonably objective, although there is substantial error of estimation associated with them and they are social as well as biologic groups. As a geneticist, I find the term "African ancestry" rather confusing in this context.

Dr. Garn: That is one of the reasons for our interest in including the Puerto Ricans, who share about the same proportion of African genes but whose European genes come from a very different sector. I won't go into it now, but it does appear that the Spanish genes of the Puerto Rican population, as well as the Carib genes, contribute to differences in body size and growth rate which distinguish them from the American Negro (formerly the "American Colored") with a comparable proportion of African genes.

Dr. Kass: We have looked at pregnant black women, psychologically as well as studying other characteristics (Harrison et al., 1968), and can show quite clearly with a variety of psychological instruments that acculturation occurs within one or two generations.

Dr. Garn: What we are after is how much the population differences have a genetic basis, and to what extent they are rooted in the underlying environment. It has been very interesting for us to show that in blacks, exactly as in whites, the higher the income the skinnier the woman and the fatter the man.

On the other hand, there are differences in hemoglobin levels, the skeletal mass, postnatal ossification timing, postnatal dental development and early psychomotor measures which are all earlier in black children than in white children (Garn and Clark, 1976).

Prof. Meyer: If you compare birth-weight-specific mortality rates for low birth weight babies, the mortality for blacks is lower than for whites. This supports the idea that their appropriate birth weight is lower and that their optimum birth weight would be lower.

Dr. Terris: That has been known for a long time. In India and other developing countries you have the same phenomenon. This again raises the question, "Is this genetic or is it environmental?" and we don't know.

DISCUSSION REFERENCES

Frisancho, A. R.; Klayman, J.; Matos, J.: Influences of Maternal Nutritional Status on Prenatal Growth in a Peruvian Urban Population. Am J Phys Anthrop 46(1977a)265-274

Frisancho, A. R.; Klayman, J.; and Matos, J.: Newborn Body Composition and its Relationship to Linear Growth. Am J Clin Nutr 30(1977b)704-722

Garn, S. M.; Clark, D. C.: Problems in the

Nutritional Assessment of Black Individuals. Am J Publ Health 66(1976)262–267

Garn, S. M.; Greaney, G.; Young, R.: Fat Thickness and Growth Progress During Infancy. Hum Biol 28(1956)232–250

Harrison, R. H.; Kass, E. M.: MMPI Correlates of Negro Acculturation in a Northern City. J Personality and Soc Psychol 10(1968)262–270

Hytten, F. E.; Leitch, I.: The Physiology of Human Pregnancy, 2nd ed. Blackwell Scientific Publications, Oxford, 1971

Weiss, W.; Jackson, E. C.; Niswander, K.; Eastman, N.: The Influence on Birthweight of Change in Maternal Weight Gain in Successive Pregnancies in the Same Woman. Int J Gynecol Obstet 7(1969)210–223

Sociobiologic Factors and Birth Weight in Great Britain

Eva Alberman, M. D.

Since 1953 local health authorities in England and Wales have returned to the Central Health Department (formerly the Ministry, now the Department of Health and Social Security) the number of live and still births notified with a birth weight of 2500 gm. (5-1/2 lb.) or less born to mothers resident in their authority. These are divided into finer weight groups, and by hospital, home delivery or transfer and the time of death within the first month. The results are summarized annually in the Report of the Chief Medical Officer (DHSS), and those from 1953 to 1972 have been published together (Alberman, 1974).

Figure 1 shows that there has been very little variation in the proportion of low-birth-weight births since 1966, and indeed between 1953 and 1975 (England only) this ratio has never varied more than between 7 and 6.4% of all live births. In contrast, the neonatal death rate of such babies has fallen sharply (Fig. 2), so that we now have an increasing proportion of survivors of low birth weight, although even now the neonatal mortality of those of 2500 gm. or less is nearly 10%. In 1975 (England only) these babies represented 6.4% of all births but 59% of all neonatal deaths.

Indeed, one important reason why Great Britain's infant mortality, like that of the United States, is still considerably higher than that of the Scandinavian countries, and now even of Japan, is because we have a higher proportion of low-birth-weight births (Chase, 1967). This is

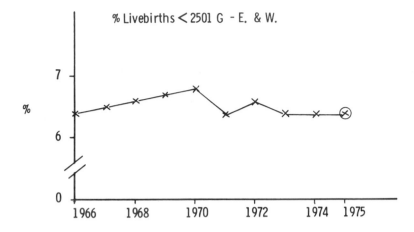

Figure 1.   **Percent Live Births Under 2501 gm., England and Wales, 1966–1975.** ⊗ =
England only.   Source: Department of Health and Social Security, various years.

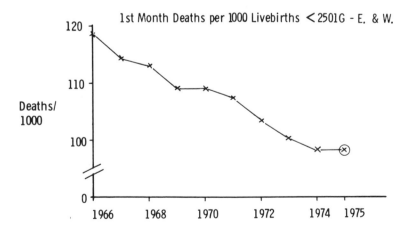

Figure 2.   **Neonatal Mortality Rate for Live Births Under 2501 gm., England and Wales,
1966–1975.** ⊗ = **England only.**   Source: Department of Health and Social Security,
various years.

shown in Table I, taken from data published by Pharoah in 1976 and with the latest US data (Chase, 1977) added.

What is difficult to explain is why the proportion of low-birth-weight babies is remaining at the same level when there is little doubt that the nutrition of the vast majority of pregnant mothers is satisfactory, their general health is probably better than 20 years ago, and we are beginning to see the beneficial effects of improved family planning on maternal age, parity and spacing of pregnancies.

An attempt has therefore been made to investigate the effects of changes in sociobiologic factors over a 12-year period (1958-70) on birth weight and rate of fetal growth. This period was chosen because two closely similar national birth studies were carried out in 1958 and 1970, thus presenting a unique opportunity to look into this problem. Both are well known, the first being the British Perinatal Mortality Study (Butler and Bonham, 1963; Butler and Alberman, 1969) and the second *British Births 1970* (Chamberlain et al., 1975). The comparisons made are only preliminary and are presented largely as a method of examining secular trends in birth weight. A more detailed examination, allowing for joint effects of related variables, is planned.

Table 2 shows the dates of the two studies, and the numbers of mothers and total births in each. Both studies included births in Scotland, and the second also included births in Northern Ireland, which comprised 3.6% of UK births in 1970. The vast majority of births in each were to mothers resident in England and Wales. Table 3 shows that the proportion of babies of 2500 gm. or less in each study was indeed very close to that notified in England and Wales in the years of each of the studies. Also evident from this table is the very small change in this proportion between the studies. This is further shown in the more detailed breakdown of birth weight of groups given in Table 4. Table 4

Table 1.   Low Birth Weight Proportion in Different Countries.

Country	Low Birth Weight as of Percentage of Live Births
England and Wales (1973)	6.5
Japan (1972)	5.3
Sweden (1971)	4.1
Finland (1970)	4.6
U.S.A. (1973)	7.5
white	6.4
black	13.2
other	7.5

Source: Chase, 1976

Table 2.   Parameters of the Two National Studies.

Date of Study	No. of Mothers	No. of Total Births	% Total Births in Study of those Notified or Registered
March 3-9, 1958	17,204	17,418	≏ 98
April 5-11, 1970	17,005	17,196	95–98

Table 3.   Low-Birth-Weight Ratios (< 2501 gm.): England and Wales, and the Two Studies, 1958 and 1970.

	Births in 1958		Births in 1970	
	% Total	% Live	% Total	% Live
England and Wales	7.8	6.9	7.5	6.8
Studies	7.9	6.9	7.8	—
		(5.7 singletons only)		(6.2 singletons only)

Table 4.   Distribution of Birth Weight of Singletons and Twins (Abortions Excluded) in 1958 and 1970 Studies.

Birth Weight (gm.)	Number		Percentage	
	1958 Study	1970 Study	1958 Study	1970 Study
1000 and under	62	73	0.4	0.4
1001–	111	125	0.6	0.7
1501–	221	255	1.3	1.5
2001–	866	894	5.0	5.2
Not weighed, but estimated under 2501	102	—	0.6	—
Sub-total under 2501	(1362)	(1347)	(7.9)	(7.8)
2501–	3182	3298	18.4	19.2
3001–	6159	6608	35.5	38.5
3501–	4591	4507	26.4	26.3
4001 and over	1587	1386	9.2	8.1
Not weighed but estimated 2501 and over	454	—	2.6	—
Total known	17335	17146	100.0	100.0
No information	71	24		

also shows that a birth weight was given for 99.9% of the 1970 and 96.4% of the 1958 babies. For the latter study, where birth weight was not known it was estimated to be over 2500 gm. in 2.6% and 2500 gm. or under in another 0.5%.

Table 5 shows the distribution of gestational age in the two studies, and the proportion in which this was not known or uncertain. The reliability of this is always problematic. In the 1958 Perinatal Mortality Study, gestational age was calculated from the date of the first day of the last menstrual period (LMP), as given by the mother and as recorded in the antenatal notes. In 7.7% this date was not known. The midwives completing the questionnaire were also asked the expected date of delivery as recorded in the notes. This is usually computed from the LMP, but occasionally changed by the obstetrician when he feels that the date as computed is incompatible with his clinical estimate of fetal maturity. For the second report of the 1958 study, the questionnaires were scrutinized further for any in which the estimated date of delivery as computed from the LMP differed from that estimated by the obstetrician by more than three days. This resulted in a further 2.9% of all cases being classified as "gestational age uncertain." In the 1970 study the persons completing the form were asked directly whether the LMP as given was recorded as being certain, uncertain or not known. In only 81.1% of the mothers of singleton children was this regarded as certain.

However, Table 5 shows that the "certain" gestational age distributions in 1958 and 1970 (after excluding deliveries before 28 weeks) were closely similar, with 5.3% of the 1958 and 5.2% of the 1970 births delivered before the 37th week. The only difference was in a slight decrease of babies with a gestational age of 42 weeks or more in 1970.

As explained above, in 10.6% of the babies in 1958 and 18.9% in 1970 it was impossible to measure birth weight by "certain" gestational age. This measure in cross-sectional form is the nearest we can get to an estimate of fetal growth. It is therefore important to note that in both the studies there was evidence that the cases excluded from the gestational age analysis because of uncertain or unknown dates included a larger than expected proportion of births of low birth weight.

Figure 3 shows the 50th percentile of birth weight from 32–42 weeks for those cases of "known" gestational age in 1958 and 1970. There is a very remarkable consistency between the findings in the two years, particularly between 37 and 41 weeks. This is very surprising in view of the fact that there had been considerable changes between 1958 and 1970 in the prevalence of sociobiological factors known to affect birth weight.

Table 6 shows the relative size of the effects on birth weight of some of these factors, based on an analysis of variance which allowed an esti-

Table 5. Distributions of "Certain" and "Uncertain" Gestational Age in 1958 and 1970 Studies, Singletons Only.

Gestational age (completed weeks)	Number				Percentage			
	1958 Study		1970 Study[1]		1958 Study		1970 Study[1]	
	"Certain"	"Uncertain"	"Certain"	"Uncertain"	"Certain"	"Uncertain"	"Certain"	"Uncertain"
28–29	36	2	39	15	0.2	0.4	0.3	0.7
30–31	70	7	62	16	0.5	1.4	0.5	0.7
32	54	10	31	21	0.4	2.0	0.2	1.0
33	70	8	60	30	0.5	1.6	0.5	1.4
34	91	10	78	36	0.6	2.0	0.6	1.6
35	158	30	136	50	1.0	6.0	1.0	2.3
36	313	29	283	92	2.1	5.8	2.1	4.2
37	654	35	511	128	4.3	7.0	3.8	5.9
38	1489	38	1396	214	9.8	7.7	10.3	9.8
39	3239	63	2770	312	21.4	12.7	20.4	14.3
40	4107	101	3809	352	27.1	20.3	28.1	16.1
41	3026	67	2937	356	20.0	13.5	21.7	16.3
42	1344	50	1033	240	8.9	10.1	7.6	11.0
43	385	35	189	122	2.5	7.0	1.4	5.6
44+	126	12	223	198	0.8	2.4	1.6	9.1
Total	15,162	497	13,557	2,182	100.0	100.0	100.0	100.0
Under 28	26	0	45	22				
No Information	1309	—	32	598				

Source: Butler and Alberman, 1969 and Chamberlain et al., 1975.
[1] Excludes 379 mothers where no information on whether LMP "certain" or "uncertain."

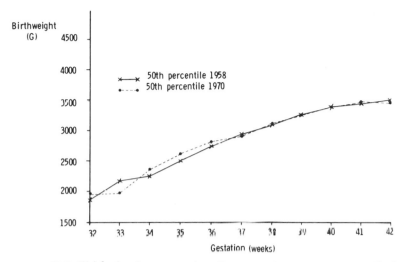

Figure 3.   Birth Weight for Gestational Age, Singletons Only, 1958 and 1970 Studies.
Source: Butler and Alberman, 1963; Chamberlain et al., 1975.

Table 6.   Fitted Constants for Analysis of Variance of Effects of Certain Characteristics on Birth Weight, 1958 Study, Singletons only.

Maternal Characteristics	Groups	Fitted Constants
Parity	0	4.71
	1	9.14
	2–3	9.89
	4+	11.46
Height	inches	inches × 1.403
Preeclampsia	none or mild	11.38
	moderate	10.89
	severe	4.13
Smoking	nonsmokers	11.74
	smokers	5.86

Source: Goldstein, in Butler and Alberman, 1969.

mate of the joint effects of the factors examined on birth weight in ounces. The size of the fitted constant gives an indication of the relative importance of each in predicting birth weight. The most important factors were, as shown, maternal height (weight was not available), a history of smoking in pregnancy, preeclamptic toxemia and parity.

Where possible, the effects of these variables on birth weight in 1970 have been compared with the 1958 findings. Perhaps the most important factor available for comparison is maternal height. Table 7 compares the distribution of three height groups in the two studies. Two changes had taken place by 1970: there were slightly more taller mothers, and slightly more short mothers, so that the "medium" group of 62-64 inches was reduced in number. The small increase of tall mothers is probably in line with the general secular increase in height between generations (Goldstein, personal communication). The excess of small mothers may be related to the increase of mothers born outside the UK in the 1970 study compared with 1958 (Table 8). However, whatever the causes of the changes seen in height distribution, the effects on birth weight were probably such as to cancel each other out. Table 9, giving the mean birth weight for each height group, keeping gestational age constant at 38-41 weeks, shows that there was relatively little difference between the two studies in view of the small numbers at the extremes, with a gradient of 245 gm. between the means of the shortest and tallest groups in 1958 and 241 gm. in 1970.

Another very important variable which changed over the period between the studies was cigarette smoking in pregnancy. Regrettably, the questions on smoking in pregnancy were not the same in the two studies. In 1958 the mothers were asked whether they had smoked after the fourth month of pregnancy, and if so, how many cigarettes a day. The results so far published from the 1970 study related to three questions:

Table 7. Percentage Distribution of Maternal Height in Singleton Births, 1958 and 1970 Studies.

Maternal Height	1958 Study		1970 Study[1]	
Group (inches)	No.	%	No.	%
Less than 62	3594	22.0	3954	23.8
62-64	7827	48.0	7302	43.9
65 or more	4884	30.0	5364	32.3
Total known	16,305	100.0	16,620	100.0
Not known	689		172	

Source: Chamberlain et al., 1975 and Butler and Alberman, 1969.
[1] 23 abortions excluded.

Table 8.   Percent Distribution of Mothers by Birth Place, 1958 and 1970 Studies.

	1958 Study	1970 Study
United Kingdom	93.3	89.2
Europe	4.4	5.2
West Indies	0.6	1.8
India/Pakistan	0.5	2.4
Other and not known	1.2	1.4
Total	100.0	100.0

Source: Chamberlain, et al., 1975 and personal communication, National Child Development Study.

Was the mother smoking at the time of the survey? If not, had she ever smoked? If so, how many cigarettes (in groups only) did she smoke per day?

Chamberlain and her colleagues suggest that the two most comparable statistics from the studies are the 65.5% of mothers who were nonsmokers after the fourth month of pregnancy in 1958, with the 55.3% who were not smoking immediately after the birth of their baby in 1970. This increase in the proportion of women of reproductive age who smoked between 1958 and 1970 is in line with other evidence available nationally.

There is also information from the birth and from other studies that in addition to the habit becoming more common, there was an increase in the number of cigarettes smoked per day. On the other hand, changes in method of manufacture and choice of tobacco meant that there was also a reduction in mean nicotine and tar content over this period.

Table 9.   Mean Birth Weight by Maternal Height Group, 1958 and 1970 Studies, Singletons of 38–41 Weeks Gestation.

Maternal Height Group	Mean Birth Weight (gm.)	
(inches)	1958 Study	1970 Study
61 and under	3241	3232
62–64	3350	3362
65 and over	3486	3473

Source: Chamberlain et al., 1975 and Butler and Alberman, 1969.

Table 10 shows that the mean birth weight of babies of mothers who smoked and those who were thought not to have smoked in pregnancy was quite remarkably similar in the two studies, with almost exactly the same mean difference (170 gm. in 1958; 176 gm. in 1970) between the smokers and nonsmokers. A very crude estimate based on the data in Table 10 suggests that if all other factors had remained constant, a 10% increase between the two studies in mothers who smoked could have reduced the overall mean birth weight by 20 gm. A reduction of this order could be brought about by an increase of 1% in the babies weighing 2500 gm. or less, at the expense of the group weighting 3501 gm. or more. This estimate is purely hypothetical and is presented only as an indication of the order of magnitude of changes in birth weight that could result from fairly major changes in factors such as maternal smoking.

In Table 4 it seems that the only reduction in birth weight achieved between the two studies was by a shift of a proportion of the heaviest babies downwards into the group between 2500 and 3500 gm.

Other changes that occurred between 1958 and 1970 were those in the distribution of birth rank. Table 11 shows that in 1970 there were both fewer first and fewer fourth or later babies than in 1958. Again, these are changes that could cancel out any effect on birth weight, the reduction in first births tending to raise the mean and that in fourth or later tending to lower it.

Finally, one very dramatic change in management that occurred between the two studies was in the medical or surgical induction of labor. No data were published for the incidence of induction in the 1958 study, but in 1970 this occurred in 31.8% of all births. In hospital deliveries in England the proportion of induced births has risen from 15% in 1964 to a provisional figure of 41% in 1974 (Department of Health and Social Security, 1976). In the 1970 study mean birth weight of babies delivered

Table 10. Mean Birth Weight of Babies by Maternal Smoking Habit, 1958 and 1970 Studies, Singletons of "Certain" Gestational Age.

Group	Mean Birth Weight (gm.)	
	1958 Study	1970 Study
Smoking (1958 after 4th month of pregnancy; 1970 at inquiry)	3205	3200
Not smoking (1958 after 4th month: 1970 never smoked)	3375	3376

Source: Chamberlain et al., 1975 and Butler and Alberman, 1969.

Table 11.   Percent Distribution of Parity in Singleton Births, 1958 and 1970 Studies.

Parity	1958 Study	1970 Study
0	36.1	35.5
1	31.2	33.2
2-3	23.8	24.2
4 +	8.9	7.1
Total	100.0	100.0

Source: Chamberlain et al., 1975.

between 38 and 41 weeks was 3376 gm. if the onset of labor was spontaneous, it was 3350 gm. if labor had been induced. This difference is very much smaller than that between birth weight in mothers who smoke and those do not, but is in the same direction.

Any comparison between induced and spontaneous births must take into account medical reasons for induction, which are themselves likely to reduce birth weight. On the other hand, with the proportion induced rising as fast as it is, a very careful watch must be kept on the effect on birth weight where induction is not for purely medical reasons.

In conclusion, the changes in variables between 1958 and 1970 that have been studied in this account would, if all other factors had remained constant, have reduced mean birth weight by something over 20 gm. In fact, the mean birth weight of singletons of "certain" gestational age was 3320 gm. in 1958 but only 10 gm. less (3310 gm.) in 1970. The finding that a decrease of the expected magnitude did not occur suggests that changes in other factors not examined here might have acted on birth weight in the opposite direction. For instance, a decrease in preeclamptic toxemia could have had such an effect, but the data are not yet available.

It was stressed at the outset of this paper that this exercise was an example of a method that might be used to examine secular trends in birth weight in some detail, and that the analysis needs to be carried out with methods that allow for multifactorial effects. In spite of its shortcomings, this preliminary crude analysis has confirmed the apparent stability of birth weight distribution, and shown that very major changes in sociobiologic variables will be needed before there are substantial changes in birth weight. Nevertheless, it is clear that a decrease in smoking in pregnancy, together with a fall in the induction rate, might have a perceptible and beneficial effect on the proportion of births of low birth weight in the United Kingdom.

TEXT REFERENCES

Alberman, E.: Stillbirths and Neonatal Mortality in England and Wales by Birth Weight, 1953-71. Health Trends, 6(1974)14

Butler, N. R.; Bonham, D. G.: Perinatal Mortality, Livingstone Ltd., Edinburgh, 1963.

Butler, N. R.; Alberman, E. D.: Perinatal Problems. Livingstone Ltd., Edinburgh, 1969

Chamberlain, R.; Chamberlain, G.; Howlett, B.; Claireaux, A.: British Births 1970, Vol. 1, The First Week of Life. William Heinemann Medical Books Ltd., London, 1975

Chase, H.: International Comparison of Perinatal and Infant Mortality. National Center for Health Statistics Series 3, No. 6. U.S. Department of Health, Education and Welfare. Public Health Service, 1967

Chase, H.: Time Trends in Low Birth Weight in the U.S. In: Epidemiology of Prematurity, ed. by D. M. Reed & F. Stanley. Urban & Schwarzenberg, Baltimore-Munich, 1977

Department of Health and Social Security. Annual Report of The Chief Medical Officer "On the State of Health of the Nation." London, HMSO. 1966-75

Pharoah, P. O. D.: International Comparisons of Perinatal and Infant Mortality Rates. Proc Roy Soc Med 69(1976)335

DISCUSSION

Dr. Rush: An interesting recent observation in Britain has been that, with an increase of the proportion of cigarettes with filters and a lowering of tar content, there has been a decrease in respiratory tract cancer and an increase in cigarette-associated coronary heart disease. This has been assumed to be due to lower tar dose, with increased combustion products, including carbon monoxide, passing freely through filters. (The increase arises from the need to smoke more cigarettes in order to sustain nicotine levels.) Thus, if high carbon monoxide is one of the causes of low birth weight among smokers, we would not expect any decrease in the rate of low birth weight, and there has been none.

Dr. Susser: Do you have a distribution of frequency of birth by social class? I wonder if that might be the distorting factor related to smoking.

Dr. Alberman: Although the classification changes between the two years, there is virtually no change in the distribution.

Dr. Mellits: As 10.6% of the 1970 population was excluded because of unknown gestations, there might be a difference due to the missing data. Missing data are very often in a disadvantaged group.

Epidemiologic Observations of Prematurity: Effects of Tobacco, Coffee and Alcohol

Bea J. van den Berg, M.D.

The main purpose of this contribution to the workshop is to describe and analyze the effect of cigarette smoking during pregnancy in relation to maternal variables and pregnancy-related factors on the incidence of prematurity in terms of low birth weight and/or short gestation. Secondly, the effects of coffee and alcohol consumption on prematurity are described, followed by some observations on infant mortality, incidence of severe congenital anomalies and utilization of medical care by the various categories of "prematures."

The data of this working paper were derived from the Child Health and Development Studies. These were designed and initiated by the late Dr. Jacob Yerushalmy. The overall objectives of the studies are to investigate the relationship of biologic, genetic, medical and environmental factors in the parents—including events in pregnancy, labor and delivery—to the normal and abnormal development of the offspring. From 1960 to 1967, pregnant women, members of a prepaid medical plan (Kaiser Health Plan), were enrolled in the studies. The population is broadly based, ethnically and socioeconomically. Data are obtained from gravida's medical record (starting before pregnancy until pregnancy termination), as well as from interviews, which include information on repro-

Supported by Grant No. HD 07256 of the National Institute of Child Health and Human Development of NIH.

ductive history, socioeconomic factors, smoking habits and beverage consumption. Among the 15,000 interviewed gravidas, 67% were white, 23% black, 3% Mexican-American, 4% Oriental and another 3% were of other ethnic backgrounds. The children were observed through their medical records for at least five years. In addition, special developmental examinations and follow-up interviews of subgroups of the cohort when the children were 5-years and 10-years old provided information on health and physical and cognitive development. Preparations are in progress for an adolescent study.

In this paper, a review of previous work on the pertinent subject is followed by a recording of ongoing studies and concluded by a few outlines for futher studies.

REVIEW OF PREVIOUS WORK

Prematurity has been the subject of several CHDS studies, and the relationship of smoking to birth weight has been extensively analyzed. A simple and practical classification of prematurity according to birth weight and gestation was proposed, utilizing as points of separation 2500 gm. and 37 weeks (Yerushalmy, 1967). Newborn infants are thus divided into four groups: 1) premature by both criteria, 2) premature by birth weight, but mature by length of gestation, 3) mature by birth weight and premature by gestation, and 4) mature by both criteria. The first group (premature by both criteria) might be further divided by birth weight, e.g., ≤ 1500 gm. and 1501-2500 gm. These categories of infants are shown to have distinct rates of neonatal mortality and morbidity.

For the purpose of research in prematurity, a special classification for infants 1501-2500 gm. was developed by constructing four groups identical for birth weight distribution but differing in length of gestation in which the birth weight was reached. The four groups were of short, intermediate short, intermediate long, and long gestation, with means of 34 weeks, 36 weeks, 38 weeks, and 40 weeks respectively. As the birth weight distributions are equal, the four groups represent decreasing rates of intrauterine growth. These groups are shown to differ considerably in placental weight, neonatal mortality and neonatal morbidity (e.g., respiratory distress syndrome, dyspnea), incidence of severe congenital anomalies, duration of initial hospitalization and need of incubator care, growth in height and weight in the first year of life, and morbidity patterns in early childhood (van den Berg and Yerushalmy, 1966; van den Berg, 1971). We also compared growth in height and weight up through age 10 years for low birth weight children in the four gestation groups with growth of children who were mature for both birth weight and gestation (Beck and van den Berg, 1975). Only the infants in the long gestation group failed to catch up in height and weight with the control group by the end of the 10-year period (Figs. 1 and 2).

The pregnancy interview provided the data on smoking habits of gravida and of her husband. Our data show the well-known higher incidence of low birth weight infants of smoking mothers as compared with those who do not smoke. This is a part of the general phenomenon that the entire distribution by birth weight of infants of smoking mothers is shifted to the side of the lower weights (Yerushalmy, 1971).

Yerushalmy (1972) developed new and complementary methodology to overcome the built-in problem of self-selection of being a smoker or nonsmoker. He tested the causal significance of smoking in low birth weight infants by comparing the birth weight of infants born before their mothers took up the smoking habit with those of mothers who smoked during pregnancy, and with those of mothers who never smoked. The result was that the percent of low birth weight infants in the first group, born before the mothers started smoking, was significantly higher than that among infants of mothers who never smoked (Fig. 3). Thus, the evidence appears to indicate that the *smoker* rather than the *smok-*

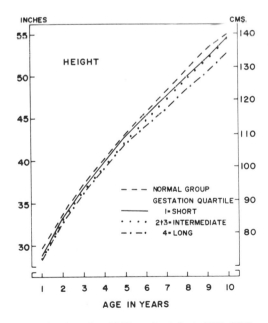

Figure 1.   **Mean Height for Ages 1 to 10 Years for Infants 1501–2500 gms Birth Weight in the Short, Intermediate and Long Gestation Quartiles, Compared with Height of Children Who Had Birth Weights above 2500 gms.**   Source: G. J. Beck and B. J. van den Berg, J of Pediat 86(1975) 504–511.

ing is involved in the increased rate of low birth weight. The author emphasized the need to investigate the problem on other and possibly larger samples of births and to include more variables for the analysis. This has not yet been done, and the observations have not been satisfactorily explained (Buck, 1975; Davies, 1975).[1]

Another approach to test the causal hypothesis is to investigate the mechanism that could explain the interference of fetal growth under the condition of cigarette smoking of the gravidas. Wingerd et al. (1976) studied the relationship of smoking and anemia among CHDS women to the placental ratio (ratio of placental weight to birth weight). The literature indicated a high placental ratio in two situations with chronic fetal hypoxia: births at high altitudes (Kruger et al., 1970) and births to women with severe anemia of pregnancy (Beischer, 1970). The placental

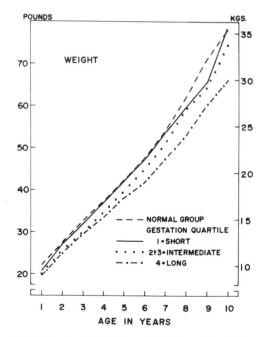

Figure 2. **Mean Weight for Ages 1 to 10 Years for Infants 1501–2500 gms Birth Weight in the Short, Intermediate and Long Gestation Quartiles, Compared with Height of Children Who Had Birth Weights above 2500 gms.**   Source: G. J. Beck and B. J. van den Berg, J of Pediat 86(1975) 504–511.

[1]After the presentation of this paper, a study was published pertaining to the issue of the *smoking* or the *smoker*, the causal hypothesis versus the self-selection hypothesis. Though the data were more consistent with the self-selection hypothesis, the findings were inconclusive and could not confirm nor deny this hypothesis (Silverman, D.T.: Maternal Smoking and Birth Weight. Am J Epid 105(1977)513–521).

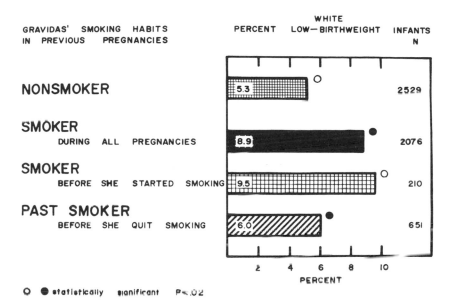

Figure 3.   Percent of Low Birth Weight Infants by Mothers' Smoking Status   Source: J. Yerushalmy, Am J Obstet Gyn 112(1972) 277-284.

ratio was also observed to be higher in pregnancies with smoking than in those without. One of the dissimilarities with the previous situations, however, is that with smoking, the birth weight is decreased but the placental weight is adequate for the length of gestation, while at high altitudes and with severe anemia, the birth weight is reduced and the placenta appears to be hypertrophied. The authors concluded that in the smoking situation the data neither totally confirm nor totally refute the hypoxia hypothesis. The placenta studies continue (Christianson, manuscript in preparation).

ONGOING STUDIES ON CIGARETTE SMOKING AND CONSUMPTION OF COFFEE AND ALCOHOL

The incidence of smoking during pregnancy, as well as the incidence of low birth weight and/or short gestation, varies widely by ethnic background. For example, the percent of women in our study cohort who smoked during pregnancy is 38% among whites, 32% among blacks, 24% among Mexican-Americans, and 14% among Oriental women. The percentages of infants weighing ≤ 2500 gm. and/or < 37 weeks gestation for these four ethnic groups are 7.5%, 15.8%, 8.3% and 10.1%

respectively. To simplify this presentation, only the data on white gravidas will be discussed.

The distribution according to the prematurity criteria of birth weight
and gestation for single (white) live born infants of women who never
smoked, who stopped smoking or who continued smoking during pregnancy is shown in Table 1. Infants of smoking women have an excess in
all categories of prematurity as compared with those of women who
never smoked or stopped smoking, but the difference is largest in the
group $\leqslant$ 2500 gm. and 37+ weeks gestation (3.1% among smokers,
1.3% among never smokers, 1.6% among past smokers). The mean
birth weight of infants of smoking women is about 200 gm. less than
that of the women who never smoked. The birth weight of infants of
past smokers is equal to that of infants of never smokers. A comparison
of women smoking less than 15 cigarettes a day and more than 15 cigarettes a day shows a definite dose effect. The first columns of the table
also show that while 38% of the mothers of the total group of infants
smoked, 55% of the mothers of low birth weight infants were smokers.

As has already been indicated in earlier presentations in this workshop,
several pre-existing maternal factors, biologic or socioeconomic, have an
increased risk of low birth weight and/or short gestation. Some of these
factors are also associated with a higher incidence of smoking, giving
rise to a certain amount of confounding. Certain of these prepregnant
maternal factors are presented in Tables 2 and 3. Table 2 shows, for
example, that very young maternal age (less than 20 years) has an increased risk of short gestation, rather than an increase in low birth
weight. In contrast, among women with low prepregnant weight (less
than 100 pounds), the risk is most increased of having infants weighing
$\leqslant$ 2500 gm. but who are not premature according to the gestation criterion.
This illustrates the necessity to use both criteria of prematurity simultaneously in establishing risk factors. The last column of Table 2 indicates the percentage of cigarette smokers among the women with the
specified characteristics. The percentages generally exceed the 38% in
the total cohort.

Table 3 compares the distributions in the four birth weight gestation
categories of live born infants of women who smoked or did not smoke
during pregnancy. (The latter includes the women who stopped smoking
before or because of this pregnancy.) The results show that for the first
four factors, the ratios of percentages (or relative risks) in the subgroups
of prematurity for smokers compared to nonsmokers are similar to the
ratios in the total cohort of Table 1. Also, the difference in mean birth
weight for smokers and nonsmokers is about 200 gm. Thus, no interaction effect is observed in these groups. However, for the gravidas with
very low prepregnant weight, and for the gravidas in the lower socioeconomic groups as indicated by level of education of gravida and hus-

Table 1. Smoking Status of Gravida: Incidence Rates Per 1000 and Percent Distributions of Live Born Infants in Four Categories of Birth Weight and Length of Gestation.

Smoking Status of Gravida During Pregnancy	Factor Incidence per 100 among:			Percent Distributions of Each Factor in Subgroups of Birth Weight and Gestation					
				≤2500 gms		>2500 gms		Number (N = 100%)	Mean Birth Weight (gms)
	All Bwt.-Gest.	Birth Weight ≤2500 gms	Gestation <37 wks	<37 wks	37- wks	<37 wks	37+ wks		
Gravida:									
Never smoked	43.4	30.9	36.7	1.8	1.3	2.8	94.1	4,249	3463.4
Stopped before pregnancy	10.7	8.8	9.6	2.0	1.6	2.9	93.5	1,051	3457.2
Stopped because of pregnancy	7.7	5.8	8.3	1.8	1.5	4.1	92.6	757	3474.4
Is current smoker	38.1	54.6	45.4	3.3	3.1	3.3	90.3	3,723	3254.9
Total	100.0	100.0	100.0	2.4	2.0	3.1	92.5	9,780	3384.1
Smokes <15 Cigarettes per Day*	16.4	17.7	17.0	2.4	2.4	3.4	91.8	1,600	3323.3
Smokes ≥15 Cigarettes per Day	21.2	36.6	27.9	4.1	3.6	3.2	89.1	2,077	3200.5

*Of 46 current smokers, the number of cigarettes smoked was unknown.

Table 2. Certain Prepregnant Maternal Factors With Increased Risk of Low Birth Weight and/or Short Gestation.

Prepregnancy Factors (Biologic and Socioeconomic)	Factor Incidence per 100 among:			Percent Distributions of Each Factor in Subgroups of Birth Weight and Gestation				Number (N = 100%)	Percent Smoking During Pregnancy
	All Bwt.-Gest.	Birth Weight <2500 gms	Gestation <37 wks	<2500 gms		>2500 gms			
				<37 wks	37+ wks	<37 wks	37+ wks		
Gravida's age: <20 years	5.7	7.1	10.0	3.2	2.3	6.5	88.0	556	41.4
Parity: ≥4 previous pregnancies	7.6	8.9	9.6	3.8	1.5	3.2	91.5	741	40.4
Birth weight of immediately preceding live birth: 2500 grams or less	3.0	11.0	5.7	8.0	8.0	2.3	81.7	299	55.5
Marital status: divorced or separated	1.6	3.5	2.6	4.8	4.8	4.1	86.3	145	63.4
Gravida's height: ≤60 inches	6.6	11.5	7.2	3.4	4.3	2.6	89.7	649	35.7
Gravida's prepregnancy wt.: <100 lbs	3.2	9.6	5.4	4.6	9.3	4.6	81.5	259	45.2
Gravida's education: less than high school graduate	15.8	21.6	21.5	3.6	3.1	4.6	88.7	1,405	49.1
Husband's education: less than high school graduate	13.6	17.4	18.6	2.9	2.8	4.6	89.7	1,315	49.7
Husband's occupation: unskilled and semi-skilled	11.3	13.8	14.5	2.7	2.8	4.3	90.2	1,086	46.9

band and occupation of husband, the ratios in the low birth weight groups are higher, and these differences in mean birth weight are about 250 gm. The smoking effect appears to be stronger in these less favorable circumstances.

Tables 4 and 5 provide information on certain obstetric observations in pregnancy and delivery. The most important factors related to prematurity are antepartum bleeding and low weekly weight gain during late second and third trimesters. Table 4 indicates that although antepartum bleeding occurs in only 3% of the pregnancies, among low birth weights the incidence amounts to 19.6% and among short gestations to 15.7%. Among the gravidas with antepartum bleeding the risk of having an infant satisfying both criteria of prematurity appears to be as high as 22.8%; this percentage in smoking and nonsmoking women is 27.2% and 19.0% respectively (Table 5). The percent of smokers among women with antepartum bleeding is disproportionately high: 46.3%, compared with 38% in the total cohort of pregnant women. This means that the risk of antepartum bleeding is higher among smoking women than among women who do not smoke during pregnancy.

Low weekly weight gain (less than 1/2 pound per week from 20 weeks of gestation until last prenatal visit before delivery) occurred in 15% of the pregnancies. However, the incidence was 26.3% among pregnancies producing low birth weight infants and was 23.2% among the pregnancies producing pre-term live born infants. The proportion of smokers is slightly higher in the low weight gain group. [The association of smoking to low weight gain is less prominent in our population than in the socioeconomically disadvantaged population discussed by Rush et al. (1976).]

Nausea and/or vomiting in the first trimester, with the exception of the very severe cases, are not related to prematurity; the proportion of smokers is low, i.e., only 29.4%, compared with 38% in our study cohort. It has been hypothesized (Hook et al., 1976) that nausea and vomiting might have the beneficial effect of producing an aversion to toxins such as cigarette smoking. This hypothesis finds some support in our data: of women with nausea and/or vomiting, 22.1% of initial smokers discontinued smoking because of pregnancy, while this percentage was 15.1% among women without that complaint. The beneficial effect of first trimester nausea/vomiting to lowered fetal and neonatal mortality has been described earlier in our study cohort (Yerushalmy and Milkovich, 1965; Brandes, 1967).

Proteinuria in pregnancy is associated with increased proportions of low birth weight infants, especially of those with 37+ weeks gestation. Glycosuria typically is associated with an increase in the subgroup of infants weighing more than 2500 gm. and born before term (< 37 weeks). The increased proportion of low birth weight infants delivered with

Table 3.   Certain Prepregnant Maternal Factors: Distributions of Single Live Births of Women who Smoked or Did Not Smoke* During Pregnancy in Four Subgroups of Birth Weight and Length of Gestation.

| Prepregnancy Factors Biologic and Socioeconomic | Percent Distribution of Each Factor | | | | Number (N = 100%) | Mean Birth Weight (gms) |
| | Birth Weight ≤2500 gms | | Birth Weight >2500 gms | | | |
	Gestation <37 wks	37+ wks	Gestation <37 wks	37+ wks		
Gravida's age: <20 years						
Smoker	4.3	3.9	7.4	84.4	230	3218.6
Non-smoker	2.5	1.2	5.8	90.5	326	3411.5
Parity: >4 previous pregnancies						
Smoker	5.0	1.3	3.3	90.3	299	3287.0
Non-smoker	2.9	1.6	3.2	92.3	442	3572.7
Birth weight of immediately preceding live births: 2500 grams or less						
Smoker	9.0	8.4	3.6	79.0	166	2911.9
Non-smoker	6.8	7.5	.8	85.0	133	3119.6
Gravida's height: ≤60 inches						
Smoker	4.3	5.2	3.5	87.4	232	3057.7
Non-smoker	2.9	3.8	2.2	91.1	417	3259.0

Gravida's prepregnancy weight: <100 lbs						
Smoker	7.7	12.0	6.0	74.4	117	2917.6
Non-smoker	2.1	7.0	5.5	87.3	142	3163.5
Gravida's education: less than high school graduate						
Smoker	4.3	4.2	4.9	86.6	739	3194.3
Non-smoker	2.9	1.8	4.4	90.9	666	3446.6
Husband's education: less than high school graduate						
Smoker	3.8	4.0	4.4	87.8	653	3196.0
Non-smoker	2.0	1.7	4.8	91.5	662	3452.3
Husband's occupation: unskilled laborer, service worker						
Smoker	3.3	3.9	4.7	88.0	509	3224.0
Non-smoker	2.1	1.7	4.0	92.2	577	3471.3

*Nonsmokers include women who stopped smoking before or because of this pregnancy.

Table 4. Certain Complications of Pregnancy and Delivery: Incidence Rates per 100 and Percent Distributions of Live Born Infants in Four Categories of Birth Weight and Length of Gestation.

Pregnancy Factors	Factor Incidence per 100 Among:			Percent Distributions of Each Factor in Subgroups of Birth Weight and Gestation					
				≤2500 gms		>2500 gms			Percent Smoking During Pregnancy
Complications of Pregnancy and Delivery	All Bwt.-Gest.	Birth Weight ≤2500 gms	Gestation <37 wks	<37 wks	37+ wks	<37 wks	37+ wks	Number (N = 100%)	
Nausea/vomiting in first trimester*	60.9	54.6	57.4	2.1	2.0	3.0	92.9	3,799	32.1
Proteinuria: two or more times ≥1+	1.8	5.2	2.1	4.5	7.9	1.7	85.9	178	37.1
Glycosuria: one or more times ≥1+	3.9	1.4	5.0	.8	.8	6.0	92.4	381	34.9
Antepartum bleeding	3.0	19.6	15.7	22.8	6.1	5.8	65.3	294	46.3
Cesarean section:									
Elective	2.3	3.5	3.9	3.6	3.2	5.9	87.3	220	38.6
Emergency	1.6	4.8	4.7	10.1	3.1	5.7	81.1	159	43.4
Weekly weight gain after 20 weeks: <0.5 pounds	15.1	26.3	23.2	3.9	3.6	4.0	88.5	1,020	39.5

*Relates to women who entered the studies before the 84th day after last menstrual period.

Table 5. Certain Complications of Pregnancy and Delivery: Distributions of Single Live Births of Women Who Smoked or Did Not Smoke During Pregnancy in Four Subgroups of Birth Weight and Length of Gestation.

	Frequency Distribution of Each Factor					
Pregnancy Factors	Birth Weight <2500 gms		Birth Weight >2500 gms		Number	Mean Birth
	Gestation		Gestation		(N = 100%)	Weight (gms)
Complications of Pregnancy and Delivery	<37 wks	37+ wks	<37 wks	37+ wks		
Nausea/vomiting in 1st trimester						
Smoker	3.3	2.9	3.0	90.8	1,218	3248.4
Non-smoker	1.5	1.6	3.1	93.8	2,581	3464.3
Proteinuria: two or more times ≥1 +						
Smoker	7.6	4.5	3.0	84.8	66	3236.5
Non-smoker	2.7	9.8	.9	86.6	112	3325.8
Glycosuria: one or more times ≥1 +						
Smoker	1.5	1.5	3.3	93.2	133	3343.3
Non-smoker	.4	.4	7.2	91.9	248	3556.9
Antepartum bleeding						
Smoker	27.2	7.4	6.6	58.8	136	2675.6
Non-smoker	19.0	5.1	5.1	70.8	158	3020.7
Cesarean section:						
Smoker	8.4	5.8	4.5	81.3	154	3141.5
Non-smoker	4.9	1.3	6.7	87.1	225	3306.5
Weekly weight gain after 20 weeks:						
<0.5 lbs						
Smoker	4.0	6.0	4.2	85.9	403	3127.7
Non-smoker	3.9	2.1	3.9	90.1	617	3313.4

Table 6. Coffee and Alcohol Consumption During Pregnancy: Incidence Rates per 100 and Percent Distributions of Live Born Infants in Four Categories of Birth Weight and Length of Gestation.

| Pregnancy Factors | Factor Incidence per 100 Among: | | | Frequency Distributions of Each Factor in Subgroups of Birth Weight and Gestation | | | | Total | Mean Birth |
| | | | | ≤2500 gms | | >2500 gms | | | |
Coffee and Alcohol Consumption	All Bwt.-Gest.	Birth Weight ≤2500 gms	Gestation <37 wks	<37 wks	37+ wks	<37 wks	37+ wks	(N = 100%)	Weight (gms)
Gravida									
Coffee:									
≤1 cup/day	39.2	29.8	32.3	1.8	1.6	2.7	93.9	3,336	3418.0
2-6 cups/day	47.8	48.8	49.0	2.5	2.1	3.2	92.2	4,073	3372.1
≥7 cups/day	13.0	21.4	18.7	4.3	3.2	3.7	88.8	1,105	3298.5
≥7 cups/day; smoker	8.5	17.0	13.6	5.1	3.9	3.7	87.3	722	3177.3
≥7 cups/day; non-smoker	4.5	4.4	5.1	2.6	1.8	3.7	91.9	383	3529.4
Alcohol:									
≤1 drink/wk	70.3	71.4	71.7	2.5	2.0	3.1	92.4	5,922	3385.4
2-6 drinks/wk	18.1	18.3	18.2	2.6	2.0	3.0	92.4	1,524	3385.9
7+ drinks/wk	11.5	10.3	10.1	1.9	2.0	2.9	93.2	980	3351.6
7+ drinks/wk; smoker	5.3	6.4	5.6	2.5	2.9	3.4	91.2	446	3253.2
7+ drinks/wk; non-smoker	6.3	3.9	4.5	1.5	1.3	2.4	94.8	534	3433.7

emergency cesarean section is largely due to an overlap with antepartum bleeding.

Table 6 provides information on coffee and alcohol consumption during pregnancy. Heavy coffee drinking ($\geqslant$ 7 cups per day) occurs in 13% of our study cohort, while the incidence among mothers of low birth weight infants was 21.4%. Increasing consumption of coffee appears to be associated with increasing rates of prematurity in all subclasses. Among heavy coffee drinkers, there is a large proportion of smokers: 722/1105, or 65.3%. The combination of these two habits results in 5.1% + 3.9% = 9% infants weighting $\leqslant$ 2500 gm. This percentage is 4.4% for women who drink $\geqslant$ 7 cups of coffee but do not smoke. As this latter percentage is equal to that of the total cohort, the coffee effect on prematurity appears to be entirely explainable by the association with smoking.

Alcohol consumption is measured in units per week, with one unit considered equal to one glass of beer or wine or one cocktail. Hardly any association is found between alcohol consumption and birth weight. Among women drinking 7+ units of alcohol per week are 45.5% smokers, who have 2.5% + 2.9% = 5.4% of their infants weighing 2500 gm. or less. This is 2.8% for the corresponding nonsmoking women.

The general conclusion of the preceding observations is that, with a few exceptions, the effect of smoking cigarettes during pregnancy on proportion of low birth weight and/or mean birth weight is additive to any effect of recognized prepregnant risk factors and obstetric complications. Many of the considered factors are interrelated and/or are related to smoking. For the unraveling of the contribution of the various factors to the variation in birth weight and proportion of prematurity, multivariate analyses are necessary. An attempt to show the main relationships is given in Table 7. It does not pretend to give more than an approximation of the associations. It shows the linear correlation coefficients for most of the discussed maternal characteristics with smoking as well as with birth weight. Noteworthy are the correlations between smoking and socioeconomic level as indicated by education and occupation. The less privileged groups have larger proportions of smokers (and smaller proportions of past smokers). The linear correlation between smoking and birth weight is 0.1904, of about the same order between prepregnant weight, weekly weight gain, or antepartum bleeding and birth weight.

The simple squared, linear correlation coefficient could be interpreted as the proportion of variance in birth weight, attributable to the linear component of each single factor, while the squared, cumulative multiple correlation coefficient stands for the combined contribution of the linear components of the so-far-entered factors to the variance of birth weight. Though the contribution of smoking is reduced when the pre-

Table 7.   Correlation Coefficients of Certain Maternal Characteristics and Pregnancy Complications with Smoking and Birth Weights.

Sample Correlation With Smoking (r)	Maternal Characteristics [1]	Sample Correlation With Birth Weight (r)	(r²)	Squared Cumulative Multiple Correlation With Birth Weight: (R²)	Increment in R²
.0380	1 Previous pregnancies	.0825	.0068		
−.0550	2 Maternal age	.0600	.0036		
−.1658	3 Gravida's education	.0617	.0038		
−.1514	4 Husband's education	.0585	.0034	.0963	.0963
.1321	5 Husband's occupation	−.0405	.0016		
.0758	6 Preceding low birthweight infants	−.1675	.0281		
.0168	7 Gravida's height	.1785	.0319		
−.0333	8 Gravida's prepregnant weight	.2276	.0518		
.1993	9 Coffee consumption	−.0706	.0050	.1026	.0063
.0580	10 Alcohol consumption	−.0204	.0004		
	11 Cigarette smoking	−.1904	.0363	.1278	.0252
−.0465	12 Weekly weight gain after 20 weeks	.1721	.0296	.1591	.0313
.0042	13 Albuminuria	−.0240	.0006		
.0306	14 Antepartum bleeding	−.1730	.0299	.1866	.0275

Notes on coding of characteristics: 1.: 4 groups: 0, 1 + 2, 3 + 4, 5+. 2.: 5 groups: <20, 20-24 25-29, 30-34, 35+ years. 3. + 4: 4 groups: less than high school, high school graduate, some college, college graduate. 5.: 4 groups: professional + manager, sales + clerical, crafts, labor + service. 6.: 5 groups: 0-4 or more previous liveborn ≤ 2500 gms. 7.: 6 groups of 2 inch intervals: < 58-67+. 8.: 6 groups of 15 lbs intervals: < 100-175+. 9.: 10 groups <1 cup-10+ cups per day. 10.: 2 groups: <7 and 7+ drinks per week. 11.: 2 groups: no-yes. 12.: 7 groups of ¼ lbs increments: < ¼-1½+ lbs per week. 13.: 2 groups: no-yes. 14.: 2 groups: no-yes.

pregnant factors are controlled, it is still among the largest identified. It appears here, as in Tables 4 and 5, that smoking and weight gain act almost independently on birth weight.

In total about 19% of the variance in birth weight may be attributed to these discussed factors. This is not different from other studies using comparable factors (Rush, 1976; Habricht et al., 1974).

The preceding discussion considered the contribution of different factors to risk of prematurity. It was demonstrated that from the viewpoint of etiology, the categorization of prematures according to the criteria of birth weight and length of gestation is useful. It is even more meaningful when infant survival and incidence of severe congenital anomalies are considered. Tables 8 and 9 provide information on infant mortality and incidence of severe congenital anomalies in the categories of birth weight and gestation, showing large differences within the prematurity group. The infants in the categories of ≤ 2500 gm. as well as < 37 weeks gestation are highest in infant mortality, while infants ≤ 2500 gm. and

Table 8.   Infant Mortality per 100 Single Live Born Infants (First Year of Life).

	Rate Per 100		
	Total	Nonsmokers	Smokers
1. By birth weight-gestation categories:			
Birth weight <1500 grams, all gestations	70.2	79.1	60.8
Birth weight 1501–2500 grams, gestation <37 weeks	15.8	23.3	9.0
Birth weight 1501–2500 grams, gestation 37+ weeks	8.0	8.1	7.9
Birth weight >2500 grams, gestation <37 weeks	2.3	2.2	2.5
Birth weight >2500 grams, gestation 37+ weeks	.7	.6	.8
TOTAL	1.5	1.4	1.6
2. By Gravida's smoking status during pregnancy:			
Never smoked	1.4		
Stopped sometime before pregnancy	1.8		
Stopped because of pregnancy	.9		
Smoked during pregnancy	1.6		
3. By Gravida's coffee consumption during pregnancy:			
<7 cups per day	1.4		
≥7 cups per day	1.7		
4. By Gravida's alcohol consumption during pregnancy:			
<7 Drinks per week	1.5		
≥7 Drinks per week	1.2		

Table 9.   Percent of Children With Severe Congenital Anomalies Diagnosed During the First Five Years of Life.

1. By birth weight-gestation categories:		
Birth weight ⩽2500 grams, gestation <37 weeks		9.7
Birth weight ⩽2500 grams, gestation 37+ weeks		13.0
Birth weight >2500 grams, gestation <37 weeks		4.3
Birth weight >2500 grams, gestation 37+ weeks		3.2
	TOTAL	3.6
2. By Gravida's smoking status during pregnancy:		
Never smoked		3.9
Stopped sometime before pregnancy		4.0
Stopped because of pregnancy		2.2
Smoked during pregnancy		3.5
3. By Gravida's coffee consumption during pregnancy:		
<7 Cups per day		3.5
⩾7 Cups per day		4.4
4. By Gravida's alcohol consumption during pregnancy:		
<7 Drinks per week		3.4*
⩾7 Drinks per week		4.7*

*Difference significant with X^2 test: $p < 0.05$.

37+ weeks gestation have the highest incidence of congenital anomalies. A comparison of mortality among the low birth weight infants of non-smoking and smoking women shows that the latter have the lower rates, as was shown earlier by Yerushalmy (1971).

Tables 8 and 9 also show the mortality rates and rates of severe congenital anomalies for infants, differentiated by maternal smoking and coffee and alcohol consumption. No significant differences are found in the mortality data. The only statistically significant difference exists between the incidence of severe anomalies of women who consume less than seven drinks per week and those who consume more. Literature exists on the so-called fetal alcohol syndrome, which is a specific set of anomalies occurring among the offspring of chronic alcoholic women. These anomalies were not found in this study group, which included only six pregnant women recognized as chronic alcoholics. The finding of an association between moderate alcohol consumption and increased risk of congenital anomalies will be studied in detail.

FUTURE STUDIES RELATED TO PREMATURITY

Beside etiologic studies in the different ethnic groups other than whites, we have planned work on sequential pregnancies of the same women.

The emphasis is on the study of the repetitive character of obstetric events, obstetric complications, and physiologic items such as blood pressure, weight gain, etc., as well as of the repetitive character of specific types of reproductive loss and the various subclasses of factors of prematurity.

Studies on chronic or acute diseases and drug treatments in relation to pregnancy outcome in terms of teratogenicity, prematurity and mortality are continuing (Milkovich and van den Berg, 1974, 1976, 1977).

We are engaged in studies on long-term effects of prematurity in terms of morbidity, utilization of medical care, and physical, mental and behavioral development. A preliminary example of utilization of medical care in the first two years of life by category of birth weight and duration of gestation is presented in Table 10. It is seen that considerable differences exist, especially in the proportion of children who were hospitalized and who obtained consultations with specialists other than their pediatricians. Equally interesting is the observation that the proportion of children with 8 + drop-in or emergency visits for acute conditions or diseases is the same in all categories. These studies are also aimed at the comparison of immediate and long-term health and development, premature infants of different etiologies (e.g., certain obstetric complications) and biologic, social and behavioral maternal factors such as those discussed in this workshop.

Table 10. Utilization of Medical Care in the First Two Years of Life of Children in Four Birth Weight-Gestation Categories.

Type of Outpatient or Inpatient Care	Birth Weight ≤2500 gms Gestation		Birth Weight >2500 gms Gestation		Total
	<37 weeks	37 + weeks	<37 weeks	37 + weeks	
Percent with:					
8 or more scheduled visits	67.6	62.8	49.4	54.9	55.1
8 or more drop-in (emergency) visits	35.9	37.8	35.6	33.6	33.8
4 or more specialists (consultations other than pediatricians)	17.9	16.0	8.5	10.3	10.5
1 or more hospitalizations	22.1	21.8	11.7	9.8	10.3
Number of children (who were health plan members more than 2 years)	145	156	247	7,363	7,911

TEXT REFERENCES

Beck, G. J.; van den Berg, B. J.: The Relationship of the Rate of Intrauterine Growth of Low Birth Weight Infants to Later Growth. J of Pediat 86(1975)504–511

Beischer, N. A.; Sivassamboo, R.; Vohra, S.; Silpisrnkosal, S.; Reid, S.: Placental Hypertrophy in Severe Pregnancy Anemia. J Obstet Gyn 77(1970)398

Brandes, J. M.: First-Trimester Nausea and Vomiting as Related to Outcome of Pregnancy. Obstet Gyn 30(1967)427–431

Buck, C.: Popper's Philosophy for Epidemiologists. Int J Epid 4(1975)159–168

Davies, A. M.: Comments on "Popper's Philosophy for Epidemiologists" by Carol Buck. Int J Epid 4(1975)169–170

Habricht, J.; Lechtig, A.; Yarbrough, C.; Klein, R. E.: Maternal Nutrition, Birth Weight and Infant Mortality, In: Size at Birth pp 353–377, ed. by K. Elliot and J. Knight. Ciba Foundation, New York, Oxford, 1974

Hook, E. B.: Changes in Tobacco Smoking and Ingestion of Alcohol and Caffeinated Beverages During Early Pregnancy: Are These Consequences, In Part, of Feto-Protective Mechanisms Diminishing Maternal Exposure to Embryotoxins? In: Birth Defects, pp. 173–183, ed. by S. Kelly, E. B. Hook, D. Janerick, I. H. Porter. Academic Press, New York, 1976

Kruger, H.; Arias-Stella, J.: The Placenta and the Newborn Infant at High Altitudes. Am J Obstet Gyn 106(1970)586

Milkovich, L.; van den Berg, B. J.: Effects of Prenatal Meprobamate and Chlordiazepoxide Hydrochloride on Human Embryonic and Fetal Development. N Engl J Med (1974)Vol. 291,1268–1271

Milkovich, L.; van den Berg, B. J.: An Evaluation of the Teratogenicity of Certain Antinauseant Drugs. Am J Obstet Gyn 125(1976)244–248

Milkovich, L.; van den Berg, B. J.: Effects of Antenatal Exposure to Anorectic Drugs. Am J Obstet Gyn, In Press (1977)

Rush, D.: Cigarette Smoking During Pregnancy: The Relationship with Depressed Weight Gain and Birth Weight; An Updated Report. In: Birth Defects, pp. 161–171, ed. by S. Kelly, E. B. Hook, D. Janerich, I. H. Porter. Academic Press, New York, 1976

van den Berg, B. J.; Yerushalmy, J.: The Relationship of the Rate of Intra-Uterine Growth of Infants of Low Birth Weight to Mortality, Morbidity, and Congenital Anomalies. J Pediat 69(1966)531–545

van den Berg, B. J.: Idiopathic Respiratory Distress Syndrome (IRDS) and Other Forms of Dyspnea (D) in a Large Cohort of Births. I. Incidence by Birth Weight and Gestation in Relation to Antepartum Bleeding, Cesarean Section, and Breech Presentation. Proc. of the International Congress of Pediatrics, Vol. XVII, 171–176, August, 29-September 4, 1971

Wingerd, J.; Christianson, R.; Lovitt, W. V.; Schoen, E. J.: Placental Ratio in White and Black Women: Relation to Smoking and Anemia. Am J Obstet Gyn 124(1976)671–675

Yerushalmy, J.: The Classification of Newborn Infants by Birth Weight and Gestational Age. J Pediat 71(1967)164–172

Yerushalmy, J.: The Relationship of Parents' Cigarette Smoking to Outcome of Pregnancy Implications as to the Problem of Inferring Causation from Observed Associations. Am J Epid 93(1971)443–456

Yerushalmy, J.: Infants with Low Birth Weight Born Before Their Mothers Started to Smoke Cigarettes. Am J Obstet Gyn 112(1972)277–284

Yerushalmy, J.; Milkovich, L: Evaluation of the Teratogenic Effect of Meclizine in Man. Amer J Obstet Gyn 93(1965)553–562

Prenatal Nutrition and Subsequent Development[1]

Mervyn Susser, M.B., B.Ch.
Zena Stein, M.B., B.Ch.

In this paper I shall discuss two studies carried out by our group at Columbia University: the Dutch Famine Study (with Drs. Zena Stein, Gerhart Saenger and the late Frank Marolla[2]) and the Prenatal Project (with Drs. David Rush and Zena Stein). These studies aim to clarify the effects of prenatal nutrition on fetal growth, on fetal viability and infant mortality and on subsequent physical and mental development.

THE DUTCH FAMINE STUDY

When the idea of this study occurred to us, it was 20 years on from Clement Smith's 1947 paper on the effects of the Dutch famine on pregnancy. We realized with excitement that the survivors among those exposed to the famine *in utero* would be in their twenties.

The Dutch famine was a tragic cadenza to World War II. The relevant aspects are fully described in our book (Stein et al., 1975), and we omit description here. The famine was unique in a number of important respects. It was sharply demarcated in time and in place, and thus permitted the identification of those exposed and those unexposed according to their

---

[1]This is a revised version of a paper presented to the International Association for the Scientific Study of Mental Deficiency, Washington, DC. August 1976
[2]Dr. Marolla died suddenly on July 27, 1976. This paper is dedicated to him.

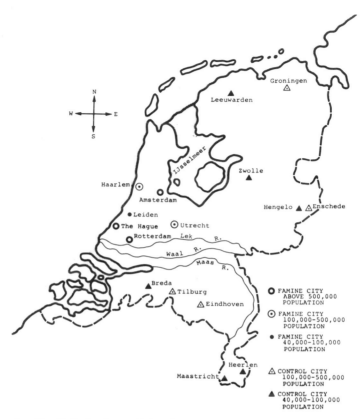

Figure 1. **The Netherlands.**   Taken from Stein, Z., M. Susser, G. Saenger, and F. Marolla. 1975. Famine and Human Development: The Dutch Hunger Winter of 1944–1945. Oxford University Press, New York p. 58.

time and place of birth. Further, the famine lasted a relatively short time—six months in all, or less than a term pregnancy. From this there followed several advantages. The extreme conditions extending over a short period of time provided the natural equivalent of a deliberate intervention. Consequently, the common difficulty of separating prenatal from postnatal malnutrition was not an obstacle, and exposure to the famine could be specified in terms of each phase of pregnancy, thus permitting a test of the critical period hypothesis (Dobbing, 1964; Winick and Noble, 1966). Finally, the country was not so disorganized that it could not maintain its excellent system of vital statistics, and extensive documentation on the famine, including nutritional intake of the population in terms of food rations, was readily available.

The design of the study rested on two prongs. Exposed and unexposed birth cohorts were assigned by time and place of birth to create two comparison groups, a place control and a time control. To achieve control by place, the exposed and unexposed cohorts were derived from total births occurring at the same time in all cities of over 40,000 population in famine and non-famine areas. The accompanying map (Fig. 1) indicates their distribution.

The time control was based on monthly births throughout the period January 1944 through December 1946. The design is illustrated in Figure 2. Each horizontal bar represents one month of births from conception to delivery. The bars are grouped according to their stages of gestation at famine exposure in order to test the critical period hypothesis. The crucial exposure in terms of maximum brain growth prenatally is during the third trimester. In the diagram, the B-2 cohort suffered the maximum at this time. The level of official rations declined to less than 500 calories at the worst period. [It should be noted from the recent work of Dobbing and Sands (1974) that the period of maximum brain growth now appears to extend through the first two years of life, an amendment that must be taken into account in assessing the ultimate effects of malnutrition on brain growth.]

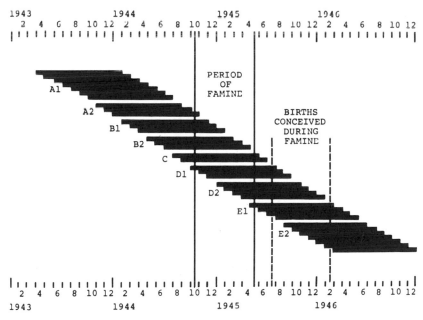

Figure 2. **Design of Study.**   Cohorts by month of conception and month of birth, in the Netherlands, 1943 through 1946, related to famine exposure. Solid vertical lines bracket the period of famine, and broken vertical lines bracket the period of births conceived during famine. Taken from Stein, Z., M. Susser, G. Saenger, and F. Marolla. 1975. Famine and Human Development: The Dutch Hunger Winter of 1944–1945. Oxford University Press, New York p. 57.

In this study we were able to examine effects of prenatal famine exposure on the following outcomes: 1) fertility, 2) fetal growth, 3) mortality
through 19 years of age, and 4) adult mental and physical health states.

Effects on fertility were profound. Here we note only that the effects
differed across social class, thus altering the social class composition of
the birth cohorts affected and requiring control of confounding in analysis.

Prenatal Famine Effects on Fetal Growth

About 6000 births in maternity hospitals were studied and allowed us to
reach the following conclusions. Growth retardation occurred in all the
fetal dimensions measured. The effects were owed solely to third trimester
exposure to the famine; thus the maximum effects were seen in the B-2
cohort. Most important, they occurred only below a threshold value of
caloric intake in the population. Below that threshold level, there was a
dose-response relationship between deprivation and fetal growth retardation. The results for birth weight are illustrated in Figure 3.

The study of mortality was based on all deaths up to 20 years of age
in the study cohorts. Age-specific death rates were developed for the
120,000 births involved. In summary, third trimester famine exposure

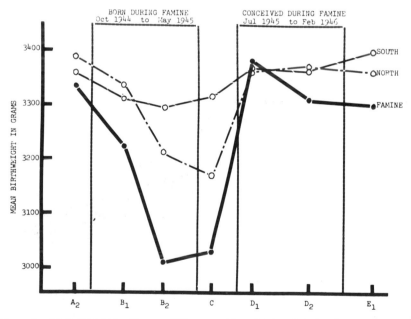

Figure 3. **Birth Weight by Time and Place.**   Mean birth weight in grams for births in
maternity hospitals for seven birth cohorts: Famine, Northern control, and Southern control areas compared for the period August 1944 to March 1946 inclusive. Taken from
Stein, Z., M. Susser, G. Saenger, and F. Marolla. 1975. Famine and Human Development: The Dutch Hunger Winter of 1944-1945. Oxford University Press, New York p. 93.

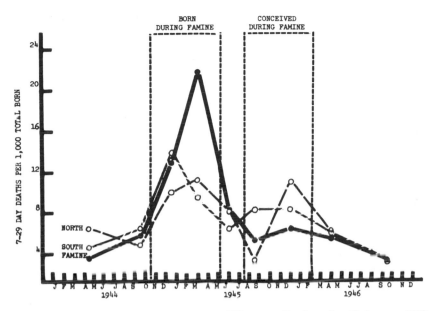

Figure 4. **Deaths at 7 to 29 Days by Time and Place.**   Deaths at 7 to 29 days per 1000 total births: famine, Northern control, and Southern control areas by cohort for births January 1944 to December 1946. Taken from Stein, Z., M. Susser, G. Saenger, and F. Marolla. 1975. Famine and Human Development: The Dutch Hunger Winter of 1944–1945. Oxford University Press, New York p. 155.

caused a sharp excess of mortality up to three months of age. These effects, while apparent in the first week of life, became marked after that stage through the first three months of life. The peak mortality in the B-2 cohort, for deaths at 7–29 days and at 30–89 days, are illustrated in Figures 4 and 5.

Prenatal Famine Effects on Adult Health State

In this part of the study, the data were taken from military induction records of examinations of 19 year old men. These data comprised virtually a total population of 120,000 men. The losses between birth and survival at 19 years that could not be accounted for by migration or mortality were an estimated 3%.

Five psychometric tests were available, of which the most sensitive was Raven's Progressive Matrices test. Figure 6 shows that there were no detectable effects of famine exposure on test performance in either the manual or the non-manual classes.

Similarly, analysis of classified diseases yielded no detectable famine effects related to third trimester exposure and fetal growth retardation.

The conditions tested included mild mental retardation, severe mental retardation and a number of psychiatric conditions, among many others.

Finally, anthropometric measures such as height, weight and Quetelet's index yielded no detectable effects of prenatal famine exposure, with one exception. Exposure in the latter part of pregnancy and early postnatal life led to a deficiency of obese individuals; exposure in the first half of pregnancy led to an excess of obese individuals. These results have considerable import for hypotheses relating to obesity.

We may conclude that third trimester prenatal exposure to famine had unequivocal somatic effects on fetal growth and infant vitality through 90 days of age. Effects persisting in adults were undetectable, with the exception of the frequency of obesity.

THE PRENATAL PROJECT

The ultimate aim of the studies we embarked on was the prevention and treatment of adverse nutritional effects. It is a logical fallacy to translate direct from ill effects of nutritional deprivation (for instance, on fetal growth and mortality, as seen in the famine study) into a presumption of benefits from nutritional supplementation. Such a presumption requires empirical tests. Hence we designed a second study based on nutri-

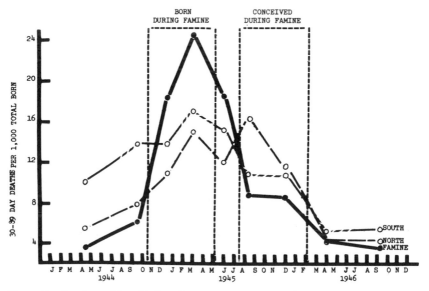

Figure 5. **Deaths at 30 to 89 Days by Time and Place.**   Deaths at 30 to 89 days per 1000 total births: famine, Northern control, and Southern control areas by cohort for births, January 1944 to December 1946. Taken from Stein, Z., M. Susser, G. Saenger, and F. Marolla. 1975. Famine and Human Development: The Dutch Hunger Winter of 1944-1945. Oxford University Press, New York p. 158.

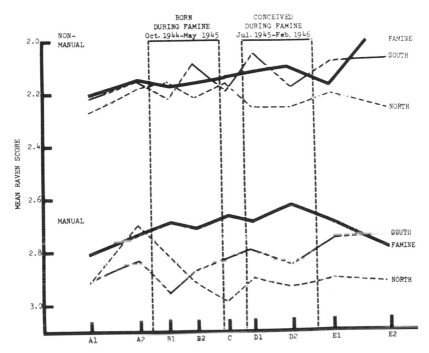

Figure 6. **Raven Scores by Area and Class.**   Mean Raven scores by cohort in famine, Northern control, and Southern control areas, comparing manual and non-manual occupational classes. Taken from Stein, Z., M. Susser, G. Saenger, and F. Marolla. 1975. Famine and Human Development: The Dutch Hunger Winter of 1944-1945. Oxford University Press, New York p. 203.

tional intervention with the object of trying to eliminate, in a population at risk of low birth weight, retardation of fetal growth owed to poor nutrition, and its subsequent effects (Rush et al., 1972).

About 1000 black women were selected from a clinic population known to be at high risk of low birth weight (about 18% vs. 5-6% in the most favored health areas of New York City). With their permission, they were assigned at random to a double-blind control trial, at different levels of nutritional supplementation. Before assignment to treatment, the women were stratified by individual attributes which placed them at particularly high risk of low birth weight (±25%), attributes which we belived might differentiate among conditions of varying sensitivity to nutritional intervention.

There were three treatment groups in all:

1. supplement (40 grams protein, 470 calories, vitamins and minerals). This constituted the high protein supplement;
2. complement (6 grams protein, 320 calories, vitamins and minerals). This constituted a balanced protein caloric supplement;

3. a sleeping control assigned to regular clinic care (routine supplements of vitamin and mineral tablets).

Results of Supplementation

Figure 7 shows an unequivocal failure to negate the null hypothesis at time of birth. There was no difference detected in birth weight, nor in other fetal dimensions, between the three treatment groups comprising about 300 women each.

Naturally, all available explanations of the absence of effect have been tested, including distributions of confounding factors that might have been biased despite the randomization of the design, the degree to which supplementation took place and the degree to which supplementation might have been substituted for the regular diet. Unfortunately, with further analysis, things got worse rather than better.

An important control variable was length of gestation, a factor intimately related with birth weight. The most proper means of controlling for length of gestation is by life table analysis. Figure 8 shows the cumulative delivery rate by stage of gestation throughout the study period. Excess of premature deliveries among the women in the high protein supplement group prior to 35-weeks gestation is evident. This excess rate of prematurity led directly to an excess of neonatal deaths. Figure 9

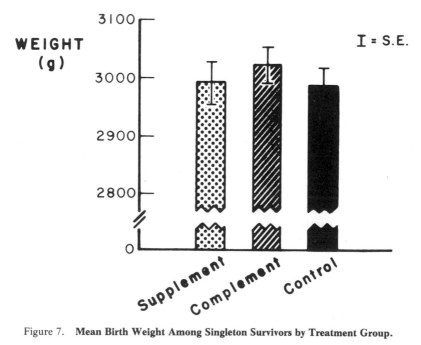

Figure 7.   **Mean Birth Weight Among Singleton Survivors by Treatment Group.**

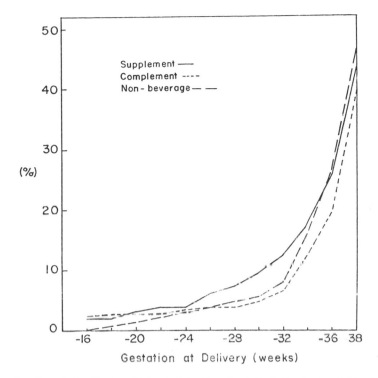

Figure 8.   **Cumulative Delivery Rates (%) by Length of Gestation for Each Treatment Group.**

shows a life table analysis of neonatal mortality by treatment group which illustrates this outcome. Further, over and above the excess of premature deliveries, the high protein supplement led to fetal growth retardation prior to 35-weeks gestation (Fig. 10).

Fortunately, the results of high protein supplementation were not adverse throughout gestation. Term pregnancies were defined as those carried beyond 37-weeks gestation. Figure 10 shows that at term there was some indication of an increased birth weight in the supplement or high protein treatment group. This result was not in itself statistically significant. A stratification of the data in accord with our initial hypotheses, however, showed that a coherent result was present. It will be recalled that at the outset a number of factors were specified because they carried a special or conditional risk of a low birth weight outcome. Without violating the conventions of hypothesis testing, therefore, we could test for nutritional effects in relation to these conditions, although at the cost of reduced power.

Analysis by these high risk conditions showed that the high protein supplement produced a significant birth weight increment at term under

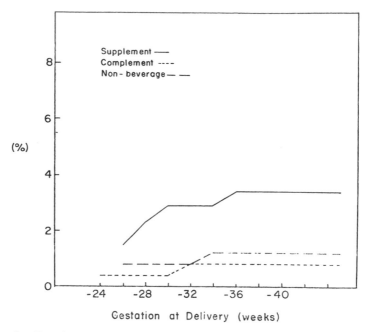

Figure 9.   **Cumulative Neonatal Mortality Rates (%) by Length of Gestation for Each Treatment Group.**

two conditions, namely, smoking and low prepregnant weight. Figure 11 illustrates this result. It also shows that these two risk conditions accounted for the total effect of high protein supplement at term. Nutritional supplementation produced no effect among nonsmokers and women of prepregnant weight above 110 pounds. A number of other outcomes measured at birth, such as maturity and neonatal behavior and also biochemical indices of placental state at birth, showed no relationship to nutritional supplementation.

At follow-up at one year of age,[3] an array of measures of physical growth, six psychometric tests, and clinical data were available. Virtually all the expected relations of measures of infant development with birth weight were present. However, none of the expected relations of development with treatment were present, with two exceptions.

On a test of visual habituation in response to a repeated stimulus, we found that those in the supplement treatment group turned their attention off sooner and when the stimulus changed, and turned their attention on again as soon as expected. In the Hunt-Uzigiris procedure for observing the infants at play, the duration of attention, as indicated by the time a child spent with each toy, turned out to be longer. The combina-

[3] Dr. Nathan Brody was our co-investigator in this aspect of the study.

tion of these two results suggests that there may be a general effect of the high protein supplement on some faculty of attention. This improved performance was unrelated to birth weight, and therefore not mediated by an accelerated rate of fetal growth or the correction of growth retardation.

In summary, the outcome of this study was ambiguous. High protein supplement led to unpredicted adverse effects on fetal growth, time of delivery and viability. The presence of three such indicators makes attribution to chance unlikely. These effects are not coherent with any known properties of the supplement. The high protein used was casein, and the beverage contained nothing that is not used in regular foods at a level within the recommended daily allowances. Hence, whether we consider undertaking new studies or whether we consider practical applications, this result cannot be ignored.

At the same time, high protein supplement has a protective effect on fetal growth coherent with the initial hypotheses of the study which, like the famine effects, was conditional. A favorable effect on a specific psy-

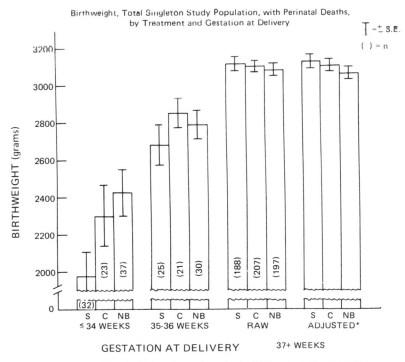

Figure 10. **Mean Singleton Birth Weight Among Survivors by Duration of Gestation for Each Treatment Group.**

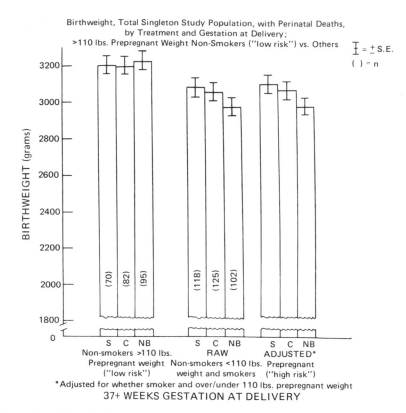

Figure 11. **Mean Singleton Birth Weight at Term, Stratified by Smoking and Prepregnant Weight for Each Treatment Group.**

chological function, e.g., attention at one year of age, was independent of fetal growth and unconditional.

DISCUSSION

These two studies—the Dutch famine study and the Prenatal Project—together with the Guatemala study (Lechtig et al., 1975; Lasky, 1974), represent the first published results of a new generation of studies that move us somewhat closer to secure causal inference about the effects of prenatal nutrition in humans than previous data could do.

Technical advances in research design, however, do not advance our capacity to reconcile conflicting and disconcerting results. How shall we conclude? In the Dutch famine a population well-nourished in previous times, when exposed to prenatal deprivation of nutrients below a threshold value during the third trimester of pregnancy, showed unequivocal but conditional effects of depressed fertility, retarded fetal growth and excess mortality up to three months of age. Among adults no effects could be detected, except on the frequency of obesity.

In the Prenatal Project the study population was at high risk of low birth weight, but only segments of it could be described as poorly nourished. In this population, too, a high protein supplement benefited growth conditionally; in that respect the result was congruent with the threshold found in the Dutch famine study. In addition, the high protein supplement benefited specific psychological test performance. This benefit, while unconditional, was not mediated by fetal growth, and it has unknown significance for later ages.

The published data of the Guatemalan study afford some reassurance with regard to supplementation. In this instance the total population suffers from chronic malnutrition, and hence the favorable effects observed on fetal growth and later test performance are subject to that condition. Data supplied elsewhere by Dr. Klein indicate, however, that even within this population the results are conditional, and that increments in fetal growth are most notable among women most likely to be malnourished.

Thus, taking together the three studies available to us:

1. We can be sure that prenatal nutrition affects fetal growth, viability and vitality, but only under certain conditions. We need to know more about these conditions and the specifics of the nutrients involved. We need also to explore the meaning of the adverse effect of the high protein supplement observed among premature deliveries.

2. We can be almost as sure that prenatal nutrition is unlikely to affect mental performance given reasonable nutritional conditions in the postnatal environment.

3. It is possible, but it is not finally established, that prenatal nutrition affects aspects of early mental development, especially where there is chronic postnatal malnutrition. Here we need to know more about the interaction and interrelations of prenatal nutrition with family and social dynamics, as well as with postnatal nutrition.

Critical pieces of the puzzle under conditions of chronic malnutrition are still missing. For example, in such populations, do effects on early cognitive function due to nutrition actually occur? Do effects on early cognitive function occur in response to the interaction of nutrition with the social environment? Or are the observed relationships of early cognitive function with prenatal nutrition solely owed to social environment? Existing studies still allow the possibility that malnutrition is a result of the social environment, separate from but confounded with cognitive performance; in other words, that a harsh social environment is the common cause of malnutrition and retarded cognitive performance.

In this respect, one may advance a unifying hypothesis to encompass the work of Chavez (1975) and of Cravioto (1974) in Mexico, and of Richardson, Birch et al. in Jamaica (Richardson, 1976; Hertzig et al., 1972), as well as the animal experiments of Frankova (1974). This work suggests that the main effect of both prenatal and postnatal nutritional supplementation on the infant may well be to promote somatic growth, while the main effect on psychological test performance is to be found in the social environment. The data taken together also suggest that supplementation improves the affective state and activity of a malnourished mother. This in turn is a likely intermediate variable in a path leading from maternal nutrition through maternal affective change to improvement in the psychological performance of their offspring. In other words, the report by Klein et al. in Guatemala of a prenatal nutritional effect on early psychological test performance (subsequently increasing with age) may in reality be due to improvements in the mother's health and affective state that influence her care of the child after birth (Klein, et al., 1976).

These three separate effects, it seems to us, may set up a dynamic interactive process.

This hypothetical process can be illustrated in a path diagram:

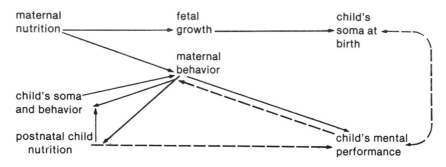

Still another generation of studies will be required to address these questions.

TEXT REFERENCES

Bergner, L.; Susser, M.: Low Birthweight and Prenatal Nutrition: An Interpretive Review. Pediatrics 46(1970)946–966

Chavez, A.: Consequences of Insufficient Nutrition and Child Character and Behavior. Cornell Conference on Malnutrition and Behavior, November 6–8, 1975, Ithaca, NY

Cravioto, J.; Delicardie, E.R.: The Relation of Size at Birth and Preschool Clinical Severe Malnutrition. Acta Paediatr Scand 63(1974)577–580

Dobbing, J.: The Influence of Early Nutrition on the Development and Myelination of the Brain. Proc Roy Soc (Biol) 159 (1964)503–509

Dobbing, J.; Sands, J.: Quantitative Growth and Development of Human Brain. Arch Dis Childh 48(1973)757-767

Douglas, J. W. B.: The Home and the School. MacGibbon and Kee, London, 1958

Frankova, S. Interaction Between Early Malnutrition and Stimulation in Animals. In: Symposia of the Swedish Nutrition Foundation XII. Early Malnutrition and Mental Development, p. 226, ed. by J. Cravioto, L. Hambraeus, and B. Vahlquist and Wilsells, 1974

Hertzig, M. F.; Birch, G. G.; Richardson, S. O.; Tizard, J.: Intellectual Levels of School Children Severely Malnourished During the First Two Years of Life. Pediatrics 49(1972)814-823

Klein, R. E.; Aruales, P.; Delgado, H.; Engle, P. L.; Guzman, G.; Irwin, M.; Lasky, R.; Lechtig, A.; Marborell, R.; Pivaral, V. M.; Russell, P.; Yarbrough, C.: Effects of Maternal Nutrition on Fetal Growth and Infant Development. PAHO Bulletin X(1976)301-316

Lasky, R. E.; Lechtig, A.; Delgado, H.; et al.: Birthweight and Psychomotor Performance In Rural Guatemala. Am J Dis Child 129(1975)566-569

Lechtig, A.; Delgado, H.; Yarbrough, C.; Habight, J.; Martorell, R.; Klein, R.: A Simple Assessment of the Risk of Low Birthweight to Select Women for Nutritional Intervention. Am J Obstet Gynec 125(1976)25-34

Ravelli, G. P.; Stein, Z. A.; Susser, M. W.: Obesity in Young Men After Famine Exposure in Utero and Early Infancy. New Eng J Med 295(1976)349-353

Richardson, S. A.: The Relation of Severe Malnutrition in Infancy to the Intelligence of School Children Having Differing Life Histories. Pediat Res 10(1976)57-61

Rush, D.; Stein, Z.; Christakis, G.; Susser, M.: The Prenatal Project: The First 20 Months of Operation. In: Malnutrition and Human Development, pp. 95-125, ed. by M. Winick. Wiley, New York, 1974

Smith, C. A.: Effects of Wartime Starvation in Holland on Pregnancy and its Products. Am J Obstet Gynec 53(1947)599-608

Stein, Z.; Susser, M.; Saenger, G.; Marolla, F.: Famine and Human Development: The Dutch Hunger Winter of 1944/45, Oxford University Press, New York, 1975

Winick, M.; Noble, A.: Cellular Response in Rats During Malnutrition at Various Ages. J Nutr 89(1966)300-306

DISCUSSION

Dr. Reed: Was the frequency of low birth weight in your control group similar to what you expected for a high risk population?

Dr. Susser: We expected about 25% below 2500 gm. in our selected clinic population. It was definitely lower than we had predicted, but there has been a decline in the frequency of low birth weight from the time we started.

Dr. Garn: What were the actual caloric and protein intakes that were consumed in the supplemented, complemented, and vitamin placebo mothers' diets?

Dr. Rush: The supplement group reported an average daily intake of about 2200 calories, the complement group 2135, and the controls 1960. While the absolute values are suspect (as are any quantitative dietary recall values), we believe that the relative differences are real. These data are based on serial 24-hour quantitative dietary recalls.

Dr. Terris: I would like to suggest a somewhat different interpretation of this so-called unfavorable result. It seems to me the rationale of supplementation is aimed not at premature labor but at low-birth-weight mature infants. In this study it may well be that the experimental and control groups were not comparable with regard to premature delivery. When you randomize, you are always taking the chance that your randomization doesn't quite work.

Dr. Mellits: We have just finished analyzing the data from Bacon Chou's study in Taiwan. The intake there was monitored closely, and the protein supplement was ingested on the spot. But even in that study, it wasn't all ingested.

   In the original analysis of the data we found no differences in either birth weight, prematurity rate or eight-month psychometric measures using the Bailey scale. However, when we took into consideration how much was actually ingested, and separated the population into those who took at least half of the supplement and those who did not, then some subtle effects of both birth weight and individual eight-month Bailey psychometric items became significant.

Maternal Urinary Tract Infections and Prematurity

John L. Sever, M.D., Ph.D.
Jonas H. Ellenberg, Ph.D.
Dorothy Edmonds, B.A.

A number of perinatal infections are known to be associated with prematurity. These include, for example, congenital rubella, toxoplasmosis and cytomegalovirus infections. Most of these diseases, however, are better known of their devastating effects on certain organ systems of the developing fetus rather than for their relation to prematurity. In the present studies, we have investigated the association between maternal urinary tract infections (UTI) and prematurity. Several previous investigations have reported an association between maternal UTI and prematurity (Savage, Jaji and Kass, 1967; Kass, 1973; Kass and Zinner, 1973; Bromfitt, 1975). Other studies have not supported these observations (Bryant et al., 1964; Little, 1976; Dixon, 1967). Our findings demonstrate an increased frequency of low birth weight children associated with maternal UTI.

MATERIALS AND METHODS

The Collaborative Perinatal Project is a longitudinal prospective investigation of approximately 56,000 pregnancies. The study was conducted at 14 university centers throughout the United States. Detailed clinical and laboratory data were obtained throughout each pregnancy and 75% of the live born children completed the 7-year follow up (Niswander and

Gordon, 1972; Broman, Nichols and Kennedy, 1975). Our analysis of UTI included only women who were symptomatic and for whom a positive urine culture was reported. Almost all cases of UTI were treated. Cases were compared to controls and matching included age of mother (± 3 years), race, institution, date of last menstrual period (± 6 weeks), socioeconomic index (computed as a weighted average of education, occupation and income as per Broman et al., 1975) and gestational age of child (± 4 weeks).

RESULTS

Among the 55,697 pregnancies studied, 1906 (3.4%) had symptomatic UTI. The proportion of white, black and "other" patients with UTI was 41%, 55% and 4% respectively. This distribution was similar to the corresponding racial distribution of the entire Collaborative Perinatal Project population.

Detailed analysis was conducted with 1524 UTI cases and an equal number of matched controls. These were pairs that could be matched and for which extensive clinical and laboratory data was available. No women were included who had multiple births or whose only UTI was in the postpartum period.

Table 1 shows that low birth weight was associated with UTI during pregnancy for all three weight groups studied ($\leq$ 1500 gm., $\leq$ 2000 gm. and $\leq$ 2500 gm.). In addition, there was a significant association between UTI and stillbirth.

A preliminary analysis of smoking as a possible indirect cause of the excess of low birth weight children among women with UTI indicated that the subject women with low birth weight children and the control women with low birth weight children were comparable with respect to smoking or non-smoking during pregnancy. While UTI thus appears to be independently associated with low birth weight, further refined analysis of degree of smoking is necessary.

DISCUSSION

The present studies demonstrate an association between symptomatic UTI during pregnancy and low birth weight and stillbirths. These associations are confined to the second and third trimesters. The absence of significant findings with first trimester UTI, however, may be due to the small number of women who registered in the first 12 weeks of gestation

Table 1.   Urinary Tract Infections During Pregnancy.

Birthweight	N[1]	Pediatric Conditions Significance[3]				Morbidity[4]		Odds Ratio[5]
		Total Gestation	First[2] Trimester 12%	Second Trimester 40%	Third Trimester 48%	Subjects	Controls	
<2500 vs. 2500–4000 gms.	1370	<.001		.019	.014	12.6	9.0	1.5
≤2000 vs. 2500–4000 gms.	1181	<.001		.005	.046	4.8	2.2	2.8
≤1500 vs. 2500–4000 gms.	1133	.006		.027		1.9	.7	4.5
Stillbirth	1516	<.001		.009		2.4	.8	3.7

[1] Number of the 1524 matched pairs included in the comparison. Pairs were excluded if, for either individual, the information concerning the condition was unknown or the classification of the case as abnormal or completely normal was not appropriate.
[2] Percentages denote approximate proportion of matched pairs where subject case had its first occurrence of UTI in indicated trimester.
[3] McNemar's Test: values indicate probability of X^2 attained.
[4] Proportion of subjects and controls having indicated outcome (Total Gestation).
[5] Defined as the odds of indicated outcome when the mother has UTI, relative to the odds of indicated outcome when the mother does not (Total Gestation).

in the Collaborative Perinatal Project.[1] Our findings are consistent with the reports by Kass and others for asymptomatic bacteriuria during pregnancy. The women in this study, however, were symptomatic and treated at university centers. For the present analysis, our matching of cases and controls included length of gestation. For this reason, the possible association between maternal UTI and length of gestation could not be determined. A further analysis of this relation is in progress. The data also showed an association between UTI and stillbirths.

In conclusion, symptomatic urinary tract infection was investigated in 55,597 pregnancies. A total of 1906 (3.4%) of the women had UTI. There was a significant association between UTI and low birth weight for all weight groups. There was also a significant association between maternal UTI and stillbirths.

TEXT REFERENCES

Broman, S. H.; Nichols, P. L.; Kennedy, W. A.: Preschool I.Q., Prenatal and Early Developmental Correlates. Lawrence Erlbaum, New Jersey, 1975

Brumfitt, W.: The Effects of Bacteriuria in Pregnancy on Maternal and Fetal Health. Kidney Int 8(1975)S-113–119

Bryant, R. E.; Wildom, R. E.; Vineyar, J. P.; Sanford, J. P.: Asymptomatic Bacteriuria in Pregnancy and Its Association with Prematurity. J Lab Clin Med 63(1964)224–231

Dixon, H. G.; Brant, H. A.: The Significance of Bacteriuria in Pregnancy. Lancet 1(1967)19–20

Kass, E. H.: The Role of Unsuspected Infection in the Etiology of Prematurity. Clin Obstet Gynec 16(1973)134–152

Kass, E. H.; Zinner, S. H.: Bacteriuria and Pyelonephritis in Pregnancy. In: Obstetric and Perinatal Infections, pp. 407–446, ed. by D. Charles and M. Finland. Lea and Febiger, Philadelphia, 1973

Little, P. J.: The Incidence of Urinary Infection in 5,000 Pregnant Women. Lancet 2(1976)925–928

Niswander, K. R.; Gordon, M.: The Women and Their Pregnancies. W. B. Saunders, Philadelphia, 1972.

Savage, W. E.; Jaji, S. N.; Kass, E. H.: Demographic and Prognostic Characteristics of Bacteriuria in Pregnancy. Medicine 46(1967)385–407

[1] The Collaborative Study of Cerebral Palsy, Mental Retardation and Other Neurological and Sensory Disorders of Infancy and Childhood is supported by the National Institute of Neurological and Communicative Disorders and Stroke. The following institutions participate: Boston Lying-In Hospital; Brown University; Charity Hospital, New Orleans; Children's Hospital of Buffalo; Children's Hospital of Philadelphia; Children's Medical Center, Boston; Columbia University; Johns Hopkins University; Medical College of Virginia; New York Medical College; Pennsylvania Hospital; University of Minnesota; University of Oregon; and University of Tennessee.

Maternal and Infant Health Factors Associated with Low Infant Birth Weight: Findings from the 1972 National Natality Survey

Paul Placek, Ph.D.

INTRODUCTION

An estimated 7%, or 197,000 out of 2,818,000, legitimate live hospital births occurring in the United States in 1972 were of low birth weight (i.e., 2500 gm. or less; 5 lbs. 8 oz. or less). This report presents percentages of births of low birth weight analyzed within four periods of gestation, according to a variety of social and demographic, maternal health, and infant health factors. The findings are based on data from the 1972 National Natality Survey, a "follow back" mail survey conducted by the National Center for Health Statistics. A number of social and demographic factors, and factors which suggest poor maternal and infant health, are found to be associated with low infant birth weight.

DATA AND METHOD

The National Natality Survey is a probability sample of one in every 500 live births in the United States, and the mothers, physicians and hospitals named on certificates of live birth were "followed back" through a mail survey. Social and demographic information provided by the mothers, and the medical information about the mother and her infant provided by hospitals and physicians, were linked with data from the birth certificate in order to expand the scope of information reported on the birth records. The one in 500 sample produced a total sample of 6505 certificates, of which 5689 were of legitimate births. Births which were reported to be illegitimate (N = 555) or inferred to be illegitimate by comparison of names of father, mother and baby (N = 261) were eliminated from this study; this represents approximately 403,000 illegitimate births not studied.

Additional information for the 5689 legitimate live births was obtained from the following sources:

1. All mothers named on the sample certificates were mailed a questionnaire to obtain a complete pregnancy history, household composition, wantedness of the sample birth, expectation of additional births, date of first and present marriage, husband's income, family income, mother's education, father's education, information regarding persons and institutions seen for prenatal care, and proportion of prenatal care, hospital bill, and doctor bill that was paid for by health insurance.

2. If the attending physician and the hospital where the birth occurred had different addresses on the birth certificate, the physician was mailed a questionnaire to obtain information regarding the mother's pregnancy history, visits for prenatal and postpartum care, complications noted during those visits, whether family planning information was given, and the method of contraception the mother may have decided to use. Also, the hospital was mailed a short questionnaire to assess the mother's pregnancy history, her admission and discharge dates, duration of labor, type of delivery, type of anesthetic used, complications of pregnancy and labor, underlying medical conditions of the mother, whether a sterilizing operation was performed, whether the mother was given family planning information, the method of contraception she may have decided to use, condition of infant at delivery, congenital malformations of the infant, birth injuries to the infant, Apgar scores, infant's condition at discharge, and birth weight.

3. If the attending physician and hospital of birth had the same address, the hospital was sent one longer questionnaire which gathered all the information on both the physician and the short hospital questionnaires.

4. If the place of delivery was not a hospital but a physician was the attendant at birth, only the physician questionnaire was mailed.

5. If the birth did not occur in a hospital and was not attended by a physician, only the mother received a questionnaire. The source document for each variable in the tables is shown in footnote form: bc = birth certificate, m = mother questionnaire and hp = hospital or physician questionnaire.

Non-hospital legitimate births (N = 42 of 5689 in the sample, representing 21,000 births nationally) are not included in this report since the hospital questionnaire was the source of information on most of the maternal and infant health information. Estimates in this report, therefore, refer to all 2,818,000 legitimate live hospital births in the United States in 1972 since the data are weighted by means of a post-stratified ratio estimation procedure for race, age and live birth order.

Response rates to the mailed questionnaires were 71.5% from the mothers, 85.4% from the hospitals and 72.2% from the physicians. Unit nonresponse (unreturned questionnaires) was treated the same as item nonresponse (some questions left blank on a returned questionnaire), and these values were imputed from a matrix of values appropriate for each birth according to certain social, demographic and medical characteristics.

The probability design of the survey makes possible the calculation of sampling errors, which measure the sampling variation that occurs by chance because only a sample rather than the entire population of births is surveyed. Approximate standard errors for estimated percentages in this report are shown in Table 1, and an example of the method by which

Table 1.   Approximate Standard Errors for Estimated Percentages Expressed in Percentage Points: 1972 National Natality Survey

Base of percentage	2 or 98	5 or 95	10 or 90	20 or 80	30 or 70	40 or 60	50
3,000	4.1	6.4	8.8	11.7	13.4	14.3	14.6
5,000	3.2	4.9	6.8	9.0	10.4	11.1	11.3
10,000	2.2	3.5	4.8	6.4	7.3	7.8	8.0
30,000	1.3	2.0	2.8	3.7	4.2	4.5	4.6
50,000	1.0	1.6	2.1	2.9	3.3	3.5	3.6
70,000	0.8	1.3	1.8	2.4	2.8	3.0	3.0
100,000	0.7	1.1	1.5	2.0	2.3	2.5	2.5
200,000	0.5	0.8	1.1	1.4	1.6	1.8	1.8
500,000	0.3	0.5	0.7	0.9	1.0	1.1	1.1
700,000	0.3	0.4	0.6	0.8	0.9	0.9	1.0
1,000,000	0.2	0.3	0.5	0.6	0.7	0.8	0.8
2,000,000	0.2	0.2	0.3	0.4	0.5	0.6	0.6
2,500,000	0.1	0.2	0.3	0.4	0.5	0.5	0.5

Example: Suppose that 20 percent of births in some category had low birth weight (2500 gms. or less), and the base of that percent is 50,000. The 20 percent column and the 50,000 row indicate that 2.9 percent is one standard error, and twice that, or 5.8 percent, is two standard errors. Therefore, the chances are about 95 out of 100 that this 20.0 percent estimate from the sample differs from the value for the entire population by less than two standard errors, and the percent of births in the population which were low birth weight ranges between 14.2 and 25.8 percent (20.0 percent ± 5.8 percent). This is a 95 percent confidence interval, and when this interval is found not to overlap with another 95 percent confidence interval which has been similarly calculated, it may be said that the difference is statistically significant at the .05 level or beyond. Interpolation may be used for percentages and base numbers which do not closely correspond to the table values shown.

sampling errors may be calculated is provided. Findings discussed are statistically significant at the 0.05 level with two-tailed normal deviate tests.

FINDINGS

Of 2,818,000 legitimate live hospital births in 1972, 7% were 2500 gm. or less. However, 32.2% of births of less than 37-weeks gestation were low birth weight, whereas only 2.4% of births of 40-weeks gestation were low birth weight (Table 2).

Only 6.2% of the infants of white mothers were low birth weight, but 12.8% of the infants of all other mothers were low birth weight. A racial difference exists for infants of all gestation groups except less than 37 weeks. Infants residing in the South are more likely to be of low birth weight than infants from other regions. Also, infants whose families have less than $4000 total family income are more likely to be of low birth weight than infants from families of higher income levels. However, differences in percent low birth weight infants for mothers and fathers of varying educational levels, for mothers of varying ages, and for births of various orders are not statistically significant. (The annual natality data collected by the states and analyzed by the Division of Vital Statistics do show birth weight variation for these factors.) If the 1972 birth was one of a multiple birth, 38.8% were of low birth weight, but intervals not involving multiple births were not significantly different.

An overview of Table 3 indicates that poor maternal health characteristics are associated with low infant birth weight. Of mothers with two or more previous fetal losses, 9.8% had low birth weight infants compared to 6.8% for mothers with no fetal losses. While 8% of the infants were low birth weight when the mother had one or more underlying medical conditions, compared to 6.8% when the mother had no such conditions, this difference is not statistically significant. The occurrence of one or more complications of pregnancy is associated with a greater probability of low birth weight; this finding is statistically significant for all births and for births of less than 37-weeks gestation.

The time of beginning and the amount of prenatal care are related to low birth weight: 10.3% of births were of low birth weight when the mother had no prenatal care from the attending physician or hospital of birth, but only 6.6% were low birth weight when prenatal care began during the first trimester. Also, mothers with no visits, 1–4 visits and 5–9 visits for prenatal care were more likely to have had low birth weight infants than mothers with the modal 10–14 visits. Maternal complications or unusual conditions noted during the first, second or third trimester are related to low birth weight. The mothers who were least likely to have low birth weight infants were those with no complications, and mothers with one, or two or more complications had higher probabilities of having low birth weight infants. Similarly, as one might expect, more trimesters with complications are associated with a greater probability of having a low birth weight infant. While this pattern is consistent, the differences are not always statistically significant. If one or more maternal complications of labor was present, 17.1% of infants were low birth weight compared to only 4.4% for mothers with no complications. This pattern holds for all periods of gestation except for infants of 40-weeks gestation.

While type of anesthetic used is not related to low birth weight, a significantly higher percentage (12.5%) of infants were low birth weight when the hospital reported the use of no anesthetics for delivery than when one anesthetic (6.4%) and two or more anesthetics (7.9%) were used. Also, 9.9% of the infants whose mothers' total duration of labor was 0-3 hours were low birth weight, which is significantly higher than for all other labor duration categories. Thus, it appears that no anesthetics used for delivery and short durations of labor are associated with low birth weight, partly because of shorter periods of gestation associated with these conditions and possible unanticipated early deliveries.

Type of delivery is related to low birth weight. Overall 28.4% of breech deliveries and 11.2% of cesarean sections are low birth weight—significantly higher than the 6.9% for spontaneous and 4.9% for forceps deliveries. This relative ranking remains and is statistically significant for births of less than 37 weeks and 37-39 weeks gestation. Cesarean section births of 40 weeks or more gestation and breech births of 41 weeks or more gestation are no more likely to be of low birth weight than spontaneous births. Cesarean section and breech deliveries are more likely to occur in the earlier weeks of gestation and hence be of low birth weight.

Hospital stay is associated with birth weight: 16.3% of the infants whose mothers' predelivery hospital stay was two or more days were of low birth weight, as compared to only 6.6% and 7.3% for infants of mothers whose stays were less than one day or exactly one day. In the case of complications to the mothers' health noted after delivery, 10.8% were of low birth weight, compared to only 6.7% if no complications were noted. Postpartum sterilization and postpartum care are not associated with infant birth weight.

In general, Table 4 reveals that poor infant health characteristics are associated with low infant birth weight, even within various gestation periods. While female infants are slightly more likely to be low birth weight, the comparison with male infants is not statistically significant. Since most plural births occur before 40-weeks gestation, it is expected that they would have a higher percent low birth weight than single births. However, even within the less than 37 weeks and 37-39 weeks gestation categories, plural births have a higher percent low birth weight (75.8%

Table 2. Estimated Number of Legitimate Live Hospital Births and Percent of Births 2500 gms. or Less[bc] by Period of Gestation According to Social and Demographic Characteristics: United States, 1972 National Natality Survey

Social and Demographic Characteristics	Total number of births in thousands by period of gestation[hp]					Percent of births 2500 grams or less by period of gestation				
	TOTAL	36 weeks or less	37–39 weeks	40 weeks	41 weeks or more	TOTAL	36 weeks or less	37–39 weeks	40 weeks	41 weeks or more
All births	2,818	273	1,093	642	810	7.0	32.2	6.1	2.4	3.3
Color of mother [bc]										
White	2,490	225	942	580	744	6.2	32.4	5.4	2.0	2.7
All other	328	48	151	63	67	12.8	31.4	10.8	6.8	9.6
Metropolitan/non-met, county of residence [bc]										
Metropolitan	1,874	184	741	408	541	6.7	30.0	6.0	2.3	3.0
Non-metropolitan	944	89	352	234	269	7.6	36.7	6.4	2.6	3.7
Region of residence [bc]										
Northeast	603	56	251	136	160	6.3	27.2	5.9	1.4	3.7
North Central	775	72	285	172	247	6.4	39.1	4.1	2.7	2.0
South	940	102	360	217	261	8.4	27.1	8.2	4.0	4.9
West	500	42	197	118	143	6.2	39.5	5.6	0.4	2.1
Total family income [m]										
Less than $4000	296	40	119	61	76	10.9	32.2	11.3	5.1	3.5
$4000 to $6999	537	48	206	126	157	7.6	38.0	5.1	3.5	4.8
$7000 to $9999	681	71	256	152	203	6.5	32.8	5.3	1.7	2.2
$10,000 to $14,999	818	69	319	192	237	6.0	29.4	5.5	1.9	3.2
$15,000 or more	487	44	193	111	138	6.5	29.4	6.3	1.7	3.2
Mother's education [m]										
None or elementary	121	15	45	32	30	9.7	27.8	8.1	4.9	8.2
1–3 years high school	475	50	187	100	137	7.2	37.7	3.7	2.1	4.4
High school graduate	1,348	129	520	305	393	6.6	29.6	6.6	2.0	2.7
1–3 years college	541	47	211	128	155	6.5	27.7	5.8	3.9	3.2
College graduate	334	31	129	78	95	8.3	44.8	7.8	1.3	2.6
Father's education [m]										
None or elementary	179	24	68	35	52	7.9	33.9	5.9	—	3.8
1–3 years high school	400	41	154	89	116	7.7	29.6	7.2	1.7	5.2
High school graduate	1,180	107	466	269	339	7.0	33.6	6.2	3.2	2.8
1–3 years college	467	47	184	105	131	6.8	29.1	6.1	2.8	3.0
College graduate	592	54	222	145	171	6.4	33.4	5.4	1.8	2.9

Age of mother[bc]									
Under 18 years	124	14	47	28	36	5.5	25.4	7.6	—	2.9
18–19 years	291	36	117	73	63	8.8	30.7	7.3	5.2	3.1
20–24 years	1,031	95	390	231	314	6.7	29.8	6.0	2.3	3.9
25–29 years	850	72	319	192	267	5.8	31.8	5.1	1.6	2.7
30–34 years	356	39	146	82	89	9.0	43.4	7.1	2.5	3.0
35 and over	166	16	74	37	39	7.7	30.2	6.6	4.0	3.8
Live birth order[bc]									
First	1,072	98	401	247	326	6.3	32.6	5.8	2.2	2.3
Second	869	78	345	208	238	6.0	25.8	5.1	2.6	3.6
Third	428	41	166	94	127	9.0	41.4	8.3	2.7	4.0
Fourth	214	27	92	42	54	5.7	29.7	4.3	2.3	2.7
Fifth or higher	236	28	90	51	66	10.5	37.5	9.4	3.0	6.2
Interval between 1972 birth and previous live birth[m]									
1972 birth was one of a multiple birth	26	*7	10	*6	*3	38.8	*	29.9	*	*
12 months or less	213	28	81	48	56	8.8	42.9	4.3	3.4	2.6
13–24 months	502	49	193	107	154	7.5	27.3	7.8	1.9	4.6
25 months or more	1,047	89	419	244	295	6.0	28.9	4.9	2.5	3.6
No previous live births	1,030	100	390	237	302	6.6	31.0	6.4	2.1	2.3

Sources of each variable:

  bc = birth certificate

  m = mother questionnaire

  hp = hospital and/or physician questionnaire

* Figure does not meet standards of reliability or
  precision

— Quantity zero

Table 3. Estimated Number of Legitimate Live Hospital Births and Percent of Births 2500 gms. or Less by Period of Gestation According to Maternal Health Characteristics: United States, 1972 National Natality Survey

Maternal Health Characteristics	Total number of births in thousands by period of gestation					Percent of births 2500 grams or less by period of gestation				
	TOTAL	36 weeks or less	37–39 weeks	40 weeks	41 weeks or more	TOTAL	36 weeks or less	37–39 weeks	40 weeks	41 weeks or more
All births	2,818	273	1,093	642	810	7.0	32.2	6.1	2.4	3.3
Previous fetal losses[m,1]										
None	2,434	236	944	560	694	6.8	31.1	6.1	2.4	3.2
One	266	25	107	55	79	7.2	36.8	5.6	2.7	3.2
Two+	119	12	43	27	37	9.8	44.2	8.2	3.7	5.3
Underlying medical conditions[hp,2]										
None	2,427	224	932	560	712	6.8	32.5	6.2	2.3	3.1
One+	391	49	161	83	99	8.0	31.1	5.6	3.2	4.5
Complications of pregnancy[hp,3]										
None	2,359	207	912	556	685	6.3	28.7	6.0	2.3	3.0
One+	459	65	182	87	125	10.8	43.4	6.6	3.4	4.9
Trimester of pregnancy that prenatal care began[hp,4]										
First trimester	1,870	157	728	431	553	6.6	34.0	5.4	2.8	3.4
Second trimester	585	75	217	137	156	7.6	28.9	7.7	1.9	2.2
Third trimester	168	18	65	36	49	5.3	16.5	6.8	—	3.3
No prenatal care	195	22	83	38	52	10.3	43.2	7.8	2.6	5.7
Number of prenatal visits reported by medical sources[hp,4]										
No visits	195	22	83	38	52	10.3	43.2	7.8	2.6	5.7
1–4 visits	204	43	82	33	46	13.5	35.1	12.2	3.0	3.5
5–9 visits	809	107	341	175	187	8.4	30.9	6.4	3.6	3.5
10–14 visits	1,306	84	505	326	391	5.4	29.5	5.3	1.8	3.2
15–19 visits	285	16	78	66	125	3.7	30.9	2.6	1.6	1.9
20+ visits	18	*1	*4	*4	*9	8.1	*	*	*	*
Complications or unusual conditions noted during first trimester[hp,4]										
No prenatal care	195	22	83	38	52	10.3	43.2	7.8	2.6	5.7
No complications	2,393	226	915	555	697	6.6	30.0	6.0	2.5	3.2
One complication	200	22	81	43	55	8.1	42.4	6.2	2.3	1.8
Two+ complications	30	*3	14	*7	*7	6.7	*	6.7	*	*

Complications or unusual conditions noted during second trimester[hp,4]									
No prenatal care	195	22	83	38	52	10.3	43.2	7.8	2.6	5.7
No complications	2,266	207	880	526	653	6.2	29.3	5.6	2.2	3.0
One complication	287	31	105	62	90	10.3	42.5	9.2	4.9	4.5
Two+ complications	70	12	26	16	15	8.5	36.0	5.5	—	—
Complications or unusual conditions noted during third trimester[hp,4]									
No prenatal care	195	22	83	38	52	10.3	43.2	7.8	2.6	5.7
No complications	2,151	195	830	496	630	6.2	31.3	4.9	2.7	3.1
One complication	398	47	152	91	108	9.4	31.5	11.5	1.1	3.7
Two+ complications	74	*8	28	18	21	7.4	*	10.2	2.8	—
Number of prenatal trimesters mother experienced complications[hp,4]									
No prenatal care	195	22	83	38	52	10.3	43.2	7.8	2.6	5.7
No trimesters	1,830	153	709	432	536	5.8	29.4	4.8	2.5	3.1
One trimester	589	78	224	122	166	3.7	30.9	8.5	2.1	3.3
Two trimesters	142	13	51	38	40	13.1	49.5	10.7	3.9	2.4
Three trimesters	62	*6	27	13	16	9.0	*	9.4	—	3.1
Complications of labor[hp,5]									
None	2,248	180	884	537	647	9.4	17.4	4.3	2.4	2.8
One+	570	93	209	105	163	17.1	60.7	14.1	2.8	5.3
Type of anesthetic used[hp]									
Inhalation									
Yes	970	89	365	230	286	6.6	25.5	7.2	2.6	3.3
No	1,848	184	728	412	525	7.2	35.4	5.6	2.4	3.3
Spinal and epidural									
Yes	661	58	264	149	190	6.4	32.3	5.5	2.0	3.2
No	2,157	214	830	493	620	7.2	32.2	6.4	2.6	3.3
Local									
Yes	653	61	254	150	188	5.7	34.2	5.7	1.8	3.1
No	2,166	211	839	493	622	7.1	31.6	6.3	2.7	3.3
Other									
Yes	660	66	255	152	187	7.?	35.4	6.2	1.7	2.7
No	2,158	206	838	490	623	7.?	31.2	6.1	2.7	3.5

Table 3.   Estimated Number of Legitimate Live Hospital Births and Percent of Births 2500 gms. or Less by Period of Gestation According to Maternal Health Characteristics: United States, 1972 National Natality Survey (Cont'd)

Maternal Health Characteristics	Total number of births in thousands by period of gestation					Percent of births 2500 grams or less by period of gestation				
	TOTAL	36 weeks or less	37-39 weeks	40 weeks	41 weeks or more	TOTAL	36 weeks or less	37-39 weeks	40 weeks	41 weeks or more
Number of anesthetics used for delivery[hp]										
None	203	29	77	39	58	12.5	44.7	7.4	7.9	6.2
One	2,296	212	898	528	658	6.4	29.9	5.8	2.1	3.0
Two+	320	31	118	76	94	7.9	35.9	7.6	2.0	3.6
Total duration of labor[hp]										
0-3 hours	647	73	271	145	158	9.9	40.7	8.6	4.2	3.2
4-7 hours	1,109	109	435	248	317	6.0	27.8	4.9	1.9	3.5
8-11 hours	565	51	212	132	170	6.4	26.8	6.4	2.6	3.3
12 + hours	497	39	175	118	165	5.9	35.5	5.2	1.3	3.0
Type of delivery[hp]										
Spontaneous	1,485	155	595	314	421	6.9	30.7	5.9	2.1	3.2
Forceps	1,038	70	374	279	315	4.9	22.9	4.5	2.4	3.7
Cesarean section	205	26	92	34	52	11.2	45.0	10.9	1.5	0.9
Breech	65	17	22	11	15	28.4	62.4	23.7	18.4	3.4
Other	26	*3	10	*5	*7	7.3	*	—	*	*
Predelivery hospital stay[hp]										
Less than one day	2,158	209	844	487	617	6.6	29.7	6.1	2.6	2.6
One day	582	45	224	142	171	7.3	37.3	5.8	1.9	5.8
Two or more days	78	18	25	13	22	16.3	48.9	11.5	3.6	2.1
Postdelivery hospital stay[hp]										
0-2 days	554	57	208	142	147	7.7	37.8	7.2	2.1	2.1
3 days	1,016	91	388	235	302	6.2	28.1	5.4	2.6	3.3
4 days	693	62	269	156	206	6.5	29.2	5.6	2.2	4.1
5 or more days	556	63	229	109	155	8.4	36.0	7.1	2.8	3.2
Total hospital stay of mother[hp]										
0-2 days	438	47	167	110	114	7.4	33.0	7.4	2.3	1.8
3 days	915	83	354	213	266	5.7	27.8	5.0	1.9	2.9
4 days	744	61	289	170	223	7.1	32.9	6.1	3.3	4.1
5 or more days	722	82	283	150	207	8.3	35.7	6.8	2.4	3.8

Complications to mother's health noted after delivery[hp]									
Yes	187	21	73	38	54	10.8	51.3	9.7	1.3	2.9
No	2,632	251	1,020	605	756	6.7	30.6	5.9	2.5	3.3
Postpartum sterilization of mother[hp]									
Yes	220	25	100	41	54	7.4	24.7	6.5	3.9	3.6
No	2,598	247	993	601	756	7.0	33.0	6.1	2.3	3.3
Interval between delivery and first postpartum visit[hp]									
Under 30 days	592	55	241	133	164	7.0	34.0	6.8	3.1	1.5
30–59 days	1,710	166	661	386	496	6.8	31.6	5.6	2.1	3.6
60–90 days	154	13	54	40	47	7.8	49.9	5.6	3.8	2.1
No postpartum visits reported	362	39	137	83	103	7.8	26.5	7.7	2.5	5.3
Reason for and number of post-partum visits[hp]									
One routine visit	887	78	348	195	265	5.3	32.5	5.7	1.8	2.6
One non-routine visit	724	78	279	162	205	7.6	34.4	5.6	2.8	3.7
Two routine visits	152	15	57	35	46	6.9	34.9	4.4	4.2	3.2
Two non-routine visits	90	*9	38	21	22	7.9	27.7	9.5	—	4.9
Two visits, one non-routine	357	34	137	81	105	7.0	26.9	7.8	3.1	2.3
Three + routine visits	30	—	10	12	*8	—	—	—	—	*
Three + visits, incl. one + non-routine	217	20	88	52	56	7.4	42.9	5.1	2.9	2.6
No postpartum visits reported	362	39	137	83	103	7.8	26.5	7.7	2.5	5.3

Sources of each variable:

bc = birth certificate

m = mother questionnaire

hp = hospital and/or physician questionnaire

* Figure does not meet standards of reliability or precision

— Quantity zero

[1] Stillbirths plus miscarriages, but not including unknown induced abortions.

[2] Diabetes, varicosity, congenital heart disease, thyroid condition, anemia, cardiovascular-renal disease asthma, other chronic pulmonary, orthopedic condition, and other.

[3] Urinary infection, hypertension, toxemia preeclampsia, eclampsia, rubella, embolism, obesity, and other.

[4] This item does not include prenatal care which may have been received from a physician who was not the attendant at birth, or care received which was unknown to the reporting hospital. These comments apply to the "no visits" and "no prenatal care" categories in other maternal health characteristics shown on Table 3.

[5] Inadequate pelvis, transverse lie, multiple birth, abnormal position of placenta or cord, premature rupture of membranes, unusual bleeding, prolonged labor, anesthesia reaction, placenta abruptio, and other.

Table 4. Estimated Number of Legitimate Live Hospital Births and Percent of Births 2500 gms. or Less by Period of Gestation According to Infant Health Characteristics: United States, 1972 National Natality Survey

Infant Health Characteristics	Total number of births in thousands by period of gestation					Percent of births 2500 grams or less by period of gestation				
	TOTAL	36 weeks or less	37–39 weeks	40 weeks	41 weeks or more	TOTAL	36 weeks or less	37–39 weeks	40 weeks	41 weeks or more
All births	2,818	273	1,093	642	810	7.0	32.2	6.1	2.4	3.3
Sex of child[bc]										
Male	1,456	143	565	329	418	6.6	31.1	5.8	2.1	2.9
Female	1,363	129	528	313	392	7.4	33.4	6.5	2.8	3.7
Number at birth[hp]										
Single	2,761	248	1,067	639	807	6.0	27.9	5.3	2.4	3.1
Plural birth	57	24	26	*3	*3	55.3	75.8	42.8	*	*
Order of presentation at birth[hp]										
Single birth	2,761	248	1,067	639	807	6.0	27.9	5.3	2.4	3.1
First	28	11	15	—	*1	46.4	70.6	32.6	—	*
Second or higher	29	13	10	*3	*2	64.1	80.4	57.7	*	*
Congenital malformations or anomalies reported on birth certificate[bc]										
No stated condition	2,647	256	1,025	605	762	6.8	31.5	5.9	2.4	3.1
Any stated condition	20	*2	*8	*3	*7	26.1	*	*	*	*
Not on state's certificate	151	14	60	35	41	8.4	35.8	6.8	2.7	6.2
Congenital malformations or anomalies noted at delivery by hospital[hp]										
No	2,686	254	1,043	610	779	6.6	30.4	5.9	2.4	3.2
Yes	133	19	51	32	31	14.5	56.8	12.1	3.3	5.0
Birth injuries noted at delivery[hp]										
No	2,757	270	1,069	623	796	7.1	32.3	6.2	2.4	3.3
Yes	62	*3	25	20	14	3.4	*	4.1	2.5	—
Unusual resuscitative efforts requires[hp]										
No	2,609	231	1,019	600	760	6.0	27.1	5.7	2.0	3.1
Yes	209	41	75	43	50	19.7	60.7	12.6	8.4	6.1

Apgar score-one minute[hp]								
Not done	467	178	112	129	7.7	37.0	6.2	1.3	4.7
0-3	41	11	*6	11	36.4	78.2	29.9	*	—
4-7	310	109	65	90	13.5	54.0	9.6	4.6	4.5
8-10	2,000	795	459	580	5.2	21.2	5.3	2.2	2.8
Apgar score-five minutes[hp]								
Not done	1,146	439	263	327	7.2	31.2	6.9	2.5	2.8
0-3	16	*7	*2	—	-2.2	*	*	*	—
4-7	52	15	*8	16	-0.8	82.4	19.7	*	6.5
8-10	1,605	632	370	467	5.7	25.8	5.1	2.2	3.5
Age when baby was first examined outside the delivery room[hp]								
One hour or less	911	347	203	261	10.5	48.3	9.3	3.5	3.1
2-6 hours	584	234	132	159	5.4	30.4	4.5	2.6	3.5
7-23 hours	655	250	154	193	5.0	22.0	4.4	0.3	4.4
24 hours or more	669	261	153	198	4.7	15.9	5.1	3.0	2.3
Birth injuries noted before discharge from hospital[hp]								
No	2,810	1,091	639	809	7.0	32.3	6.2	2.5	3.3
Yes	*8	*3	*4	*1	*	*	*	*	*
Congenital malformations or anomalies noted before discharge[hp]								
No	2,803	1,088	641	804	7.0	32.0	6.2	2.5	3.3
Yes	15	*5	*2	*6	0.3	*	*	*	*
Any other illnesses noted before discharge[hp]								
No	2,806	1,089	641	804	7.0	32.1	6.1	2.5	3.3
Yes	13	*5	*1	*6	10.7	*	*	*	*
Infant discharged from hospital alive[hp]								
Yes	2,791	1,088	641	807	6.4	28.6	5.9	2.4	3.2
No	27	*6	*1	*4	69.5	85.7	*	*	*

Sources of each variable:
bc = birth certificate
m = mother questionnaire
hp = hospital and/or physician questionnaire

* Figure does not meet standards of reliability or precision
— Quantity zero

compared with 27.9% and 42.8% compared with 5.3%, respectively). Second or higher order of presentation in a plural birth is more often associated with low birth weight than first order of presentation (64.1% compared with 46.4%).

Low birth weight characterized 26.1% of infants with a congenital malformation or anomaly reported on the birth certificate and 14.5% of infants with a congenital malformation or anomaly noted at delivery by the hospital. An interesting observation is that low birth weight does not characterize infants with birth injuries. In fact, the opposite is true; infants with birth injuries tend to be large babies. However, 19.7% of infants for whom unusual resuscitative efforts were required were low birth weight—significantly higher than the 6% among infants for whom no unusual resuscitative efforts were required. This pattern remains statistically significant for all births except those of 41 weeks or more gestation.

Low infant Apgar score at one minute is associated with low birth weight since, overall, 36.4% with Apgar 0-3, 13.5% with Apgar 4-7, but only 5.2% of infants with Apgar 8-10 were of low birth weight. This pattern persists for infants of less than 37-weeks gestation and for infants of 37-39 weeks gestation. The pattern is similar for five minute Apgar scores: 42.2% of infants were of low birth weight when Apgar was 0-3, but only 5.7% were of low birth weight when Apgar was 8-10. Infants first examined outside the delivery room at the age of one hour or less are more likely to be of low birth weight than infants examined two or more hours after birth. It is probable that the health of low birth weight infants is determined to be in greater immediate jeopardy and the infants are therefore given more immediate attention. Infants with birth injuries, congenital malformations and any other illnesses noted before discharge are not significantly different in percent low birth weight from infants without such medical problems since small numbers of sample births in these categories have larger standard errors. However, 69.5% of the infants who were not discharged from the hospital alive were of low birth weight, compared to only 6.4% low birth weight for infants discharged alive from the hospital, reflecting the strong association between low birth weight and early infant mortality.

SUMMARY AND DISCUSSION

Low infant birth weight (2500 gm. or less) characterized 7% of legitimate live hospital births in 1972; however, 32.2% of births occurring at 36 weeks or less gestation were low birth weight. Births to all other mothers, to mothers residing in the South, to families with less than $4000 total family income, and multiple births are more often of low birth weight.

The following factors which suggest poor maternal health are associated with low infant birth weight: previous fetal losses, complications of pregnancy, no prenatal care, fewer prenatal visits, complications or unusual medical conditions noted during pregnancy, complications of labor, no anesthetics used for delivery, short durations of labor, breech and cesarean section deliveries, longer maternal predelivery hospital stay, and complications to mother's health noted after delivery. Finally, the following characteristics which suggest poor infant health are also associated with low birth weight: plural births (especially those of second or higher order presentation), infants with congenital malformations or anomalies, infants for whom unusual resuscitative efforts were required, infants with low Apgar scores, infants examined one hour or less after birth, and infants who were not discharged from the hospital alive.

In interpreting the statistics in this report, three points must be kept in mind. First, the patterns observed here of percent low birth weight for 2,818,000 legitimate live hospital births may differ from patterns for the estimated 403,000 illegitimate and 21,000 non-hospital legitimate births which occurred in 1972. Second, the percent of low birth weight infants has been declining slowly in recent years, and some of the relationships discussed here may change as the characteristics of women who give birth change. Finally, some of the maternal health factors associated with low birth weight may be related to social and demographic factors, and some of the infant health factors associated with low birth weight may be related to maternal health factors.

Thus, more complex multivariate procedures of analysis may help in unravelling the epidemiology of prematurity.

DISCUSSION

Dr. Rush: This has been very interesting, particularly Table 2, which presented data relative to trimester when prenatal care was begun. With gestation at delivery controlled, there was no relationship of time of registration for prenatal care and low birth weight. These results again fail to support a simple relationship between prenatal care and outcome, and underscore the need to evaluate the efficacy of specific elements of prenatal care.

Dr. Placek: I concur with that. There is a report being prepared in the Natality Statistics Branch on the effect of prenatal care on low birth weight and it suggests basically what you have said. There is no clear straight line relationship between amount of prenatal care and the health of the infant.

Dr. Kass: We are discussing the epidemiology of prematurity, but the problem that one addresses oneself to is not prematurity but the things that are associated with it. It may be that being small is a problem, and smaller infants tend to have higher mortality, and therefore it has adverse consequences. However, a number of risk factors affect mortality in the infants, out of all proportions to the effect of birth weight or gestational age.

Dr. Rush: There is a methodologic problem. Because death is an infrequent event, if it is the projected end point, studies may demand impractically large numbers of subjects.

Dr. Susser: It certainly is true, as Dr. Rush said, that you get into problems of numbers very quickly when you try and refine your dependent variable. But I support Dr. Kass' point that you really do need to be more specific and refined about outcome variables. Deaths in the Dutch famine study related to different antecedent factors according to age at death (Stein et al., 1975), and in our New York intervention study fetal growth related to different antecedents more than did psychological functions.

Dr. Hardy: Lula Lubchenco in Colorado made a very profound comment to me. She said that we should be concerned about making good babies better rather than putting all our efforts into salvaging bad babies. I want to make the point that there is value to focusing on the continuum of birth weight rather than just on prematurity.

Dr. Morton: An example from genetics may be helpful. Every chromosomal abnormality except for sex chromosome aneuploids is associated with low birth weight. Now clearly the disease is a sickly child and birth weight is only a symptom, but it is a most useful symptom for certain statistical purposes.

DISCUSSION REFERENCES

Stein, Z.; Susser, M.; Saenger, G.; Marolla, F.: Famine and Human Development: The Dutch Hunger Winter of 1944/45. Oxford University Press, New York, 1975

Genetic Aspects of Prematurity

Newton E. Morton, Ph.D.

Prematurity may be defined in terms of gestation time and/or birth weight, two variables which are ordinarily given in hospital records and birth certificates. If the objective is to predict survival, other measures like crown-rump length might be useful and a composite could be created as a discriminant between deaths and survivors, but these refinements have seldom been practiced. I shall therefore discuss two nearly continuous traits (gestation time in days and birth weight in grams) and their conventional dichotomies (less than 37 weeks and less than 2500 gms., respectively), although the latter have received little attention from geneticists.

SYNDROMES

At least one genetic entity (hyper-β-alaninemia), many birth defects (e.g., spina bifida) and the grossly abnormal chromosomal aberrations (like triploidy) are associated with low gestation time through high fetal mortality. Low gestation time interacts with the African allele for glucose-6-phosphate dehydrogenase deficiency to cause hyperbilirubinemia. A few diseases (notably some gigantism and transposition of great vessels) have elevated birth weight at term. Pituitary, hypothalamic and adrenal

PGL paper no. 162. This work was supported by research grant GM 17173 from NIH.

hypoplasia are associated with prolonged pregnancy, which is part of the evidence that time of birth near and after term is governed by the unborn child (Liggins, 1974).

A large group of birth defects is associated with "small for date" babies of normal gestation time. These include some autosomal dominants (like snubnose dwarfism) and recessives (e.g., lissencephaly), congenital rubella, conditions of obscure etiology like the de Lange syndrome and many chromosomal anomalies.

While the total incidence of syndromes among premature live births is small, gestational disorders are frequent in severe birth defects and mental retardation. Some of these cases are due to hypoxia and other complications of premature birth. In other cases the defect existed prenatally and might cause prematurity or postmaturity (by weight or date) as well as malpresentation, dystocia or perinatal distress. The category of "gestational disorders" in the AAMD manual on terminology and classification of mental retardation (Grossman, 1973) is therefore a nightmare for epidemiologists and should be revised.

FAMILY RESEMBLANCE

Robson (1955) reported on birth weight in British cousins. There is no significant resemblance except for children of sisters (Table 1). This suggests that maternal constitution has an important effect on birth weight, but does not tell us whether the genotype or environment is relevant.

Morton (1955) analyzed birth weight of Japanese half-sibs, twins and sibs (Table 2). Maternal half-sibs show the same resemblance as full sibs, whereas paternal half-sibs are much less similar. Like-sexed twins (mostly monozygous in Japan) are no more similar than unlike-sexed dizygous twins. Resemblance of sibs declines with the number of intervening births. These observations demonstrate that maternal constitution is largely responsible for sibling resemblance in birth weight, and that the effect is at least partly due to transient environment.

Several attempts have been made to estimate relative variance compo-

Table 1.   Intraclass Correlations for Birth Weight of Cousins.

Sibling type	Number N	Correlation r
Brother-brother	576	.015
Brother-sister	675	.013
Sister-sister	1108	.135

Source: Robson, 1955

Table 2.   Intraclass Correlations for Birth Weight of Half-Sibs, Twins and Sibs.

Relationship	Number N	Correlation r
Maternal half-sibs	30	.581
Paternal half-sibs	168	.102
Like-sexed twins	220	.557
Unlike-sexed twins	40	.655
Adjacent sibs	367	.523
One sib intervening	654	.425
Two sibs intervening	1215	.363

Source: Morton, 1955

nents from such data. Defining maternal factors common to sibs with three births intervening as "permanent," most of the variance is due to random environmental and temporary maternal factors, with the genotype of the fetus accounting for the smallest proportion of variance (Table 3).

In Brazilian families, Rao et al. (1975) found that heritability of weight increases to a maximum at maturity and declines thereafter. The maternal effect persists throughout childhood into maturity (Tanner and Israelsohn, 1963). In childhood about half the covariance of sibs is due to common environment (Table 4), which diminishes with increasing age difference (Fig. 1). Persistence of maternal effects is supported by several studies which reveal that obesity is more frequent among mothers than among fathers of obese probands (Seltzer and Mayer, 1966).

Similar evidence has accumulated from other mammals. Lush, Hetzer and Culbertson (1934) found in swine that heredity of the offspring, including breed and sex differences, accounts for no more than a small

Table 3.   Estimates of Relative Variance Components for Birth Weight.

Source	Morton (1955)	Penrose (1959)	Rao et al. (1974)	Lush et al. (1934) swine	Chapman and Lush (1932) sheep
Genotype of fetus	− .09	.16	.08	.06	< .30
Permanent maternal factors	.28	> .20	.49	.47	> .30
Temporary maternal factors	.37	< .32			
Random environment	.44	.32	.43	.47	> .40
Total	1.00	1.00	1.00	1.00	1.00

Table 4.   Variance Components for Weight of Brazilian Children Adjusted for Age and Sex.

Source	Path analysis	Segregation analysis
Genotype	.416	.363
Common environment	.181	.180
Random environment	.403	.457

Source: Rao et al., 1975

percentage of the variance of birth weight, environment common to litter mates and random environment accounting equally for the rest (Table 3). At 180 days, the heritability of pig weight has increased to about 0.3. In beef cattle, heritability has been estimated as 0.3 at birth, 0.2 at weaning and 0.8 at 15 months (Tyler, Chapman and Dickerson, 1947). The latter value is substantially above human estimates, which are based on age-adjusted measurements at different ages when both gene action and environmental effects are different. Reciprocal matings of large and small breeds produce offspring more nearly resembling the maternal breed in horses and rabbits (Cawley, McKeown and Record, 1954).

I am not aware of critical data on the causes of family resemblance for gestation time in man. Shibata and Ishihara (1948) reported recessive

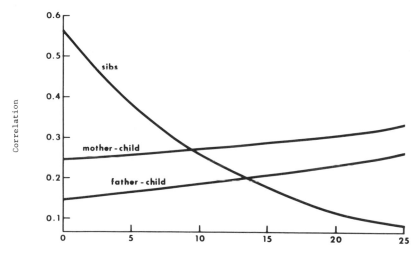

Figure 1.   **Temporal Trends in Familial Correlations for Normalized Weight.**   Abcissa is the age of child (for parent-child pairs) or absolute difference in age (for sibs). Source: Rao et al., 1975.

inheritance of prolonged gestation time (more than 309 days) in dairy cattle, all affected fetuses resulting from inbreeding of animals that could be traced back to one bull. Jafar et al. (1950) estimated that 29% of variance in gestation length of singleton, live born dairy cattle is due to sex of calf. Of the remainder, 45% is due to genotype of calf within sexes, 8% to maternal genotype and 21% to permanent maternal environment. De Fries et al. (1959) adjusted for sex of calf and concluded that about 42% of the remaining variance is due to genotype of the calf and 5% to maternal genotype. The correlation of gestation time and birth weight was 0.4. No effect of sex on gestation time was observed in sheep and swine (reviewed in Jafar, Chapman and Casida, 1950).

CAUSAL ANALYSIS

Minot (1891) suggested that the relation of birth weight and litter size in live born guinea pigs was due to premature parturition of large litters rather than depression of fetal growth. Wright (1921) applied his new technique of path analysis and came to the opposite conclusion (Fig. 2). He was able to infer four paths from three correlations by assuming complete linear determination of birth weight. Fetal growth rate appears to account for more than six times as much of the variance of birth weight as does gestation time. As far as I know, a comparable analysis has not been carried out for man in the 55 years since Wright showed how it could be done.

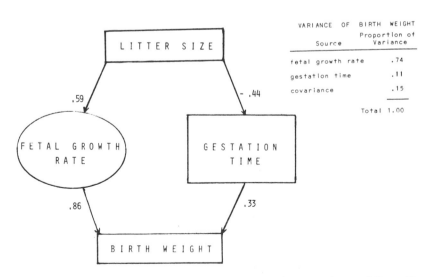

Figure 2. **Path Analysis of Correlations of Birth Weight, Gestation Time and Litter Size in Guinea Pigs.**   Rectangles represent measured variables. Source: Wright 1973.

However, progress has been made in the theory of path analysis through the z transform to justify normality and the likelihood ratio test to disprove causal hypotheses (Rao, Morton and Yee, 1974; Rao et al., 1977). Many aspects of prematurity, in addition to family resemblance, lend themselves to this kind of analysis (e.g., the effects of race, socioeconomic status, maternal age and unfavorable gestational factors).

We have seen that there is a large effect of fetal genotype on gestation time (at least in cattle), a rather low correlation between birth weight and gestation time, and low heritability of birth weight. Fetal hormonal activity appears to be the explanatory variable, since it determines gestation time. Many syndromes which include perinatal respiratory distress have an elevated incidence of malpresentation. Here the etiology is much less clear, but it may depend on fetal activity. Figure 3 shows an untested model for simultaneous determination of live birth weight, gestation time, and presentation. With four observed variables there are six correlations and so one residual degree of freedom if birth weight is completely determined. It has the interest of distinguishing between complications of pregnancy which affect fetal growth rate and gestation time. While we can have no confidence in an untested hypothesis, it illustrates a direction in which causal analysis might profitably be pursued. Determination of gestation time by the unborn child was demonstrated by analysis of family resemblance long before modern work on fetal hormones established the mechanism (Liggins, 1974).

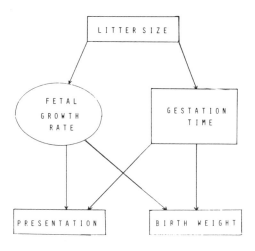

Figure 3.   **Untested Model for Simultaneous Determination of Live Birth Weight, Gestation Time and Presentation.**

INBREEDING AND OUTCROSSING EFFECTS

Morton (1959) found that consanguineous marriage had no effect on gestation time in nearly 60,000 Japanese live births. With the exception of an inferred recessive gene for prolonged gestation time in dairy cattle (Shibata and Ishihara, 1948), there is no evidence to suggest that gestation time in mammals is affected by inbreeding or outcrossing despite the large variance due to fetal genotype (Jafar et al., 1950). This is really no paradox since control of gestation time by fetal hormones makes it unlikely that homozygous for recessive genes would curtail gestation except through fetal death.

On the contrary, in a sample of more than 70,000 Japanese babies the regression of birth weight on the inbreeding coefficient was -540 ± 120 gm., which is highly significant (Morton, 1959). This effect corresponds to 1.29 standard deviations, in striking contrast to the small proportion of variance due to fetal genotype, and is comparable to the inbreeding depression observed for quantitative traits in domestic and laboratory animals (Falconer, 1960). There was no significant effect of inbreeding on variance of birth weight. Inbreeding depression of weight persists in childhood (Schull and Neel, 1965), but there is no evidence that adult weight is appreciably affected by inbreeding (Barrai, Cavalli-Sforza, and Mainardi, 1964). Evidence in farm animals has been summarized as follows (Shreffler and Touchberry, 1959): "The effect of inbreeding is to decrease heterozygosity and decrease rate of growth; the effect of crossbreeding is to increase heterozygosity and to increase rate of growth. In neither situation, however, is the size at maturity significantly affected."

Morton, Chung, and Mi (1967) studied birth weight of more than 160,000 live births in Hawaii. There was no significant effect of fetal or maternal hybridity in these interracial crosses. This is part of the evidence that genetic differentiation of racial groups is small for genes affecting morbidity, equivalent to inbreeding of 0.0005 for minor races and 0.0009 for major ones. Much larger equivalent inbreeding coefficients (0.014 for minor races, 0.129 major races) are found for isozymes, blood groups and other polymorphisms, suggesting that they have been subject to weaker or more divergent selection. In either case, nonsignificance of outcrossing effects in this large material is impressive and is supported by other studies (Trevor, 1953; Krieger, 1966).

Population geneticists do not agree on the interpretation of inbreeding effects, which to some are evidence that polygenes are not strictly additive, while others emphasize rare recessive genes that are part of the genetic load. Table 5 shows that a completely recessive gene ($d = 0$) contributes appreciably to resemblance of relatives and twice as much to the additive variance as to the dominance variance when the gene frequency is inter-

Table 5. Dominance Deviations under Two Hypotheses.

Source	General	Polygenic $(q = \tfrac{1}{2})$	Rare recessive $q \to 0$
Additive (H)	$2q(1 - q)\,t^2[q + (1 - 2q)d]^2$	$t^2/8$	$2qt^2(q + d)^2$
Dominance (D)	$[q(1 - q)\,t\,(1 - 2d)]^2$	$t^2(1 - 2d)^2/16$	$q^2t^2(1 - 2d)^2$
D/H	$\parallel$	$(1 - 2d)^2/2$	$q(1 - 2d)^2/2(q + d)^2$
D/H when d = 0		$\tfrac{1}{2}$	$\tfrac{1}{2}q$

mediate, but virtually nothing to resemblance of relatives or to the additive variance if the gene frequency is small. Consequently, we may ignore inbreeding effects and dominance deviations in studying resemblance of relatives if and only if significant deviations from additivity are restricted to rare genes, and in that case we may infer major gene effects if significant dominance deviations are observed.

The best evidence on this question comes from IQ (Morton et al., 1976). The inbred load for mental defect:

$$B = \Sigma qs = .83 \pm .21,$$

where q is the frequency of a gene producing mental defect (IQ < 70), s is its penetrance and the summation is over all loci. The mean gene frequency is $Q \leq 0.0024$, the mean displacement of homozygotes is $t = 52.5$ IQ points, and the number of loci which produce mental retardation is $k \geq 351$. Schull and Neel(1965) estimated the regression of IQ on inbreeding as -39.5. The contribution of a completely recessive gene to inbreeding depression is:

$$b \equiv qt \doteq .126 \text{ IQ points.}$$

The observed decline of IQ with inbreeding corresponds to

$$k = 39.5/.126 = 313$$

loci, in almost perfect agreement with the estimate of 351 from mental retardation. Thus the decline of IQ with inbreeding appears to be due entirely to rare recessive genes, and not to dominance deviations of polygenes. This justifies omission of dominance deviations from analysis of family resemblance.

For birth weight the essential estimate of the inbred load B for prematurity (say, < 2500 gm.) is lacking, and so we cannot be certain that the same conclusion holds. However, we may make a heuristic calculation as follows. The standard deviation of live birth weight was estimated by Morton et al. (1967) as 560 gm. in Hawaii (including late fetal deaths) and by Morton (1958) as 418 gm. for live births in Japan. If rare recessives have the same frequency and effect on IQ and birth weight in standard deviation units, the mean effect of homozygosis for a single gene would be:

$$b \doteq qt = (.0024) (500) (3.5) = 4.2 \text{ gm.}$$

Then the observed inbreeding decline would correspond to:

$$k = 540/4.2 = 129$$

loci at which recessive genes occur with large effects on birth weight. Some of these may also cause mental retardation and infant death. This is a modest number, which gives us no reason to suppose that the inbreeding effect on birth weight is due to any other cause than rare recessive genes.

The dominance deviation generated by this number of rare recessive genes could account for only:

$$kq^2t^2 = (129) (.0024)^2(3.5)^2 = .009,$$

or less than 1% of the phenotypic variance. By this argument we are not only completely justified in neglecting dominance deviations for analysis of family resemblance, but we would be unwise to attempt the exercise, which confounds environment common to sibs with dominance (Nance and Corey, 1976).

Because of segregation of rare recessive genes, as well as other megaphenic effects (both genetic and environmental) at the extremes of the distribution of birth weight, we would not expect different truncations to give the same estimates of variance components. This may explain the results of Trimble (1971), who experimented with Falconer's method for quasi-continuity in a large body of human birth weight data. However, his conclusion that "uncritical application of the models is likely to lead to very poor predication of sib risks" is illogical. Since the model is fitted to data, it cannot describe those data badly, although extrapolation should be cautious. His error was in assuming that etiology is the same over the range of birth weight and in using Edwards' square root prediction, which is reliable only for familial correlation in the neighborhood of 0.5. Morton et al. (1976) have shown that heterogeneity of mental retardation is no bar to genetic analysis.

SECULAR TRENDS

During the last century there has been an appreciable increase in birth weight. Takahashi and Oshio (1938), comparing babies born at the Red Cross Hospital, Tokyo, in 1926–27 and again in 1937–38, observed an increase in birth weight of 74 ± 8 gm. During the postwar period non-inbred babies studied by the Atomic Bomb Casualty Commission increased by 6.9 ± 1.2 gm. per year within parity and city (Morton, 1959).

These secular trends, which are paralleled by anthropometrics during childhood, are certainly not due to genetic effects of "isolate-breaking," which are not likely to exceed 5 gm. for birth weight (corresponding to an inbreeding coefficient of 0.01). Temporal changes of greater magnitude than this must be due to changes in nutrition, infection, maternal size, complications of pregnancy and labor or other environmental factors.

PREMATURITY AND FITNESS

Penrose (1954) suggested that "the majority of so-called 'premature' infants are perfectly normal though small, like adults of short stature." The problem is to distinguish these normal variations from high risk infants.

Karn and Penrose (1951) found that perinatal mortality is at a minimum for English births averaging 379 gm. more than the mean. Morton et al. (1967) reported that the optimum birth weight in Hawaii is:

$$1.061 \, \mu \, + \, 195 \text{ gm.}$$

where μ is the mean birth weight (Mi and Yamashita, 1976). For Caucasian infants the mean birth weight was 3281 gm., corresponding to an optimum 395 gm. greater, in good agreement with the English data (Table 6). Filipino infants with a birth weight of 2200 gm. have about the same mortality as Caucasian infants that weigh 2500 gm. A less arbitrary definition of prematurity might help to reduce perinatal mortality and later morbidity by directing intensive care to babies most at risk.

The consistent difference between optimum and mean birth weight is a puzzle to evolutionary geneticists. In the absence of some countervailing selection, we might suppose that mean birth weight would coincide with the optimum. Perhaps the difference is due to noxious environmental effects. Perhaps there is (or was in the past) postnatal selection in favor of children whose birth weight had been below the optimum with respect to neonatal death. For example, fetal hormonal activity may be correlated

Table 6. Mean and Optimum Birth Weight (gm.) with the Corresponding Criteria for Prematurity.

Race	Mean	Optimum	Prematurity
Caucasian	3281	3678	2500
Hawaiian	3252	3646	2500
Puerto Rican	3141	3529	2400
Japanese and Chinese	3116	3502	2300
Filipino	2981	3358	2200

Source: Morton et al., 1967

both with gestation time and subsequent level of physical activity. Questions in evolutionary genetics are seldom answered, but we might hope that this will be an exception.

PATERNAL EFFECTS ON PREMATURITY

Inbreeding effects and studies of family resemblance show that the father exerts an effect on birth weight. For gestation time there does not seem to be any appreciable effect of rare recessive genes, but data from other mammals consistently show a genetic effect of the father on gestation time.

The evidence is just as clear that the uterine environment exerts an effect on birth weight independent of the genotype of the fetus. In part, this depends on maternal size, perhaps operating through size of the placenta (Cawley et al., 1954). However, inequality of the parental effects remains even after covariance adjustment for size of the other parent (Table 7).

Paternal effects are not exclusively genetic. Birth weight in Hawaii is influenced as much by paternal race as maternal race (Morton et al., 1967); in this population there is no correlation within maternal race between maternal size and father's race. In view of the data on family resemblance within race, which demonstrate a preponderant maternal effect, the effects of paternal race must be largely determined through social, behavioral and environmental factors during pregnancy such as maternal diet, health, smoking habits and other characteristics. There are no critical observations to determine what part, if any, of the maternal effect on birth weight is genetic.

The small effect of paternal size on birth weight partly accounts for the absence of any effect of interracial crosses on complications of labor and birth injury (Morton et al., 1967). Other causes are the smallness of

Table 7. Correlations Between Birth Weight and Parental Height, Corrected for Height of the Other Parent.

Parent	Sample size N	Corrected r	Uncorrected r
Mother	1534	.17	.20
Father	1534	.07	.12

Source: Cawley et al., 1954

racial differences and the capability of the bony pelvis, even of races with small pelvic girths, to accommodate rather large fetuses.

SUGGESTIONS FOR FURTHER RESEARCH

Before making suggestions for further research, it is appropriate to ask whether the kind of information which genetic epidemiology provides is interesting and useful. Feldman and Lewontin (1975) give a resounding negative. Their credentials are that one is a compiler of *Drosophila* gene frequencies, and the other a dabbler in biology who has spent the last few years describing cultural inheritance by a genetic locus with two alleles. As to their arguments, they use the rhetoric with which Lyssenko destroyed genetics in Russia. They point out that the latest development in genetic epidemiology (the mixed model which includes a major locus, polygenes and cultural inheritance) has seen little use in genetic counseling (Feldman and Lewontin, 1976). That is hardly surprising, since the theory was published only two years ago (Morton and MacLean, 1974) and applications must follow collection and analysis of suitable bodies of data. This endeavor is not advanced by their doctrinaire rejection of genetic epidemiology, which for several years has been represented on the Genetics Study Section only by its two most rabid and ill-informed opponents. I shall not discuss their arguments in detail, since they derive from dialectical materialism rather than genetics.

Let me instead give a formal definition of *genetic epidemiology* as a science that deals with the etiology, distribution and control of disease in groups of relatives or with inherited causes of disease in populations. "Inherited" is used here in a broad sense to include both biologic and cultural inheritance. The proposition that genetic epidemiology is interesting and important requires no defense. I hope that the small effort so far devoted to the genetic epidemiology of prematurity is not irrelevant to its understanding and prevention. In summary, I would like to make the following suggestions for future research:

1. In future research there is an advantage in retaining birth weight and gestation time as separate variables. A discriminant based on both variables is more useful as an indicator of neonatal risk.

2. However prematurity is defined in studies of family resemblance and inbreeding effects, it should be analyzed both as a continuous and discrete trait. This is especially important for interpreting inbreeding effects.

3. Although in the past cousins, twins and half-sibs have been informative, nuclear families should be the focus of attention.

4. Inbreeding effects should be examined for segregation of major genes.

5. The Institute of Medicine of the National Academy of Sciences has recommended that "all pregnant women should be evaluated in the first trimester and classified by risks that would adversely affect the survival of their infants." In addition to the usual social and medical risks, recurrence risks for prematurity, derived from segregation analysis of family resemblance, may be a useful guide to intensive care of later born children.

6. Sibships inferred to be segregating for a major gene or chromosomal aberration affecting birth weight are valuable for recognizing new syndromes, which may or may not have increased morbidity.

7. Path analysis has unexplored potential to clarify prematurity. For example, consider the causal diagram in Figure 4. Mortality is the frequency of neonatal deaths. Prematurity is a discriminant of mortality based on birth weight and gestation time. Social risk is a discriminant of mortality based on socioeconomic class, medical risk is similarly defined on unfavorable characteristics of the pregnancy and X is any factor (like race) to be tested for its direct effect on prematurity and mortality. There are 15 observed correlations and parameters, of which three (the paths from X) are null on the hypothesis that X has no direct effect. The likelihood ratio test is appropriate. In a particular case X might be an intervention strategy. Many similar causal models are worth considering. The utility of path analysis has been much discussed; criticism was formulated largely against earlier usage which emphasized estimates rather than tests

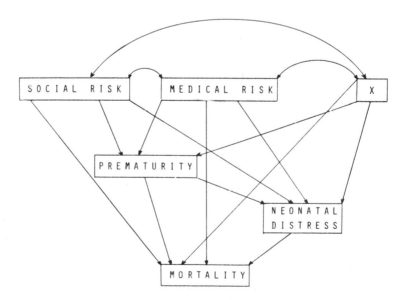

Figure 4. **Causal Model for Prematurity and Mortality.**

of hypotheses. With the new developments path analysis should be a powerful tool in epidemiology (Morton et al., 1976).

8. While the primary objective in genetic studies of prematurity is to contribute knowledge relevant to disease control, their value to basic science is by no means negligible. Genetic epidemiology is a new discipline, and it will take much effort and ingenuity to develop it through methodological advances and application to specific health problems. In the evolution of science this is as important as any advance in molecular genetics. For example, interpretation of inbreeding effects on quantitative traits has been heavily influenced by the controversy between Mendelian and biometrical genetics at the beginning of this century. At a mathematical level this was settled by accommodating any degree of dominance. However, biochemical data have failed to support any appreciable dominance for quantitative effects of isozymes; red cell acid phosphatase in man has been particularly instructive. At the same time biometrical genetics has conspicuously failed to demonstrate dominance or epistasis for polygenic traits within nearly panmictic populations. Apparently these phenomena, while they certainly exist, have negligible effects on family resemblance for polygenic traits. It is not surprising that small effects should be nearly additive. Some of the critical evidence comes from IQ data discussed above. The supporting evidence from prematurity could be made rigorous by further studies. If those who deplore the present state of genetic epidemiology were sincere, they would be the first to advocate such critical tests.

Genetic epidemiology is so easily and efficiently combined with other epidemiologic studies that it should be considered in any serious program to understand and control prematurity. The results may have immediate practical utility. Even if they do not, they help to provide the understanding necessary for intelligent intervention. In the words of Francis Bacon: "Nor can nature be commanded, except by being obeyed, and so these twin objects, human knowledge and human power, do really meet in one; and it is from ignorance of causes that operation fails."

TEXT REFERENCES

Barrai, I.; Cavalli-Sforza, L. L.; Mainardi, M.: Testing a Model of Dominant Inheritance for Metric Traits in Man. Heredity 19:(1964)651–668

Cawley, R. H.; McKeown, T.; Record, R. G.: Parental Stature and Birth Weight. Am J Hum Genet 6(1954)448–456

Chapman, A. B.; Lush, J. L.: Twinning, Sex Ratios, and Genetic Variability in Birth Weight in Sheep. J Hered 32(1932) 473–478

Falconer, D. S.: Introduction to Quantitative Genetics. Harper & Row, New York, 1960

Feldman, M. W.; Lewontin, R. C.: Letters: Re Heritability of IQ. Science 194(1976) 12–14

Grossman, H. J.: Manual on Terminology and Classification in Mental Retardation

Revised. AAMD Special Publication Series No. 2. Garamond/Pridemark Press, Baltimore, 1973

Jafar, S. M.; Chapman, A. B.; Casida, L. E.: Causes of Variation in Length of Gestation in Dairy Cattle. J Animal Sci 9(1950)593–601

Karn, M. N.; Penrose, L. S.: Birth Weight and Gestation Time in Relation to Maternal Age, Parity and Infant Survival. Ann Eugen 16(1951)147

Krieger, H.: Inbreeding Effects in Northeastern Brazil. Ph.D. Thesis. U. Hawaii, Honolulu, 1966

Liggins, G. C.: Parturition in the Sheep and the Human. In: Physiology and Genetics of Reproduction, Part B, pp. 423–444, ed. by E. M. Coutinho, and F. Fuchs. Plenum Press, New York, 1974

Lush, J. L.; Hetzer, H. O.; Culbertson, C. C.: Factors Affecting Birth Weights of Swine. Genetics 19(1934)329–343

Mi, M. P.; Yamashita, T.: Birth Weight and Neonatal Survival in Sibs. Presented at the 5th International Congress on Human Genetics, Mexico City, 1976

Minot, C. S.: Senescence and Rejuvenescence. J Physiol 12(1891)97–153

Morton, N. E.; MacLean, C. J.: Analysis of Family Resemblance. III. Complex Segregation of Quantitative Traits. Am J Hum Genet 26(1974)489–503

Morton, N. E.; Chung, C. S.; Mi, M. P.: Genetics of Interracial Crosses in Hawaii. Karger, Basel, 1967

Morton, N. E.; Rao, D. C.; MacLean, C. J.; Bart, R. C.; Lang-Brown, H.; Lew, R.: Colchester Revisited: A Genetic Study of Mental Defect. J Med Genet (1977)1–9

Morton, N. E.: The Inheritance of Human Birth Weight. Ann Hum Genet 20(1955) 125–134

Nance, W. E.; Corey, L.: Genetic Models for the Analysis of Data from the Families of Identical Twins. Genetics 83(1976) 811–826

Penrose, L. S.: Genetical Factors Affecting the Growth of the Foetus. La Prophylaxie en Gynecologie et Obstetrique. Int. Congr. Gynaec. Obstet. (Geneva) Vol. I, 1– , 1954

Rao, D. C.; Morton, N. E.; Yee, S.: Analysis of Family Resemblance. II. A Linear Model for Familial Correlation. Am J Hum Genet 26(1974)331–359

Rao, D. C.; MacLean, C. J.; Morton, N. E.; Yee, S.: Analysis of Family Resemblance. V. Height and Weight in Northeastern Brazil. Am J Hum Genet 27(1975) 509–520

Rao, D. C.; Morton, N. E.; Elston, R. C.; Yee, S.: Causal Analysis of Academic Performance. Behav Genet (in press), 1977

Robson, E. B.: Birth Weight in Cousins. Ann Hum Genet 19(1955)262–268

Schull, W. J.; Neel, J. V.: The Effects of Inbreeding on Japanese Children. Harper and Row, New York, 1965

Seltzer, C. C.; Mayer, J.: A Review of Genetic and Constitutional Factors in Human Obesity. In: The Biology of Human Variation, pp. 688–695, ed. by J. Brozek. Annals of the New York Academy of Science, Vol. 134, Art. 2, New York, 1966

Shibata, S.; Ishihara, M.: Studies on Hereditary Defects in Japanese Native Cattle. Zootach Exp Sta Res Bull 54 (1948)42–100

Shreffler, D. C.; Touchberry, R. W.: Effects of Cross Breeding on Rate of Growth in Dairy Cattle. J Dairy Sci 42(1959) 607–620

Takahashi, K.; Oshio, R.: Concerning the Distinct Increase in Height and Weight of the Newborn of Today. Sanka to Fujinka 6(1938)617–623

Tanner, J.; Israelsohn, W.: Changes in Parent-Child Correlations for Body Measurements During Growth of Children Followed Individually from One Month After Birth to Seven Years. In: Proceedings 2nd International Congress of Human Genetics, Rome, September 1961, Vol. 1, p.460. Instituto. G. Mendel, Rome, 1963

Trevor, J. C.: Race Crossing in Man. The Analysis of Metrical Characters. Eugen Lab Mem 36(1953)45

Trimble, B. K.: An Empirical Simulation of Quasi-Continuous Inheritance (Abstract #48) In: International Congress Series No. 233, 4th International Congress of Human Genetics, Paris, September 1971, ed. by J. de Grouchy, F. J. H. Ebling, I. Henderson, and J. Francois. Exerpta Medica, Amsterdam, 1971

Tyler, W. J.; Chapman, A. B.; Dickerson, G. E.: Sources of Variation in the Birth Weight of Holstein-Friesian Calves. J Dairy Sci 30(1947)483–498

Wright, S.: Correlation and Causation. J Agric Res 20(1921)557–585

Wright, S.: The Origin of the F-Statistics for Describing the Genetic Aspects of Population Structure. In: Genetic Structure of Populations, pp. ed. by N. E. Morton. University Press of Hawaii, Honolulu, 1973

DISCUSSION

Dr. Garn: I would like to add a note to Dr. Morton's parent, child and sibling correlations because our most recent studies using *adopted* parent-child pairs, and both singly and doubly adopted sibling pairs, quite duplicate what is traditionally found in the genetic literature—namely, parent-child correlations of 0.25, sibling correlations of about 0.3, correlations between parent and child rising with age to adulthood and sibling correlations decreasing as the number of years between them increases (Garn, Bailey and Higgins, 1976; Garn, Bailey and Cole, 1976; Garn, Cole and Bailey, 1977). So we can quite duplicate what has been conventionally presented in the literature, although with adopted pairs rather than with parents and their own children, which perhaps shows that "heritability" is less important than "*housability*." Should we not be studying the progeny of crossracial marriages which are occurring now in increasing numbers? (Table 8).

Dr. Morton: We have done this with birth weight for 170,000 births in Hawaii, and there are several conclusions (Morton et al., 1967). One of them is that outcrossing by itself doesn't increase or decrease birth weight. Secondly, the maternal effects are what you would expect, but also there are suprisingly large paternal effects. Since the analysis within racial groups is quite convincing that the paternal effect is small on birth weight, it seems clear that any large paternal effects must be mediated through

Table 8.   Intraracial and Crossracial Prevalence of Gestational Prematurity

Parental combination		Total series		Parity > 1	
Mother	Father	N	Percent ≤ 37 weeks	N	Percent ≤ 37 weeks
Black	Black	9,901	26.2	7,100	26.4
Black	White	34	20.6	26	19.2
White	Black	98	17.3	65	16.9
White	White	9,433	11.7	6,107	12.0

Source: Garn and Bailey, 1977.

the maternal diet and environment. That is substantially the evidence from such interracial crosses so far.

Dr. Stein: I was interested in Table 6 in Dr. Morton's presentation on mean and optimum birth weights and prematurity. I just wondered what the optimum meant.

Dr. Morton: The criterion is perinatal mortality. We followed Karn and Penrose (1951) in finding that it is quadratic on birth weight. The optimum occurs at about 1.06 times the mean plus 200 grams. So in England, for example, it is roughly 400 grams above the mean.

Dr. Stein: So the optimum might be revised year by year, the mean staying the same but the optimum changing.?

Dr. Stanley: Because smaller babies are surviving with improvements in medical care.

Dr. Morton: Yes, although we were surprised that the excess of the optimum over the mean was consistent in Hawaii and England.

DISCUSSION REFERENCES

Garn S. M.; Bailey, S. M.: Genetics of Maturational Processes. In: Human Growth, eds. F. Falkner and J. M. Tanner. Plenum Publishing Corp., New York, 1977

Garn, S. M.; Bailey, S. M.; Higgins, I. T. T.: Fatness Similarities in Adopted Pairs. Am J Clin Nutr 29(1976)1067-1068

Garn, S. M.; Bailey, S. M.; Cole, P. E.: Similarities between Parents and their Adopted Children. Am J Phys Anthrop 45(1976)539-543

Garn, S.M.; Cole, P. E.; Bailey, S. M.: Effect of Parental Fatness Levels on the Fatness of Biological and Adoptive Children. Ecol. Food Nutr. 6(1977)in press

Karn, M. N.; Penrose, L. S.: Birth Weight and Gestation Time in Relation to Maternal Age, Parity and Infant Survival. Ann Eugen 16(1951)147

Morton, N. E.; Chung, C. S.; Mi, M. P.: Genetics of Interracial Crosses in Hawaii. Karger, Basel. 1967

The Risk of Repeated Preterm or Low Birth Weight Delivery

Leiv S. Bakketeig, M.D.

Many studies have shown an association between low birth weight and previous history of low birth weight deliveries (Karn et al., 1951; Ounsted, 1965; Collaborative Perinatal Study, 1972; Habicht et al., 1974; Fedrick and Anderson, 1976; Kaltreider and Johnson, 1976). Most of these studies have been done retrospectively. The authors have not or only to a limited extent been able to obtain information on gestational age of previous births. Thus the authors have mostly been unable to take into account both gestational age and birth weight when studying the tendency of repeating low birth weight or preterm births.

It has now become possible to carry out prospective studies based on routinely collected information on all births in Norway. Information on all births with gestational age 16 weeks or more is provided by *Medical Registration of Births* (Bjerkedal and Bakketeig, 1972 and 1975), which was introduced in Norway in 1967. All information on the birth, the parents, labor and delivery is kept on computer files at the Medical Birth Registry of Norway, where both child and parents are identified by unique identification numbers. This permits easy record linkage between mother and child and makes it possible to study subsequent births to the same mother. This paper presents some preliminary results from an analysis based on this source of data.

MATERIALS AND METHODS

During the seven-year period 1967–1973, a total of 464,067 births were registered in Norway to mothers resident within the country. This study is based on 81,400 mothers who had their first and second single births during this time period. For 5002 (6.6%) of these mothers, birth weight or gestational age are not known for either their first or second birth, or for both. These mothers are excluded from the analysis, which is limited to the 76,398 mothers where birth weight and gestational age are known for both first and second births.

The results are presented for mothers in groups according to birth weight and gestational age of their first birth. Three different outcomes of their next pregnancies are studied: low birth weight (LBW), defined as a birth weighing 2500 gm. or less; preterm delivery, defined as delivery before 37 completed weeks (16–36 weeks of gestation); and "growth retardation," based on an operational definition for birth weight being below the 10th percentile for gestational age. The combinations of birth weight and gestational age used for grouping of the mothers based on their first birth are based partly on recommendations by WHO (1974) and on contour distributions of birth weight and gestational age (Hoffman et al., 1974). A total of 64 combinations of the following eight weight groups and eight gestational age groups is being used:

Birth weight:	*Gestational age:*
1000 gm. or less	less than 28 weeks (less than 196 days)
1001–1500 gm.	28–30 weeks (196–216 days)
1501–2000 gm.	31–33 weeks (217–237 days)
2001–2500 gm.	34–36 weeks (238–258 days)
2501–3000 gm.	37–38 weeks (259–272 days)
3001–4000 gm.	39–41 weeks (273–293 days)
4001–4500 gm.	42–44 weeks (294–314 days)
4501 gm. or more	45 weeks or more (315 days or more)

Gestational age is based on the number of days between first day of last menstrual period and time of birth.

RESULTS

The overall risk of having a second birth with low birth weight was 3.5% for the 76,398 mothers included in the study. Table 1 shows the distribution of the mothers according to the birth weight and gestational age of their first birth, and the proportion of mothers in the different

Table 1. Risk (Percent) of Low Birth Weight (<2500 gm) of Second Birth for 76,398 Mothers By Birth Weight and Gestational Age of First Birth.

Birth Weight (gm)	Gestational Age (weeks)							
	16	28	31	34	37	39	42	45
>4500	—	—	1	8	30	622 (1.3)	370 (0.8)	22
4001–4500	4	—	5	51	195 (1.0)	4878 (1.1)	1911 (1.3)	151 (2.0)
3001–4000	35	17	107 (6.5)	845 (3.1)	4847 (3.0)	37135 (2.1)	8638 (1.7)	795 (2.1)
2501–3000	14	14	99 (2.0)	1040 (8.6)	2489 (7.5)	6330 (6.0)	1083 (5.7)	139 (4.3)
2001–2500	7	22	246 (13.8)	728 (14.1)	534 (.2)	812 (11.2)	112 (13.4)	29
1501–2000	20	90 (21.1)	296 (17.2)	235 (14.5)	15 (13.4)	108 (13.0)	9	8
1001–1500	74 (27.0)	196 (19.9)	106 (24.5)	98 (14.3)	40	12	—	
0–1000	397 (21.2)	75 (16.0)	42	19	4	3		2

groups whose second birth was a low birth weight baby. Mothers whose first birth had a gestational age 39 weeks or more and weighed more than 3000 gm. had a 2% or lower chance of having a LBW second birth. If, on the other hand, the first birth weighed 2000 gm. or less and the gestational age was less than 34 weeks, the risk of a LBW second birth was about 20%. The risk of a LBW second birth was more than 30 times as high for mothers whose first birth had the least favorable combination of birth weight and gestational age, compared to mothers with a first birth whose birth weight and gestational age was the most favorable one. By studying Table 1, it appears that the risk of a LBW second birth decreases as the birth weight of the first birth increases. For example, where the gestational age of the first birth was 39–41 weeks, the risk of subsequent LBW birth decreased from 13 to slightly more than 1% as the birth weight increased from below 2000 gm. to above 4000 gm.

A similar relationship seems to be present, to some extent, between gestational age of the first birth and the risk of a LBW second birth. For example, if the birth weight of the first birth was between 3000–4000 gm., the risk decreased from 6.5 to about 2% as the gestational age of the first birth increased from 31 to 44 weeks and more. However, the risk does not change as dramatically by gestational age as by birth weight, particularly if the birth weight of the first birth is below 2500 gm.

In Table 2, the risk of a preterm second birth is shown for the mothers grouped by birth weight and gestational age as in Table 1. The overall risk of having a preterm second birth was 4.9% for these mothers. If the first birth weighed more than 4000 gm. and the gestational age was 39 weeks or more, the risk of a preterm second birth was less than 3%. If, however, the birth weight of the first birth was 2500 gm. or less and the gestational age less than 34 weeks, the risk was over 20%. The ratio of the highest and lowest risk was slightly less than twenty times. The risk of a preterm second birth seems to decrease both as birth weight and gestational age of first birth increases. Gestational age seems to be more powerful in predicting a preterm second birth than predicting a LBW second birth. For example, if the first birth weighed between 2000–2500 gm., the risk of a preterm second birth decreased from 23.6 to 5.4% as the gestational age of the first birth increased from 31–33 to 42–44 weeks.

A growth retarded birth is defined here as one where the birth weight falls below the 10th percentile for gestational age (Battaglia and Lubchenko, 1967). The solid line in Table 3 represents an operational definition of the 10th percentile, which is relatively close to the 10th percentile of birth weights of single births at different gestation periods for Norwegian births (Bjerkedal, Bakketeig and Lehmann, 1973). When

Table 2. Risk (Percent) of Preterm (<37 Weeks) Second Birth for 76,398 Mothers by Birth Weight and Gestational Age of First Birth.

Birth Weight (gm)	16	28	31	34	37	39	42	45
>4500	—	—	1	8	30	622 (2.1)	370 (2.4)	22
4001–4500	4	—	5	51	155 (6.2)	4878 (2.7)	1911 (1.8)	151 (2.0)
3001–4000	35	17	107 (7.5)	845 (3.9)	4847 (5.2)	37135 (3.6)	8638 (2.6)	795 (3.9)
2501–3000	14	14	99 (10.1)	1040 (15.7)	2483 (10.2)	6330 (5.6)	1083 (3.8)	139 (5.0)
2001–2500	7	22	246 (23.6)	728 (16.4)	584 (11.8)	812 (8.6)	112 (5.4)	29
1501–2000	20	90	296 (24.4)	235 (22.3)	149 (15.3)	108 (4.7)	9	8
1001–1500	74 (33.8)	196 (23.0)	106 (21.7)	98 (11.2)	40	12	—	2
0–1000	397 (28.2)	75 (13.3)	42	19	4	3	—	—

Gestational Age (weeks)

growth retardation is defined as having a combination of birth weight and gestational age which falls below the solid line in Table 3, 7.9% of the second births in this study can be classified as growth retarded.

The risk of having a growth retarded second birth is shown in Table 3 for the mothers grouped according to birth weight and gestational age of their first birth. If their first birth weighed more than 4000 gm., the risk of the second birth being growth retarded was 1.5% or less. If, however, the first birth was growth retarded (e.g., weighing 2001–2500 gm. with gestational age 39–44 weeks), the risk was around 30%. Within the weight groups below 3000 gm., there seems to be a tendency of increased risk of the second birth being growth retarded as the gestational age of the first birth increases. This would indicate that the more growth retarded the first birth is, the greater the increase in risk.

The obtained prediction of the three different outcomes of second births is shown in Table 4, using as selection criteria birth weight, gestational age and combinations of birth weight and gestational age of the first birth. The table shows, for each subgroup of mothers, the risk of subsequent LBW, preterm and growth retarded births. The relative risk of each outcome is calculated as the ratio of the risk within the subgroup to the risk of the mothers not included in the subgroup. The columns showing the predicted proportion of all second births being LBW, preterm and growth retarded contain information on what proportion of all second births that are LBW, preterm and growth retarded are produced by mothers within each subgroup. For example, of all LBW second births, 26% were delivered by mothers whose first births weighed 2500 gm. or less.

The findings may be summarized as follows: birth weight of the first birth seems to be the best predictor of low birth weight of the second birth; gestational age of the first birth is a good predictor of a preterm second birth; and growth retardation of the first birth is the best predictor of growth retardation of the second birth.

It is possible to predict a substantial part of subsequent LBW, preterm or growth retarded births using as selection criteria a combination of birth weight and gestational age of the first birth. Thus, by selecting pregnant women whose first births weighed 3000 gm. or less or had a gestational age below 39 weeks, it may be estimated that these mothers (28.6% of all) will give birth to 60% of LBW second births, more than 50% of preterm second birth and more than 50% of the growth retarded second births.

DISCUSSION

A total of 5002 mothers have been excluded from the analysis, due to incomplete information on either birth weight or gestational age of their

Table 3. Risk (Percent) of Growth Retarded* Second Birth for 76,398 Mothers by Birth Weight and Gestational Age of First Birth.

Birth Weight (gm)	16	28	31	34	37	39	42	45
>4500	—	—	1	8	50	622 (1.0)	370 (0.5)	22
4001–4500	4	—	5	51	155 (1.3)	4878 (1.5)	1911 (1.5)	151 (1.3)
3001–4000	35	17	107 (9.4)	845 (3.8)	4840 (4.9)	37135 (5.7)	8688 (6.2)	795 (8.6)
2501–3000	14	14	99 (9.1)	1040 (9.2)	2489 (14.3)	6330 (20.6)	1083 (21.2)	139 (15.1)
2001–2500	7	22	246 (6.5)	728 (15.4)	584 (24.8)	812 (31.0)	112 (29.5)	29
1501–2000	20	90 (12.2)	296 (15.2)	235 (26.0)	149 (28.9)	108 (25.9)	9	8
1001–1500	74 (13.5)	196 (12.2)	106 (32.1)	98 (27.6)	40	12	—	2
0–1000	397 (13.6)	75 (14.7)	42	19	4	3	—	—

Gestational Age (weeks)

*"Growth retarded" here defined as being below the 10th percentile, approximated by being below the solid line in the table.

Table 4. Prediction of Low Birth Weight, Preterm (<37 Weeks) and Growth Retarded Second Birth Based on Birth Weight and Gestational Age of the First Birth*.

1st Birth (BW/GA)	Prop. of Total Number of Mothers (%)	Risk of Second Birth Being (%):			Relative Risk of:			Predicted prop. of all second births being (%):		
		LBW	Preterm	Growth Retarded	LBW	Preterm Birth	Growth Retarded	LBW	Preterm	Growth Retarded
<2500 gm	5.9	15.2	15.4	20.5	5.6	3.7	4.1	26.0	18.7	15.3
<3000 gm	20.6	9.0	9.7	18.7	4.5	2.7	3.7	53.5	41.1	48.6
<37 weeks	6.4	11.8	16.4	11.5	4.1	4.0	1.5	21.9	21.5	9.3
<39 weeks	17.3	7.7	11.0	10.2	3.0	3.1	1.4	38.7	39.0	22.2
<2500 gm and/or <37 weeks	8.9	12.0	14.3	16.0	4.6	3.6	2.2	30.8	26.0	17.8
<3000 gm and/or <39 weeks	28.6	7.3	8.9	14.8	3.8	2.7	2.8	60.4	52.2	53.3
Growth retarded	13.1	7.7	6.6	22.1	2.8	1.4	3.9	29.4	17.7	36.7

*) Based on 76,398 mothers in Norway who had their 1st and 2nd single births during the 7 year period, 1967–1973.

births. Exclusion of these mothers might have influenced the results, since these mothers are likely to differ to some extent from those mothers included in the analysis. For 2049 of these mothers, birth weight was known for both first and second births. LBW births were more common among these mothers, thus 9.1% had a LBW first birth compared to 5.9% of the mothers included in the analysis. However, the tendency of repeating a LBW birth seemed to be much the same among the two groups of mothers. Of the mothers excluded from the analysis, 17.2% had a LBW first birth and a LBW second birth, compared to 15.1% among the mothers included in the analysis. This indicates that excluding mothers of births with unknown birth weight and/or gestational age may have introduced only a limited amount of bias in the results of this analysis.

In order to avoid confounding effects of parity and to some extent age, this analysis has been limited to mothers having their first and second births. The measures of outcomes have been made for all single births, and have not been made separately for subgroups of deliveries such as spontaneous and non-spontaneous births.

The study has shown a substantial variation in the risk of subsequent LBW, preterm or growth retarded births between groups of mothers with different combinations of birth weight and gestational age of their first births.

Other studies have indicated that the risk of a subsequent LBW birth is 3-4 times for those mothers who have delivered a previous LBW birth compared to those who have not (Collaborative Perinatal Study, 1972; Habicht et al., 1974; Fedrick and Anderson, 1976; Kaltreider and Johnson; 1976). In this study the relative risk is found to be slightly higher (5.6). The overall risk of LBW, however, is far below that reported in these studies.

A high relative risk of repeating LBW births indicates that a large proportion of LBW births are produced by mothers who repeatedly give birth to LBW babies ("repeaters"). Thus, of the growth retarded second births included in this study, more than one-third were delivered by mothers whose first births were also growth retarded.

In a country like Norway, where the LBW rate is low, it might be that some of the environmental factors such as those associated with poverty (e.g., insufficient diet, poor health conditions and lack of medical care) affecting the greater part of the population of pregnant women have been reduced. It might be, however, that there exists a subgroup of women who for some "intrinsic" reason carry a high risk of LBW births, and as the risk of LBW in the majority of the population is being reduced, this would imply that the "high risk group" of mothers would contribute a relatively greater proportion of all LBW births. This could be one possible explanation for the relatively strong tendency of repeating LBW, preterm and growth retarded births shown in this study.

Information on repeated pregnancy outcomes to the same mothers represents a valuable basis for research. For example, mothers who tend to repeat events like LBW, preterm or growth retarded births can be compared to mothers who do not repeat such events. Studies of "repeaters" ought to be carried out in different populations, and such studies might provide some clues to causation.

SUMMARY

The study is based on births in Norway between 1967–1973. Information on births is provided by *Medical Registration of Birth*, covering all births (gestational age 16 weeks or more) within the country. Due to record linkage, it has become possible to study subsequent births to the same mothers.

This analysis is based on 76,398 mothers who had their first and second births (singletons only) during the seven-year period, and where birth weight and gestational age are known for both births.

Mothers are grouped according to birth weight and gestational age of their first births and the outcomes of their second births have been studied within each group. The following three outcomes were used: low birth weight (LBW), defined as 2500 gm. or less; preterm birth, defined as gestational age less than 37 weeks; and growth retardation, defined as below an operational definition of the 10th percentile of birth weight for known gestation.

Birth weight of first birth seems to be the most powerful predictor of LBW for the second birth. Gestational age of the first birth, on the other hand, seems to be a better predictor of preterm second birth. Growth retardation of the second birth seems to be most effectively predicted by growth retardation of the first birth. As the birth weight and gestational age of the first birth change from the most favorable to the least favorable combination, the risk of all three outcomes of second birth increases 20–30 times.

ACKNOWLEDGEMENTS

The author wishes to express his gratitude to Tor Bjerkedal and his staff at the Medical Birth Registry of Norway, Institute of Hygiene and Social Medicine, University of Bergen, for having made these data available for analysis. Daniel G. Seigel and Howard Hoffman have given valuable advice and assistance in the analysis of the data. Finally, the author wants to express gratitude to Ernest Harley for his skillful conduct of the computer programming of the data.

TEXT REFERENCES

Battaglia, F. C.; Lubchenko, L. O.: A Practical Classification Of Newborn Infants by Weight and Gestational Age. J Pediat 71(1967)159-163

Bjerkedal, T.; Bakketeig, L. S.: Medical Registration of Births in Norway, 1967-1968. Some Descriptive and Analytical Aspects. Univ. of Bergen, Bergen, Norway, 1972

Bjerkedal, T.; Bakketeig, L. S.: Medical Registration of Births in Norway During the 5-year Period, 1967-71, Univ of Bergen, Bergen, Norway, 1975

Bjerkedal, T.; Bakketeig, L. S.; Lehmann, E. H.: Percentiles of Birth Weights of Single, Livebirths at Different Gestation Periods, Based on 125485 Births in Norway, 1967 and 1968. Acta Paediat Scand 62(1973)449-457

Collaborative Perinatal Study of the National Institute of Neurological Diseases and Stroke: The Women and their Pregnancies. U.S. Dept. of Health, Education and Welfare, Public Health Service, Publ. no. (NIH) 73-379, Washington, D.C. 1972

Fedrick, J.; Anderson, A. B. M.: Factors Associated with Spontaneous Pre-term Birth. Brit J Obstet and Gynecol 83 (1976)342-350

Habicht, J. P. et al: Maternal Nutrition, Birthweight and Infant Mortality. In:

Ciba Foundation Symposium 27 (new series) Size of Birth. Amsterdam, Associated Scientific Publishers, 1974

Hoffman, H. J., Lundin, F. E. Jr., Bakketeig, L. S. and Harley, E. E.: Classification of Births by Weight and Gestational Age for Future Studies of Prematurity: Some Demographic and Statistical Perceptions Based on Bivariate Distribution. In: Epidemiology of Prematurity, ed. by D. M. Reed and F. J. Stanley. Urban and Schwarzenberg, Baltimore, 1977

Hoffman, H. J., Stark, C. R., Lundin, F. E. Jr. and Ashbrook, J. D. Analysis of Birthweight, Gestational Age, and Fetal Viability, U.S. Births, 1968, Obstet and Gynec Survey 29(1974)651-681

Kaltreider, D. F.; Johnson, J. W. C.: Patients at High Risk of Low Birth Weight Delivery. Am J Obstet Gynec 124 (1976)251-256

Karn, M. N. et al: Birthweight, Gestation Time and Survival in Sibs. Ann Eugen 15(1951)306-322

Ounsted, M.: Maternal Constraint on Foetal Growth in Man. Develop Med Child Neurol 7(1965)479-491

World Health Organization: Report on Methodology Related to Perinatal Events, 1974, (document ICD/74.4)

A Simple Model for the Interpretation of Low Birth Weight Repeater Data

Daniel G. Seigel, Sc.D.

Dr. Bakketeig[1] has demonstrated that women with low birth weight babies in their first pregnancy are at considerably greater risk of low birth weight in their second births than are women whose first babies were not low birth weight. This result is summarized in Table 1. The risks obtained are 0.152 and 0.027, respectively, with a relative risk of 5.6. Moreover, he has discussed the opportunities available for taking advantage of this statistic as a screening index for selecting women whose pregnancies are at high risk for low birth weight deliveries.

The data are also of interest insofar as they can be used to suggest the extent to which subgroups of women are diverse in the probability that their pregnancies terminate with a low birth weight baby. Table 1 provides no direct information on this, but can nevertheless be helpful to us in generating some estimates as to the extent of such diversity.

Table 2 postulates an extremely simple population model with two subgroups of women, one of which (group a) is at little risk of LBW in either pregnancy. The second group (b), amounting to 5% of the population, has a very sizable risk, fifteen times greater than group a in births one and two. The model provides for lower rates of low birth weight in the second birth for both groups, to reflect the 40% decrease in such rates in the Norwegian data.

---

[1] Preceding chapter.

Table 1.   Birth Weight of First and Second Births in Norwegian Data Set.

		Second Baby		
		LBW	Not LBW	
First Baby	LBW	.0090	.0504	.0594
	Not LBW	.0254	.9152	.9406
		.0344		

Probability of LBW in second pregnancy in women with LBW in first = .0090/.0594 = .152.

Probability of LBW in second pregnancy in women without LBW in first = .0254/ .9406 = .027.

Relative Risk = .152/.027 = 5.6.

Such a population would yield the four-fold table (Table 3) of low birth weight babies in first and second pregnancies. An example of how the entries in the cells are computed is provided at the bottom of Table 3. The primary assumption is that the risks in the two pregnancies are independent. The distribution of pairs of pregnancies in Tables 1 and 3 are nearly identical. That is, the model succeeds in reproducing the observed data, as all models strive to do.

Consider the distribution of risks required to reproduce the observed data. It was necessary to assume a high risk group with a probability of low birth weight in the first birth at approximately one-half and that this high risk group constitutes 5% of the population. It is impressive to note that this group's risk of low birth weight was fifteen times greater than that of the "normal" group.

I would hasten to add that the data in Table 1 are compatible with other models using other assumptions. Indeed, Table 5 also reproduces the Norwegian data, assuming this time a high risk group making up 15% of the population. To make this model fit the data, however, one has to assume that a relative risk of 20 prevails (Table 4). It is in fact possible to fit these data with these simple models using proportions of

Table 2.   A Simple Model With Two Risk Groups, to Reproduce Norwegian Data Set.

Population Group	Proportion In Population	Risk of LBW First Baby	Risk of LBW Second Baby
Low Risk (Group a)	.95	.035	.021
High Risk (Group b)	.05	.525	.315

Risk of LBW in Group b/Risk of LBW in Group a = 15.
Risk of LBW First Baby/Risk of LBW Second Baby = .6.

Table 3.   Distribution of LBW in First and Second Births for Population in Table 2.

		Second Baby		
		LBW	Not LBW	
First Baby	LBW	.0090	.0506	.0596
	Not LBW	.0268	.9138	.9406
		.0351		

Probability of LBW in second pregnancy in women with LBW in first = .0090/.0596 = .151.

Probability of LBW in second pregnancy in women without LBW in first = .0268/.9406 = .028.

Relative Risk = .151/.028 = 5.4.

Note: .0090 is calculated from Table 2a as .0090 = (.035) (.021) .95 + (.525) (.315) .05. Analogous calculations yield .0506, .0268, .9138.

high risk groups ranging from 0.02 to 0.20. To do so requires assuming the risk of low birth weight at these two ends of the range to be 0.82 and 0.28 respectively.

Both of the models in Tables 2 and 4 are almost undoubtedly false representations of the population. But then, this is true of virtually all models. These are patently false in that they postulate two risk groups— one high and one low—whereas the population is almost certainly distributed along a scale of risk that is more nearly continuous. It is unlikely, however, that analysis of a more elaborate model would alter the basic finding that the data in Table 1 imply a sizable proportion of the population of pregnant women to have extraordinary levels of risk which they carry to each of their pregnancies.

Dr. Bakketeig and I have, in a preliminary way, examined the question of whether known risk factors for low birth weight such as smoking, height and socioeconomic level could produce variation in the popula-

Table 4.   A Second Simple Model With Two Risk Groups, To Reproduce Norwegian Data Set.

		Risk of LBW	
Population Group	Proportion in Population	First Baby	Second Baby
Low Risk (Group a)	.85	.015	.009
High Risk (Group b)	.15	.300	.180

Risk of LBW in Group b/Risk of LBW in Group a = 20.
Risk of LBW First Baby/Risk of LBW Second Baby = .6.

Table 5.   Distribution of LBW in First and Second Births for Population in Table 4.

		Second Baby		
		LBW	Not LBW	
First Baby	LBW	.0082	.0495	.0577
	Not LBW	.0264	.9158	.9422
		.0346		

Probability of LBW in second pregnancy in women with LBW in first = .0082/.0577 = .14.

Probability of LBW in second pregnancy in women without LBW in first = .0264/.9422 = .028.

Relative Risk = .14/.028 = 5.

tion to an extent sufficient to explain the relative risk of five seen in Table 1. We concluded that such risk factors were not nearly sufficient to generate the observed tendency of repeating LBW. The implication, then, is that there are other major factors whose roles are not yet fully appreciated that play a major role in determining the risk of LBW. It strikes us that studies of "repeaters" to determine what such risk factors might be constitute a relatively unexplored research opportunity.

DISCUSSION

Dr. Stein: I wonder if in New York we could come up with results similar to the Norwegian data which Dr. Bakketeig presented. I am sure others have been struck by the difference in the range of birth weights within the socioeconomic status in Britain, compared to New York City, where the range is much wider between a good suburb and a bad suburb than it is right across Britain.

The Norwegian prematurity rate for first births was 5.9%; this would be much higher in Harlem, but not all that different in some of the middle class New York suburbs. In Norway the factors contributing to low birth weight might be thought to be immovable.

I was going to ask Dr. Bakketeig if he has available in his data set things like maternal weight, SES and smoking, and if so, wouldn't it be much better to use this information in the prediction?

Dr. Bakketeig: Unfortunately, we don't have information on smoking in our data set, and we don't have information on mother's height, prepregnancy weight and weight gain during pregnancy, and that is the reason for not being able to adjust for these factors directly.

Dr. Alberman: In the culture of spontaneous abortions, there are apparent differences in cell division rates, certainly between the chromosomally abnormal and the normal. I suspect there are families where actual cell division—and this is before nutrition comes into it—is inherently slow.

Saugstad (1972) showed that the siblings of phenylketonuric children have a higher birth weight than expected for controls, and suggested that heterozygotes had some genetic advantage which sped up their growth and birth weight. I think this may answer some of Dr. Seigel's points. There is an enormous area that we just dont't know anything about which obviously contributes. And Margaret Ounstead's work, too, has shown that there is a material repeatability of low birth weight from generation to generation, which I suspect may be the same sort of thing.

DISCUSSION REFERENCE

Saugstad, L. F.: Birth Weights in Children with Phenylketonuria and in their Siblings. Lancet 1(1972)809-813

Obstetric Factors Related to Prematurity

Kenneth R. Niswander, M.D.

There are many factors well recognized by the obstetrician which relate to, or perhaps predispose to, prematurity, but which are not specifically obstetric influences. I refer, for example, to social background of the patient, race of the patient and her parity, and these relationships and many others have been discussed already. There are, however, a number of factors of specific interest to the obstetrician and which can be identified as "obstetric" in nature. Many, perhaps most, are irremediable with present medical knowledge. This need not discourage the obstetrician, however, since the risk of perinatal mortality in the gravida with one of these diseases has been reduced and probably can be reduced further by applying currently available techniques for patient observation and care.

As I review these obstetric factors related to prematurity, you may notice from the language I use, if I am unable to hide it, our continuing confusion over the terms "low birth weight," "prematurity," and "intrauterine growth retardation." Most of the obstetric literature has related the obstetric factors in question to low birth weight, but the term usually used by authors to describe this outcome has been not low birth weight, but rather prematurity. Only in recent years have obstetric authors spoken of the birth weight/gestation relationship, and one of the major needs in this field of study is to categorize each of the obstetric factors I am going to list according to whether the disease is related to premature birth or to intrauterine growth retardation (IUGR). Does the factor precipitate premature labor? Does it interfere with intrauterine growth? Or does it operate in both ways? Where data are available on this matter, I have tried to bring them to your attention.

It is possible to divide the obstetric factors related to prematurity into five categories: 1) obstetric history; 2) cogenital malformations of the female reproductive tract; 3) medical disease during pregnancy; 4) diseases peculiar to pregnancy; and 5) iatrogenic disease and miscellaneous factors.

OBSTETRIC HISTORY

It is well known that a poor prior obstetric history, manifested by one of a number of bad outcomes, is related to a poor outcome in the present pregnancy (Niswander et al., 1971). On Table 1 we have illustrated this point using material from the Collaborative Perinatal Project (CPP) (Niswander et al., 1971). In this table, as in most of those which follow, the outcome we have illustrated is birth weight under 2501 gm., subsequently called low birth weight. Other adverse outcomes, such as fetal or neonatal death, frequently accompany this effect on birth weight, but since our topic is the epidemiology of prematurity, we have resisted the urge to proliferate tables. As an example, if the last prior child born of a white mother was living at the time of the present pregnancy, the risk of the pregnancy under study terminating in a low birth weight baby was only 6.6%. If the last prior pregnancy had ended in neonatal death, there was a 21.8% risk of a low birth weight infant in the present pregnancy. Similar trends are seen for black patients.

On Table 2 we have illustrated material which is more pertinent to our present discussion. If the birth weight of the last prior child was in the low birth weight range, there was a 24.8% incidence of low birth weight infants noted in the present pregnancy among white patients. In contrast,

Table 1.   Influence of Prior Perinatal or Infant Loss.

Survival State of Last Prior Child	Birth Weight of Study Child: Percentage under 2501 Gms.	
	White	Black
Fetal Death	9.5 (163)	15.6 (316)
Neonatal Death	21.8 (39)	30.5 (98)
Child Death	9.2 (10)	19.2 (28)
Living	6.6 (605)	11.2 (1189)

Source: Niswander et al., 1971.

Table 2. Influence of Prior Delivery of Low Birth Weight Infant.

Birth Weight of Last Prior Child	Birth Weight of Study Child: Percentage Under 2501 Grams	
	White	Black
Under 2501 gms.	24.8 (233)	31.2 (590)
Over 2500 gms.	5.8 (507)	8.9 (833)

Source: Niswander et al., 1971

if the birth weight of the last prior child was in the mature range, there was only a 5.8% risk of a low birth weight infant in the present pregnancy. Similar figures can be noted among blacks.

Kaltreider and Johnson (1976) have reported a similar experience from Baltimore, and their data are illustrated in Table 3. The greater the number of previous term deliveries, the lower the risk of a low birth weight infant in the present pregnancy. Similarly, the greater the number of previous low birth weight deliveries, the higher the risk of the occurrence of a low birth weight infant in the present pregnancy.

CONGENITAL MALFORMATIONS OF THE GENITAL TRACT

Congenital malformations of the genital tract clearly predispose to low birth weight. Blair (1960), for example, noted a low birth weight rate of 31.2% among 68 patients with a congenital malformation. That this is not a major contributor numerically to the frequency of low birth weight, however, is suggested by the fact that Blair noted congenital malformations in only 0.13% of his large population of gravidas. Zabriskie (1962) recorded 92 congenital abnormalities of the uterus among 29,539 deliveries, an incidence of 0.31%. The overall incidence of low birth weight among these patients was 30%.

Table 3. The Incidence of LBW Delivery According to Past Obstetric Performance.

Previous Term Deliveries	Previous LBW Deliveries			
	0	1	2	3 +
0	19.3	35.3	54.1	59.7
1	15.1	28.4	36.4	45.2
2	11.0	21.6	27.0	46.2
3	9.2	16.9	39.7	50.0
4 +	9.8	14.7	20.6	23.1

Source: Kaltreider and Johnson, 1976

Kaufman et al. (1977) have recently reported an interesting complication of *in utero* diethylstilbestrol (DES) exposure which is germane to our discussion. Among 60 young women exposed to DES *in utero*, 40 were found to have substantial changes in the uterus as documented by hysterosalpingogram. These changes consisted of a T-shaped appearance of the uterus, a hypoplastic uterus or one of a number of other less frequent abnormalities. The common demonimator of the various abnormalities noted was a decrease in size of the uterine cavity. Twelve of the patients had had prior pregnancies, and five of these were terminated intentionally while one was an ectopic pregnancy. Two women aborted spontaneously. Of the four women who had live births, the one term delivery occurred in a woman with a normal uterus. Of the three premature deliveries, two occurred in abnormal uteri. While the ultimate effect on reproduction of this fascinating new abnormality remains unknown, it could have an important numerical impact on the national prematurity rate.

MEDICAL DISEASE DURING PREGNANCY

Many nonobstetric diseases occurring during pregnancy have been related at one time or another to an increased incidence of low birth weight. In the CPP any disease of significance which was recognized during pregnancy was coded, and it is thus possible to report an incidence of low birth weight with each of a number of diseases (Niswander et al., 1971). A word of caution is necessary, however, before an etiologic relationship between a disease and low birth weight can be assumed. The form on which the medical diagnosis was entered was a "flagging" form, i.e., the medical editor was asked to record the disease even when the diagnosis had not been made with absolute certainty. Some overcoding must certainly have occurred, but such overdiagnosis may have minimized an apparent relationship rather than exaggerated it. Secondly, the tables which I am about to present are uncontrolled except for race. With these limitations in mind, you may be interested in the findings.

Pneumonia, diabetes mellitus, hypothyroidism and convulsions not due to eclampsia showed no relationship to the incidence of low birth weight (Table 4). Patients with bronchial asthma, hyperthyroidism, glomerulonephritis, genitourinary infection with a temperature of 100.4 °F or higher, alcoholism, drug habituation, appendicitis and organic heart disease experienced a higher than expected risk of delivery of a low birth weight infant.

What is perhaps more important than listing these relationships is to determine whether the diseases that were associated with low birth weight

Table 4.   Incidence of LBW with Maternal Disease.

Disease	White		Black	
	With	Without	With	Without
Pneumonia	104	71	140	133
Asthma	105	71	159	133
Diabetes	114	71	118	133
Hypothyroidism	70	72	183	133
Hyperthyroidism	244	71	281	133
Glomerulonephritis	267*	71	259	133
GU infect. T. 100.4	121	72	186	132
Convulsions (not eclamptic)	62	71	136	133
Alcoholism	375*	71	167	133
Drug habituation	187	71	294	133
Appendicitis	143	71	273*	134
Organic heart disease	176	70	189	133

* Rate based on less than 20 cases.

Source: Niswander et al., 1971.

were related to premature labor, to intrauterine growth retardation or to both. In the CPP asthmatic patients, Gordon et al. (1970) were unable to demonstrate intrauterine growth retardation. Similarly, when we simultaneously plotted the birth weight and gestational age of each baby born to a mother with organic heart disease on an appropriate graph based on the entire CPP population, we were unable to show delayed intrauterine growth in these patients (Niswander and Berendes, 1968). When the patients who suffered heart failure were analyzed separately, again no intrauterine growth retardation could be demonstrated. It should be noted, however, that this particular finding is not in accord with the findings of others. Barnes (1963), for example, noted delayed intrauterine growth in patients with congenital heart disease severe enough to cause polycythemia. We have no information regarding birth weight/gestational age relationships on any of the other diseases reported on Table 4.

DISEASES PECULIAR TO PREGNANCY

Certain diseases which may be labelled as exclusively obstetric have also been implicated as potential etiologic agents with low birth weight (Table 5). In the CPP data, neither hyperemesis gravidarum nor uterine dysfunction was associated with the likelihood of delivery of a low birth weight infant. A diagnosis of incompetent cervix was, as expected, associated with an extremely high incidence of low birth weight delivery. Vaginal bleeding

Table 5.   Incidence of LBW with OB/GYN Disease.

Disease	White		Black	
	With	Without	With	Without
Hyperemesis	67	72	118	134
Incompetent cervix	614	70	679	132
Vaginal bleeding				
First Trimester	95	60	156	123
Second Trimester	163	60	184	123
Third Trimester	98	60	155	123
Placenta previa	328	69	529	130
Abruptio placentae	263	67	477	129
Premature rupt.				
membranes (>48 hrs)	506	58	514	107

in any trimester related to a slight increase in low birth weight delivery. More will be said of these diseases shortly. The high rate of low birth weight delivery with premature rupture of the membranes of greater than 48 hours is at least partially due to the well-known clinical fact that the earlier in pregnancy that rupture of the membranes occurs, the more likely is the onset of labor to be delayed. It is unusual for a patient near term to experience rupture of the membranes without labor ensuing within 24 hours (Burchell, 1964). More will be said of this later. There is little epidemiologic information on any of these obstetric diseases. What information is available has helped little in elucidating etiologies.

Placenta Previa

The incidence of placenta previa increases with increasing parity (Record and McKeown, 1956), but increasing maternal age *per se* seems to have no similar effect. Repetition of the disease in the same patient has been noted. Hellman and Pritchard (1971) report that if a pregnancy is carried to viability in a patient who has experienced a previous placenta previa, the risk of a repeat placenta previa is about 6%, or about 12 times the expected incidence in their population. Although placenta accreta is a rare disease, it occurs more frequently in association with placenta previa than without placenta previa (Malkasian and Welch, 1964). This observation supports the theory that placenta previa may be due to defective vascularization of the decidua due to inflammation, atrophy or repeated pregnancies, thus necessitating a larger area of placental attachment.

We plotted the birth weight/gestational age of each of the white infants born following placenta previa on a birth weight/gestation age chart of the entire white population of CPP (Niswander, unpublished data). No evidence of intrauterine growth retardation was seen. Others have reported a similar absence of IUGR (Gabert, 1971).

Abruptio Placentae

Abruptio placentae is directly related to increasing parity but not to increasing maternal age (Hibbard and Jeffcoate, 1966). As with placenta previa, severe abruptio placentae has a recurrence rate of 11% compared to an initial incidence of less than 1%(Pritchard, 1970). Hibbard and Jeffcoate (1966) have reported that a woman who has twice experienced abruptio placentae incurs a 25% chance of experiencing the disease with her next pregnancy.

The relationship between abruptio placentae and preeclampsia or other hypertensive disease of pregnancy has been studied by innumerable investigators. The CPP data, for example, showed that abruptio placentae was about twice as common in toxemic patients as in non-toxemic patients (Niswander et al., 1966). Most investigators feel that there is little relationship between hypertensive disease and abruptio placentae unless the placental separation is extensive enough to kill the fetus. In this case, 40% of the abruptions are complicated by hypertension (Pritchard, 1970). Hellman and Pritchard (1971) say that "we cannot conclude that chronic hypertension or preeclampsia plays a significant role in abruptio placentae."

Hibbard and Jeffcoate (1966) reported that the predisposing factor in 97.5% of patients with abruptio placentae is defective folate metabolism. Other authors have been unable to corroborate any relationship whatsoever between abruptio placentae and folic acid metabolism (Whalley, Scott and Pritchard, 1969). Trauma to the mother's abdomen accounts for about 1% of cases of abruptio placentae (Pritchard, 1970). Obstruction of the vena cava has irregularly produced abruptio placentae (Mengert et al., 1953).

As with placenta previa, when the CPP data on white infants born following abruptio placentae were plotted on a birth weight/gestational age graph of the entire CPP white population, no evidence of intrauterine growth retardation was uncovered (Niswander, unpublished data). Apparently abruptio placentae is associated with premature labor, not with IUGR.

Multiple Pregnancy

Multiple pregnancy is another cause for low birth weight delivery. The mechanism for this relationship may be similar to that theorized for patients with congenital abnormalities of the uterus, i.e., the uterus can enlarge only to a certain point. McKeown and Record (1952) in 23,000 births listed the mean birth weight of singleton, doubleton, triplet and quadruplet fetuses (Table 6). They also reported mean pregnancy durations for each of these types of pregnancies. It is evident from their data that fetal growth is indeed retarded in multiple pregnancy and that this occurs during the last weeks of gestation. They reported that up to 27 weeks, the mean fetal weight seemed independent of the litter size. Furthermore, their data suggested that the increment in the mean weight of the entire litter from the time that fetal growth is retarded is about the same for every litter size. They felt that these facts suggest that the restriction on the litter size is probably a function of uterine crowding.

Premature Rupture of the Membranes

Premature rupture of the membranes has had various definitions attached to it, but by whatever standard, premature rupture clearly is directly associated with an increased risk of low birth weight. Burchell (1964), for example, made the diagnosis when labor did not ensue within one hour following rupture. In his series, 23% of cases resulted in a low birth weight delivery, while only 12.9% of his entire obstetric population was similarly affected. Taylor et al.(1961) diagnosed premature rupture of the membranes when more than 12 hours ensued between rupture and the onset of labor. These authors reported that 32.6% of the population was delivered of a low birth weight infant compared to a 13% incidence among the entire obstetric population.

The cause of the "accident" remains obscure. A number of authors have suggested a socioeconomic factor, and this is illustrated by a report from New York Medical College that 6.3% of ward deliveries were complicated by premature rupture of the membranes while only 2% of private deliveries were so complicated (Gordon and Weingold, 1974). Russell and Cheung (1974) reported a number of conditions which contribute to premature rupture of the membranes (multiple pregnancy, hydramnios, vaginal infections, incompetent cervix, placenta previa, breech presentation, genetic abnormality and amnionitis), but they did not provide bibliographic support for this statement. Most authorities simply say that the etiology of premature rupture of the membranes is unknown

Table 6.   Multiple pregnancy.

	Singleton	Twins	Triplets	Quadruplets
Mean Birth Weight (lbs.)	7.43	5.27	4.00	3.07
Pregnancy Duration (days)	280.5	261.6	246.8	236.8

Source: McKeown and Record, 1952.

(Douglas and Stromme, 1976). Danforth, McElin and States (1970) studied the tensile strength of the membranes to determine if there might be a local cause for the premature rupture. These authors concluded that premature rupture of the membranes is not due to any inherent weakness of the membranes as evidenced by bursting strength. They further stated that membranes are apparently constructed to withstand pressures which exceed those of normal labor.

There is an especially strong association between premature rupture of the membranes of greater than 48 hours and increased incidence of low birth weight as demonstrated by the CPP data. All that can be concluded from these data, however, is that if rupture of the membranes occurs well before term gestation is reached, a much longer delay before the onset of labor is experienced by the gravida.

Hypertensive Disease of Pregnancy

There are some interesting new data culled from the CPP data by Friedman and Neff on hypertensive disease of pregnancy and its relationship to low birth weight delivery. The data I will present are from a book by these men (Friedman and Neff, 1977), and I am grateful to Dr. Friedman for allowing me to extract material from that book for our purposes.

That hypertensive disease of pregnancy is related to low birth weight delivery and to an increase in perinatal mortality is unquestioned. Determination of the degree to which this relationship extends, however, has been hampered by confusion over the criteria necessary to make the diagnosis of hypertensive disease of pregnancy. Friedman and Neff (1977) have chosen a logical approach to the diagnosis by determining the level of diastolic blood pressure and the level of proteinuria above which bad fetal outcomes result. Blood pressure and/or proteinuria above these levels thus, by definition, constitute "disease." In the data we are presenting, we will note the effect of various levels of diastolic blood pressure and various degrees of proteinuria on fetal outcomes.

In Table 7, it is evident that a diastolic blood pressure of 85 mm Hg or greater is associated with an increased incidence of low birth weight delivery. For example, if the high diastolic pressure was recorded in the gestational interval of 28-32 weeks, the risk of low birth weight delivery was between 10-11% and only 8½% with a lower diastolic pressure. Similar differences are noted in other epochal weeks. A relationship of similar magnitude with proteinuria is illustrated in Table 8. If no proteinuria was noted between 28-32 weeks, the incidence of low birth weight delivery was between 8-9%. If the proteinuria was 3+ or 4+, almost a third of the infants experienced low birth weight.

Dr. Friedman pursued the problem further, however, since he wished to learn whether the observed low birth weight was due to premature

Table 7.   Incidence of LBW by Diastolic BP.

Epochal Weeks	Diastolic BP Grouping (mm Hg)		
	75 – 84	85 +	Total
28–32	84	106*	88
33–34	71	102*	74
35–36	57	90*	62
37–38	42	67*	48
39–41	25	40	34

*Significant (P < 0.01).
Source: Adapted from Friedman and Neff, 1977.

Table 8.   Incidence of LBW by Proteinuria.

Epochal Weeks	Proteinuria		
	None	1 +	3 + and 4 +
28–32	87	106	304 *
33–34	73	109	283 *
35–36	61	87	203 *
37–38	49	63	141 *
39–41	34	37	85 *

*Significant (P < 0.01).
Source: Adapted from Friedman and Neff, 1977.

Table 9.   Fetal Mortality by Diastolic BP.

Epochal Weeks	Diastolic BP Grouping (mm Hg)		
	75 – 84	85 +	Total
28–32	9.4	21.2*	9.0
33–34	8.2	19.3*	7.7
35–36	6.4	16.6*	6.6
37–38	5.4	9.0*	5.4
39–41	5.0	9.0*	5.1

*Significant (P < 0.01)
Source: Adapted from Friedman and Neff. 1977.

Table 10.   Neonatal Mortality by Diastolic BP.

	Diastolic BP Grouping (mm Hg)		
Epochal Weeks	75 – 84	85 +	Total
28–32	8.2	11.6	8.2
33–34	7.1	5.1	6.3
35–36	4.5	10.9*	5.8
37–38	5.1	6.7	5.4
39–41	4.0	8.6*	4.9

*Significant (P < 0.01).
Source: Adapted from Friedman and Neff, 1977.

delivery or to delayed intrauterine growth. He wished to learn as much as possible about the mechanism by which hypertensive disease exerts its ill effects on the fetus. That the disease increases the perinatal mortality is well known and is illustrated in the CPP material by the next two tables. A diastolic blood pressure of 85 mm Hg or greater was associated with a fetal mortality about two-fold higher than with a lower diastolic blood pressure grouping (Table 9). The neonatal mortality was also higher with diastolic hypertension, but to a smaller degree (Table 10).

Dr. Friedman studied the risk of delivery of a small-for-gestational-age (SGA) infant with various blood pressure and proteinuria recordings. The SGA infant was defined as that infant falling below the fifth percentile on the birth weight/gestational age curve developed for the CPP population by race. As Table 11 demonstrates, an increase in diastolic blood pressure was associated with an increased risk of delivery of an SGA infant. Similarly, increasing proteinuria was directly related to an increased risk of IUGR. When both factors were present, the risk was greater than the sum of the risks of each individual factor. There seems no question then that hypertensive disease of pregnancy is related to IUGR.

Table 11.   Risk of SGA for Proteinuria: Diastolic BP Combinations.

Diastolic BP (mm Hg)	Proteinuria maxima			
	None	1 +	3 +	4 +
75–84	3.8	3.8	3.4	—
85–94	4.6	4.9	15.6*	—
95–104	6.8*	8.7*	15.6*	42.9*
105 +	6.5	18.6	37.6*	27.7*

*Significant (P < 0.01).
Source: Adapted from Friedman and Neff, 1977.

Table 12.   Frequency of Perinatal Death as Related to SGA.

	Percentage	
Outcome	Normal	SGA
Fetal death	0.68	8.57*
Neonatal death	0.79	3.37*

*Significant (P < 0.01).
Source: Adapted from Friedman and Neff, 1977.

What remained to be shown was, first, whether IUGR is associated with an increased perinatal mortality risk and, secondly, whether the increase in perinatal mortality associated with hypertensive disease is due to IUGR. Tables 12 and 13 well illustrate the enormously higher perinatal death rates associated with SGA infants when compared to those without growth retardation. This is especially noticeable among fetal deaths. In Table 14, similarly high perinatal death rates are noted among SGA babies for each level of diastolic blood pressure. You will note the marked increase in fetal death rates as higher diastolic blood pressure readings are recorded. Little change in neonatal death rates is observed with higher diastolic blood pressure readings.

Dr. Friedman concluded that the deleterious effect of high diastolic blood pressure and proteinuria on the fetus is exerted primarily through an effect on fetal growth. This is an important new finding and may in the future help us reduce the fetal death rate with hypertensive disease of pregnancy. Unfortunately, methods of determining fetal size clinically are currently neither inexpensive nor universally available. Moreover, many inaccuracies continue to be reported in determining fetal size by these methods (Thompson, 1974).

Table 13.   Perinatal Death Rates Associated with SGA.

Delivery	Percentage			
	Fetal		Neonatal	
Epochal Weeks	Non SGA	SGA	Non SGA	SGA
28–32	6.4	36.8*	10.8	36.8
33–34	2.0	37.9*	2.0	17.2
35–36	1.6	32.5*	1.1	8.4*
37–38	0.7	11.3*	0.7	4.2*
39–41	0.3	3.3*	0.4	1.2

*Significant (P < 0.01).
Source: Adapted from Friedman and Neff, 1977.

Table 14.   Perinatal Deaths With SGA Related to Diastolic BP Maxima.

Diastolic BP (mm Hg)	Percentage			
	Fetal		Neonatal	
	Non SGA	SGA	Non SGA	SGA
75–84	0.5	5.8 *	0.7	3.4 *
85–94	0.6	9.7 *	0.6	4.9 *
95–104	1.4	16.0 *	0.3	—
105 +	1.6	19.0 *	0.5	3.2

Significant (P < 0.01).
Source: Adapted from Friedman and Neff, 1977.

Dr. Friedman divided his population of gravida with hypertension and/or proteinuria into various groupings (Table 15). We have discussed two of these groupings—those with diastolic hypertension only, and those with a combination of diastolic hypertension and proteinuria. Dr. Friedman searched for positive predictors of the likelihood of development of hypertension and/or proteinuria. Table 16 illustrates the results of this study. Among white patients with diastolic hypertension only, the gravida is likely to be a nullipara of advanced age with heavy prepregnancy weight. She is liable to be a nonsmoker and to have either a urinary tract infection or a neurologic or psychiatric disorder. The strongest factors useful in predicting diastolic hypertension are nulliparity and heavy prepregnancy weight. The black gravida also tends to be a heavy, elderly nullipara.

Combined hypertension and proteninuria has a tendency to develop in single white gravidas who are elderly and heavy in body weight. They have often had several prior pregnancy losses. Diabetes mellitus is an especially strong predictor among these women, along with obesity. Vaginitis is also common among such patients. Similarly, many have demonstrated

Table 15.   Classification of Hypertensive Disease of Pregnancy.

Group I	Gravidas presenting with the single factor of diastolic blood pressure elevation of 95 mm Hg or greater.
Group II	Gravidas shown to possess synergistic combinations of diastolic blood pressure elevation and proteinuria, with diastolic pressures of 85 mm Hg or greater, together with proteinuria of 1 + or greater.
Group III	Gravidas presenting with proteinuria of 2 + or greater without diastolic blood pressure elevation.

Source: Adapted from Friedman and Neff, 1977.

Table 16.   Profiles of Gravidad Likely to Develop Hypertensive Disease of Pregnancy.

	WHITE	BLACK
Diastolic Hypertension (> 95 mm Hg)	Nulliparous * Older Obese * Nonsmoker Neuro-psychiatric disorder Genitourinary infection	Nulliparous Older * Obese * Thyroid surgery
Diastolic Hypertension (> 85 mm Hg) and Proteinuria (> 1 +)	Older Poor obstetrical history Obese * Single Diabetes * Glomerulonephritis Vaginitis * Hepatitis	Nulliparous* Older Obese* Genitourinary infection Hydramnios Neuro-psychiatric disorder

* Especially strong predictive factor.
(Source: Adapted from Friedman and Neff, 1977).

glomerulonephritis and/or hepatitis in the course of the index pregnancy. The black gravida who develops this disorder is often an obese nullipara of advanced years. The black woman who develops genitourinary infection, a neurologic or psychiatric disorder, or hydramnios is also at risk in this regard.

Dr. Friedman suggests, and I agree, that this list of predictive factors is of little clinical use at the present time. It is included in today's presentation to demonstrate the type of data that can be collected when studying obstetric factors leading to prematurity.

IATROGENIC AND MISCELLANEOUS CAUSES

A listing of obstetric causes of low birth weight would be incomplete without including certain iatrogenic causes, notably repeat elective cesarean section and elective induction of labor. We should not include either cesarean section or induction of labor performed for indication in our discussion, since here it is the underlying disease that demands premature labor or delivery.

Diddle, Gibbs and Lambeth (1959) reported a prematurity incidence of about 10% with repeat cesarean section. This report reflected the general experience of that era. Recent advances in diagnostic techniques, notably determination of the lecithin/sphyngomyelin ratio of the amniotic fluid, have substantially reduced the risk of delivery of a low birth weight infant with elective cesarean section.

With proper patient selection, there should be no low birth weight infants among electively induced patients, yet the literature reports incidences of low birth rate varying from 1.8% to 3.5% (Niswander, 1969). That this error in judgement is not innocuous is supported by the fact that in our personal series of 2862 elective inductions, we experienced 15 perinatal deaths among 100 low birth weight babies. Fortunately, the recent advances in diagnostic techniques mentioned above for determining fetal birth weight and maturity have greatly reduced, if not eliminated, this cause for low birth weight.

A final factor of unknown importance in the etiology of premature labor is maternal orgasm during late pregnancy. Goodlin, Keiler and Raffin (1971) reported that the incidence of maternal orgasm after 32 weeks of pregnancy was significantly higher in patients who subsequently delivered prematurely than in those who delivered at term. These authors think that it is the orgasm *per se* which induced uterine contractions rather than the possible effect of prostaglandins contained in semen. How important this factor will prove to be in the initiation of premature labor remains uncertain.

SUMMARY AND CONCLUSIONS

We have discussed the obstetric causes of prematurity under five headings: 1) obstetrical history; 2) congenital uterine abnormalities; 3) medical disease complicating pregnancy; 4) diseases peculiar to pregnancy; and 5) iatrogenic and miscellaneous causes.

A major shortcoming of the obstetric literature is the infrequency with which each of the various obstetric causes of prematurity is identified with premature labor, low birth weight or intrauterine growth retardation. By what mechanism does each obstetric cause of prematurity act? We have illustrated an approach to this problem in the case of hypertensive disease of pregnancy. A recent publication showed that the primary pathway in the etiology of fetal death in the hypertensive gravida is through delayed intrauterine growth. A plea is made for similar work on other obstetric causes of prematurity.

TEXT REFERENCES

Barnes, A.: Discussion of paper by D. Cannell and C. Vernon, Congenital Heart Disease and Pregnancy. Am J Obstet Gynec 85(1963)749

Blair, R.: Pregnancy Associated with Congenital Malformations of the Reproductive Tract. J Obstet Gynaecol Br Emp 67(1960)36

Burchell, R.: Premature Spontaneous Rupture of the Membranes. Am J Obstet Gynec 88(1964)251

Danforth, D.; McElin, T.; States, N.: Bursting Tension of Fetal Membranes. Am J Obstet Gynec 65(1970)480

Diddle, A.; Gibbs, V.; Lambeth, S.: Fetal Mortality and Prematurity with Repeat Abdominal Delivery. Am J Obstet Gynec 77(1959)719

Douglas, R.; Stromme, W.: Operative Obstetrics, 3rd ed. Appleton-Century-Crofts, N.Y., 1976

Friedman, E.; Neff, R.: Pregnancy Hypertension: A Systematic Evaluation of Clinical Diagnostic Criteria. Publishing Sciences Group, Acton, Mass., 1977

Gabert, H.: Placenta Previa and Fetal Growth. Obstet Gynec 38(1971)403

Goodlin, R.; Keller, D.; Raffin, M.: Orgasm During Late Pregnancy. Obstet Gynec 38 (1971)916

Gordon, M.; Niswander, K.; Berendes, H.; Kantor, A.: Fetal Morbidity Following Potentially Anoxigenic Obstetric Conditions. Am J Obstet Gynec 106(1970)421

Gordon, M.; Weingold, A.: Premature rupture of the membrane—a rational approach to management. In: Controversy in Obstetrics and Gynecology II, ed. by D. Reid, and C. Christian. W. B. Saunders, Philadelphia, 1974

Hellman, L.; Pritchard, J.: Williams' Obstetrics, 14th ed. Appleton-Century-Crofts, N. Y., 1971

Hibbard, B.; Jeffcoate, T.: Abruptio Placentae. Obstet Gynec 27(1966)155

Kaltreider, B.; Johnson, J.: Patients at High Risk for Low-Birth-Weight Delivery. Am J Obstet Gynec 124(1976)251

Kaufman, R.; Binder, G.; Gray, P.; Adam, E.: Upper Genital Tract Changes Associated with In Utero Exposure to Diethylstilbestrol. Am J Obstet Gynec (1977)

Malkasian, G.; Welch, J.: Placenta Previa Percreta Obstet Gynec 24(1964)298

McKeown, T.; T.; Record, R.: Observations on Foetal Growth in Multiple Pregnancies in Man. J Endocrin 8(1952)386

Mengert, W.; Goodson, J.; Campbell, R.; Haynes, D.: Observations on the Pathogenesis of Premature Separation of the Normally Implanted Placenta. Am J Obstet Gynec 66(1953)1104

Niswander, K.; Berendes, H.: Effect of Maternal Cardiac Disease on the Infant. Clin Obstet Gynec 11(1968)1026

Niswander, K.: The value and danger in the conservative management of placenta previa. In: Controversy in Obstetrics and Gynecology, II, ed. by D. Reid and C. Christian. Saunders, Philadelphia, 1969

Niswander, K.; Friedman, E.; Hoover, D.; Pietrowski, H.; Westphal, M.: Fetal Morbidity Following Potentially Anoxigenic Obstetric Conditions. Am J Obstet Gynec 95(1966)838

Niswander, K.; Gordon, M.; et al: The Women and their Pregnancies. Saunders, Philadelphia, 1971

Pritchard, J.: Genesis of Severe Placental Abruption. Am J Obstet Gynec 108 (1970)22

Record, R.; McKeown, T.: Investigation of Foetal Mortality Associated with Placenta Praevia. Brit J Prev Soc Med 10(1956)25

Russell, K.; Cheung, J.: The management of premature rupture of the fetal membrane—a continuing controversy. In: Controversy in Obstetrics and Gynecology II, ed. by D. Reid, and C. Christain. Saunders, Philadelphia, 1974

Taylor, E.; Morton, R.; Bruns, P.; Drose, V.: Spontaneous Premature Rupture of the Fetal Membranes. Am J Obstet Gynec 82(1961)1341

Thompson, H.: Evaluation of the Obstetric and Gynecologic Patient by the Use of Diagnostic Ultrasound. Clin Obstet Gynec 17(1974)1

Whalley, P.; Scott, V.; Pritchard, J.: Maternal Folate Deficiency and Pregnancy Wastage. Am J Obstet Gynec 105(1969) 670

Zabriskie, E.: Pregnancy and the Malformed Uterus—Report of 92 Cases. West J Surg Obstet Gynec 70(1962)293

DISCUSSION

Dr. Janerich: With Dr. Niswander's report on DES, we have an example whereby an environmental agent operates not in the generation exposed and not in the next generation, but in the third generation. To what extent this kind of environmental factor might explain some of the familiar contributions to low birth weight has to be considered. I think that we also have to consider not only environmental factors such as drugs or other environmental toxins, but the possibility of maternal disease such as preeclamptic states which might also be in some way determined to be a recurrence or a familiar tendency for birth weight to cluster in these families.

Dr. Stanley: What was the frequency of taking DES by US women?

Dr. Berendes: It has been estimated that from one to two million pregnant women may have been exposed to DES. Use was most frequent during the late 1940s and 1950s and less frequent during the 1960s. We are currently conducting a study which involves the tracing and evaluation of about 2000 young men and women who were exposed to DES *in utero* as a part of a controlled clinical trial of the efficacy of DES conducted in Chicago from 1951 to 1953 (Dieckmann et al., 1953; Gill, Schumacher and Bibbo, 1976). The preliminary results show no pronounced effect on subsequent progeny (Bibbo et al., 1977). There is, however, an effect on the male offspring which may have consequences for subsequent fertility.

Dr. Susser: There is, however, a confounding factor. One should be concerned that DES is given for problems of reproduction in the first instance. With vaginal carcinoma, such a bias would not matter. It is important to control for the existence of the antecedent of reproductive disorder for which DES was given.

Dr. Berendes: This bias, however, does not operate in the study which we are involved in. The controlled clinical trial of the efficacy of DES in preventing perinatal loss and morbidity involved normal middle class pregnant women who were included into the study early in pregnancy, at the time of registration for prenatal care. They were randomly assigned to DES treatment or placebo group and retained in these groups until delivery.

Dr. Reed: If we added up the total burden of low birth weight and pre-term delivery, could you give us an estimate of what proportion of this group would be due to complications of pregnancy and delivery?

Dr. Niswander: Something less than 1% of pregnancies are complicated by abruption, 1% by placenta previa and the risk of low birth weight in each of those is about 40%. Thus there is a low birth weight rate of about 1% due to those two factors alone. Hypertensive disease—acute and chronic—accounts for perhaps another 0.5%. That would account for one-sixth or one-seventh of low birth infants just from those three factors alone.

Dr. Stanley: I don't think it is helpful to lump low birth weight and pre-term deliveries together. Probably the important obstetric factors in each are going to be different.

Dr. Emanuel: I would like to ask Dr. Niswander what role induction may play in prematurity. Dr. Alberman pointed out that the data on birth weights of the induced babies in *British Births 1970* (Chamberlain et. al., 1975) were those for whom gestational duration was certain, and there are as yet no data on the 19% of induced babies whose gestational age was not certain. Induction is another possible obstetric cause of pre-maturity.

Dr. Niswander: There is no doubt that elective induction of labor has in the past exerted a substantial impact on the low birth weight inci-dence, in this country at least. Obstetricians have finally become aware of this and, at least in good medical centers, methods are now being used to determine fetal maturity before the induction is done. So I doubt if it is going to be a very large contributing factor in the next five years.

Dr. Stein: I want to ask Dr. Niswander if prenatal care reduces the consequences for the fetus and for the mother of preeclamptic toxemia, because you showed us quite convincingly the association of diastolic blood pressure and proteinuria in prematurity. What role does prenatal care play in reducing preeclamptic toxemia?

Dr. Niswander: Dr. Baird can perhaps answer that better than I.

Dr. Baird: The perinatal mortality rate from preeclampsia (for practical purposes, a disease of first pregnancies) in the city of Aberdeen was unchanged at about 5 per 1000 births from 1948 to 1964. In that year (1964) a number of changes occurred which started a decline in the death rate to 2.2 per 1000 by 1969. They were 1) a substantial increase in the incidence of induction of labor, 2) steady improvements in the techniques of assessing fetal well being *in utero*, 3) more liberal use of cesarean section, primarily for fetal indications, and 4) the use of chlormethiazole as an anticonvulsant in labor in place of sedative drugs which had a depressant effect on the baby. The primigravida's aged 25-29 and 30-34 in 1958-64 were born between 1929 and 1939 and between 1924 and 1930 respectively, when the economic depression was at its worst. By 1965 onwards these women were replaced by a younger and healthier cohort of primigravida. The induction policy was changed in 1964 because safer and more efficient methods of induction of labor became available. The fact that a fall in the perinatal mortality rate occurred in the same years in other centers in Scotland points to the importance of the improved standnard of health of primigravida and their youth and the fact that the undernourished and elderly primigravida of the previous generation had by this time had their first child (Scottish Health Bulletin, in press).

Dr. Niswander: In terms of recent developments in prenatal care, we have "discovered" two methods of evaluating fetal condition that we have felt were distinctly going to reduce the perinatal mortality rate. One was the appearance of such tests as urinary estriol, and the other was fetal heart rate monitoring. Obstetric care has become extremely complex, primarily because of the availability of these two tests. Now we hear that two very good double-blind controlled studies suggest that neither evaluative tool has any measurable effect on the perinatal mortality rate whatsoever (Duenhoelter, Whalley and MacDonald, 1976; Haverkamp et al., 1976).

DISCUSSION REFERENCES

Bibbo, M.; Gill, W. B.; Azizi, F.; Blough, R.; Fang, V. S.; Rosenfield, R. L.; Schumacher, G. F. B.; Sleeper, K.; Sonek, M. G.; Wied, G.L.: Follow-up Study of Male and Female Offspring of DES-Exposed Mothers. Obstet and Gynec 49(1977)1

Chamberlain, R.; Chamberlain, G.; Howlett, B.; Claireaux, A.: Bristish Births 1970 . Volume I: The First Week of Life. A survey under the Joint Auspices of the National Birthday Trust Fund and the Royal College of Obstetricians and Gynecologists. William Heinemann Medical Books, London, 1975

Dieckmann, W. J.; Davis, M. E.; Rynkiewicz, L. M.; Pottinger, R. E.: Does the Administration of Diethylstibesterol During Pregnancy Have Therapeutic Value? Am J Obstet Gynec 66(1953)1062-1075

Duenhoelter, J.; Whalley, P.; MacDonald, P.: An Analysis of the Utility of Plasma Immunoreactive Estrogen Measurements in Determining Delivery Time of Gravidas with a Fetus Considered at High Risk. Am J Obstet Gynec 125(1976)889

Gill, W. B.; Schumacher, G. F. B.; Bibbo, M.: Structural and Functional Abnormalities in the Sex Organs of Male Offspring of Mothers Treated with Diethylstilbesterol (DES). J Reprod Med 16 (1976)147-153

Haverkamp, A.; Thompson, H.; McFee, J.;
    Cetrulo, C.: The Evaluation of Continuous
    Fetal Heart Rate Monitoring in High-Risk
    Pregnancy. Am J Obstet Gynec 125
    (1976)310

Scottish Health Bulletin (1977) In press

Medical Care of the Fetus and the Risk of Prematurity

Fiona J. Stanley, M.B., B.S., M.Sc., M.F.C.M.

INTRODUCTION

This workshop has amply documented the considerable amount of knowledge of the significance of the antenatal environment on birth weight. I will address myself to the question of whether prenatal care affects the percentage of infants born who are low birth weight. The function of prenatal care is often no more than educational and selective. In a majority of cases prenatal care consists of little more than a routine screening for the early detection of preeclampsia, multiple pregnancy and other complications, following an initial appraisal of the likelihood of hazards associated with delivery.

Potentially, however, if the knowledge was available, prenatal care is the vehicle through which women at high risk of delivering either preterm or other low birth weight infants will be identified and intervention and prevention perhaps carried out. However, at the moment, the evidence of prenatal care having an effect on these two outcomes is not at all clear. If an association of prenatal care with outcome is observed, e.g., improved mortality, lowered incidence or severity of complications of pregnancy, etc., it is certainly most difficult to sort out whether prenatal care is the important factor or if other factors associated with the mother are the significant variables.

The effects of prenatal care on low birth weight are difficult to evaluate; the many social and biological factors which have already been discussed at this workshop tend to dominate any effect of prenatal care. Because prenatal care is rarely defined or separated into its various components, it is also impossible to tell from recent studies which of these components may be responsible for the beneficial effects which have been reported. Many of the factors which affect birth weight, as I have mentioned, may in the future be delivered through prenatal care, and it is important to know what an individual procedure is achieving.

The majority of the studies which I have reviewed for this paper do not define prenatal care at all, and this is important. In a developing country or poor urban environment of a developed country where general nutrition, health and hygiene may be poor, prenatal care programs which provide nutritional supplements, health education, etc. may be more effective in reducing the low birth weight rate than the routine taking of blood pressure and recording of maternal weight. The studies reviewed here have all used either the week or month of the first prenatal visit or the total number of prenatal visits as an index of care, which has then been related to the level of prematurity. Prematurity has usually been defined in the "old" way as any birth under 2500 gm., irrespective of the gestational age, ignoring the fact that some babies under this weight can be term, some over this weight can be preterm, and the causes of their low birth weight may be different.

Therefore, in investigating the effect of prenatal care on either low birth weight or mortality associated with low birth weight, allowance should be made for many other factors which are probably more important than prenatal care.

In Table 1, I have listed some factors which are associated both with low birth weight and with either decreased or increased prenatal care attendance. In order to determine the difference in low birth weight or

Table 1.   Factors Associated With Low Birth Weight and Prenatal Care Attendance (No. of Visits and Week of First Visit.)

Prenatal Care Attendance	
Decreased	Increased
Low gestational age at delivery	Maternal disease
Low social class—small stature	Pregnancy complications
—poor weight gain	Poor previous obstetric history
—illegitimacy	(previous low birth weight, etc.)
—smoking	
High parity	
Maternal age ($<$20 years, $>$40 years)	

preterm rates of mothers with and without prenatal care, the two groups should be comparable with regard to at least those other factors which influence the occurrence of low birth weight.

GESTATIONAL AGE

The length of the pregnancy is probably the most important factor, especially if the total number of prenatal visits is being used as the index of prenatal care. Women who deliver at 34 weeks or sooner are obviously far less likely to attend prenatal care as often as women who deliver at 40 weeks. They are also more likely to have a fetal death, or a live birth dying in the neonatal period, hence at least part of the association of prenatal care and mortality if the effect of gestational age is not considered. This is shown in Table 2, taken from the 1958 British Mortality Survey (Butler and Bonham, 1963). Figure 1 shows a similar relationship for infants of very low birth weight in a study which I undertook in southeast London in 1975 (Stanley, 1976). This relationship of mortality and prenatal care disappears when allowance is made for gestational age, as was shown by Dr. Placek yesterday in his paper on the NCHS Natality Survey Data. There was no relationship of prenatal care and mortality when gestational age was included.

Studies which allow for the shorter gestational age of premature infants have done so using simple but elegant techniques. Terris and

Table 2. Distribution of Population and Deaths by Number of Prenatal Visits With Mortality Ratio.

Number of Prenatal Visits	Population		Deaths		Mortality Ratio
	No.	%	No.	%	
None	100	0.6	225	3.2	502
1	77	0.4	132	1.9	409
2	144	0.8	228	3.2	378
3–4	571	3.4	754	10.6	315
5–9	4853	28.6	2570	36.1	126
10–14	6830	40.2	1917	26.9	67
15–19	2812	16.5	682	9.6	58
20–24	905	5.3	219	3.1	58
25–29	266	1.6	87	1.2	78
≥ 30	170	1.0	87	1.2	122
No Information	266	1.6	216	3.0	199
Total	16994	100.0	7117	100.0	100

Source: Butler and Bonham, 1963

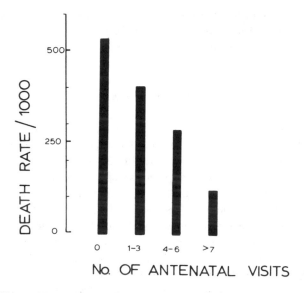

Figure 1.   **Neonatal Death Rates by Number of Antenatal Visits.**   Source: Stanley, 1976.

Gold (1969) calculated an expected number of prenatal visits for both the premature and control groups in their study if they had both followed the recommended schedule at the hospital where the study was undertaken. The ratios of observed to expected visits were 43% and 46% for the premature and control groups respectively, and this is not significantly different. The infants were matched by sex, birth order, race, social class, maternal age and marital status. They also showed no difference in the time of the first prenatal visit between premature and mature controls, as shown in Table 3.

Schwartz and Vineyard (1965), and Terris and Glasser (1974), used modified life table analysis to allow for the effect of gestational age. The

Table 3.   Week of Pregnancy at the Time of First Prenatal Visit.

Week of Pregnancy	PREMATURE		CONTROL	
	No.	%	No.	%
< 13	9	4.7	8	4.1
13–20	45	23.3	39	20.2
21–28	86	44.6	84	43.5
≥ 29	47	24.4	59	30.6
No Visits	6	3.1	3	1.6
Total	193	100.1	193	100.0

Source: Terris and Gold, 1969

Table 4. Month of First Prenatal Visit, Premature and Mature Matched Black Single Births, New York City 1961.

Month of First visit	Premature (≤ 2500 g)		Mature (> 2500 g)	
	No.	%	No.	%
Total	3,902	100.0	3,902	100.0
1–3	319	8.2	336	8.6
4–6	1,531	39.2	1,689	43.3
7–9	1,243	31.9	1,547	39.6
None	809	20.7	330	8.5

Source: Terris and Glasser, 1974.

Table 5. Life Table Analysis of Month of First Prenatal Visit by Mothers of Premature and Mature Matched Black Single Births, New York City 1961.

Interval since conception (months)	"Effective" no. of mothers at risk of having first prenatal visit at start of interval.	No. of mothers having first prenatal visit during interval.	% of mothers not having first prenatal visit before or during interval
	Premature Births		
0–1	3902	23	99.4
1–2	3879	73	97.5
2–3	3,803.5	223	91.7
3–4	2,559.5	370	82.2
4–5	3138	530	68.3
5–6	2513	631	51.2
6–7	1,748.5	659	31.9
7–8	932.5	400	18.2
8–9	335	133	11.0
	Mature Births		
0–1	3902	19	99.5
1–2	3883	85	97.3
2–3	3798	232	91.4
3–4	3566	412	80.8
4–5	3,153.5	533	67.1
5–6	2619	744	48.0
6–7	1,870.5	720	29.5
7–8	1,132.5	522	15.9
8–9	481.5	192	9.6

Source: Terris and Glasser, 1974.

month of the first prenatal visit for a large number of premature and mature black single births in New York City is shown in Table 4. From this table one could conclude that fewer of those women with premature births attended for any prenatal care than those with mature births. However, using a modified life table analysis, as shown in Table 5, they calculated for each monthly interval since conception the percentage of women not having a first prenatal visit before or during the interval, based on the effective numbers of mothers at risk of having a first prenatal visit (i.e., those who had not delivered or had a visit previously). As shown, the percentage is similar for both premature and control groups.

Some differences, however, do appear in the attendance for prenatal care in those women (in both of the above mentioned studies) who delivered after 36 weeks with uncomplicated deliveries, i.e., the small-for-date infants. This association was independent of maternal age, parity, race and income level. However, the effect even if causal, on the overall incidence of prematurity in the study populations was shown to be negligible.

Drillien (1957) compared a group of premature and full term births and assessed the adequacy of prenatal care in the two groups. The results are shown in Table 6, and if we compare the percentage who attended by the 16th week and thereafter, no significant differences are

Table 6.   Attendance at Antenatal Clinic.

Week of First Attendance	Cumulative Percent of Mothers							
	No Complications				All Births			
	Para 0		Para 1 & 2		Para 0		Para 1 & 2	
	Prem	Mat	Prem	Mat	Prem	Mat	Prem	Mat
≤8	17.8	24.8	18.2	25.0	24.7	29.3	20.2	23.3
9–12	66.4	70.5	63.3	72.4	73.1	75.1	63.9	72.6
13–16	83.2	84.2	85.4	89.6	87.0	87.5	83.2	89.3
17–20	90.7	93.3	94.5	95.6	93.7	95.1	90.8	95.3
21–24	96.3	96.7	98.1	96.4	96.8	97.3	95.0	96.6
25–28	98.2	98.6	99.9	97.2	98.4	99.1	97.5	97.9
29–32	98.2	98.5	99.9	98.0	98.4	99.1	98.3	98.6
33–36	99.1	99.2	99.9	99.9	98.9	99.5	98.3	99.9
≥37	99.1	99.9	99.9	99.9	98.9	99.9	98.3	99.9
None	100.0	99.9	99.9	99.9	99.9	99.9	99.9	99.9
Total Number	107	153	55	116	194	225	119	150

Source: Drillien, 1957.

observed between the premature and control groups. The two groups were not controlled for differences in social class or other factors.

Another approach to the study of the effects of prenatal care on prematurity has been to compare the low birth weight rates between countries or within certain areas of one country, or to attempt to relate changes in the low birth weight rate over time to prenatal care practice. This approach is fraught with dangers.

Wynn and Wynn (1974) compared the low birth weight rates between England and Wales and Finland in the late 1960s. England and Wales had a rate of 6.7% and Finland of 4.7%. They commented on the dramatic lowering of perinatal and neonatal mortality in Finland and on the tremendous effort of that country in increasing its maternal and child health services, particularly prenatal care. Table 7 shows the percentage of women who reported for prenatal care in Finland from 1938–1968. What we don't have for comparison is the low birth weight rate for all those years, nor do Wynn and Wynn comment on many of the other changes which must have been occurring in postwar Finland. They then compared (Table 8) the percentage of women reporting for prenatal care before the 16th week of pregnancy in certain regions of the studied countries. Apart from the years being different, can we honestly compare these two percentages without considering all the other factors involved? I feel it is too difficult. Prenatal care differs as do the women; their social and biological characteristics were not described, and we have no idea of how comparable they are in these respects.

One country in which the low birth weight rate has been changing is Japan. Gruenwald et al. (1967) presented data on the secular changes in mean birth weight for each gestational age in Japan since World War II. The most dramatic change appeared to have been an increase in the birth weight at each gestational age but particularly after 37 weeks, with

Table 7. Coverage of Pregnant Women for Antenatal Care: All Births, Finland 1939–1968.

Year	% of Women Delivered who were Registered at Maternal Health Centres
1938	11.0
1944	31.3
1949	82.4
1950	95.4
1960	96.6
1964	97.5
1968	99.3

Source: Wynn and Wynn, 1974.

Table 8.   Percentages of Pregnant Women Reporting for Antenatal Care Before the 16th Week of Gestation: England and Wales and Finland.

England and Wales		Finland	
Local Health Authority	1962–66	Province	1968
Merthyr Tydfil	19.2	Undenmaan	92.2
Sunderland	56.2	Turun-Porin	90.1
Blackburn	42.2	Hameen	90.5
Anglesey County	17.7	Kymen	93.3
Cumberland County	42.7	Mikkelin	91.6
Lindsey County	52.7	Kuopion	90.8
York	48.5	Pohjois-Karjalan	91.8
Great Yarmouth	79.1	Vaasan	92.7
Oxford	74.9	Keski-Suomen	89.9
Oxford County	71.5	Oulun	90.9
		Lapin (Lapland)	88.5

Source: Wynn and Wynn, 1974.

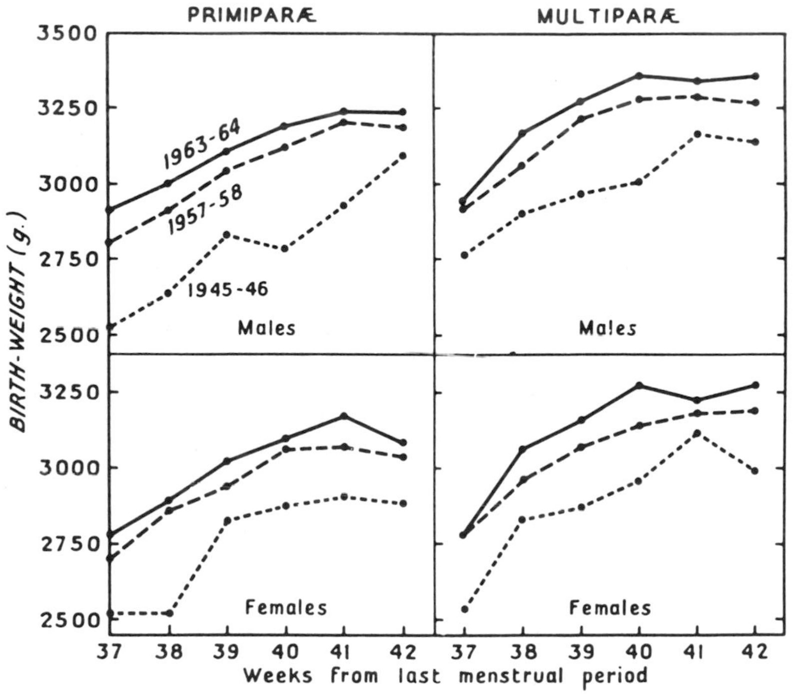

Figure 2.   **Growth Curves of Japanese Fetuses Derived From Birth Weights During the Years Indicated by Sex and Maternal Parity.**   Source: Gruenwald et al., 1967.

Table 9. Neonatal Mortality Rates by Birth Weight and Gestational Age (Excluding those with unknown or uncertain gestational age).

Neonatal Mortality Rates			
Birth Weight (gms)			
1751 2000	267	82	87	36
1501–1750	400	196	250	53
1251–1500	459	292	200	200
1001–1250	620	333	143	1000*
< 1000	954	1000*	500*	1000*
	< 30	30–32	33–36	≥ 37
	Gestational Age (weeks)			

Numbers of Infants			
1751–2000	15	49	115	83
1501–1750	25	46	44	19
1251–1500	37	24	20	5
1001–1250	50	12	7	4
< 1000	65	4	2	2
	< 30	30–32	33–36	≥ 37
	Gestational Age (weeks)			

*Rates based on less than 5 deaths.
Source: Stanley, 1976.

fewer small-for-date infants (Fig. 2). Dramatic changes, however, have occurred in national diet, economic (and therefore obviously social) conditions and medical expenditure per capita. The data on the changes in parity and maternal age of births, which must have occurred and which affect birth weight, were not given. To sort out the effect of pre-natal care is impossible. Although both Finland and Japan have had positive policies of improving maternal and child health care, one can-not attribute the differences in the low birth weight to prenatal care when so many other factors have been changing.

CONCLUSIONS

Because of the many factors involved in low birth weight, its relationship to prenatal care can be evaluated only in specially designed and an-alyzed studies. National and international comparisons may provide clues but no proof. These specially designed studies must take into account all the other factors associated with low birth weight—at least gestational age, social class, race, parity and maternal age. Studies which do fulfill these criteria tend to show little or no effect on low birth weight as defined. Prenatal care should also be clearly defined and its components described.

Obviously some prenatal care freely available to all pregnant women is desirable for many reasons other than its effect on the prematurity rate. If it is important to evaluate specifically its importance in reducing the proportion of births which are preterm or low birth weight, then we need to instigate further study of this relationship. And we need to do it so that the effect on the total birth weight/gestational age distribution can be measured. Table 9 illustrates this approach. If two procedures or populations with different exposures are to be compared, then this is best done by comparing the two birth weight/gestational age distributions or contours (see Hoffman, of this volume) and observing the effects of prenatal care on the distribution (or on mortality) as shown.

TEXT REFERENCES

Butler, N. R.; Bonham, D. G.: Perinatal Mortality. The First Report of the 1958 British Perinatal Mortality Survey. Churchill-Livingstone, Edinburgh and London, 1963

Drillien, C. M.: The Social and Economic Factors Affecting the Incidence of Premature Birth. Part I—Premature Births Without Complications of Pregnancy. J Obstet Gynaecol Brit Emp 64(1957) 161-184

Gruenwald, P.; Funakawa, H.; Mitani, S.; Nishimura, T.; Takeuchi, S.: Influence of Environmental Factors on Foetal Growth in Man. Lancet 1(1967)1026-1028

Schwartz, S.; Vineyard, J. H.: Prenatal Care and Prematurity. Publ Health Rep 80(1965)237-248

Stanley, F. J.: Infants of Very Low Birth-weight: The Effect of some Perinatal Factors. MSc. Thesis, London University, 1976

Terris, M.; Gold, E. M.: An Epidemiologic Study of Prematurity. II. Relation to Prenatal Care, Birth Interval, Residential History and Outcome of Previous Pregnancies. Am J Obstet Gynec 103(1969) 371-379

Terris, M.; Glasser, M.: A Life Table Analysis of the Relation of Prenatal Care to Prematurity. Am J Public Health 64 (1974)869-875

Wynn, M.; Wynn, A.: The Protection of Maternity and Infancy. A Study of the Services for Pregnant Women and Young Children in Finland with Some Comparisons with Britain. Council for Children's Welfare, 1974

DISCUSSION

Dr. Emanuel: In our Taiwan study of neural tube malformations, (Emanuel, 1975), we also found a relationship to prenatal care. These defects are, of course, very strongly related to socioeconomic factors and aren't likely to be influenced by prenatal care since they are established between the third and fourth weeks of embryonic development. Our finding is additional evidence that prenatal care experience or maternal care seeking behavior, which is really what is described in most of these studies, may be largely a social indicator.

DISCUSSION REFERENCES

Emanuel, I.: Some Observations on Pre natal Health Practices in an Urban Chinese Community. In: Medicine in Chinese Cultures: Comparative Studies of Health Care in Chinese and Other Societies, pp. 551–558, ed. by A. Kleinman, P. Kunstadter, E. R. Alexander and J. L. Gale. Department of Health, Education and Welfare Publication No. (NIH) 75-653, Washington, D.C. 1975

Methods of Family Planning and the Risk of Low Birth Weight

Heinz W. Berendes, M.D., M.H.S.

A current consideration of variables which have an impact on low birth weight or on preterm delivery has to include the modern methods of family planning. In theory at least, these practices may have a direct effect on the maternal or the fetal organism and thereby result in alterations in the risk of prematurity. The relevance of this hypothesis will be explored with data reported in the literature.

Furthermore, the adoption of modern methods of family practice may affect patterns of reproduction of various segments of the population. This in turn may result in changes in the overall rate of low birth weight. Examples from published reports will be used to demonstrate this effect.

Therapeutic abortion has become one of the most commonly used methods of fertility regulation. This has come about through the liberalization of laws governing the use of therapeutic abortion or through a change in mores which has resulted in acceptance of this practice, although still illegal and without amendment of the law in certain countries. Not enough is known about the medical effects of induced abortion, particularly regarding long-term effects. A substantial concern exists about a possible adverse effect on subsequent pregnancies. There are indeed numerous reports in the literature which attempt to deal with the question and are derived from data reflecting the experience of different countries. They are largely based upon data in certain hospitals or geographic areas, combine different abortion techniques, include divergent population groups and approach the problem in different ways methodologically. Some of these reports suggest a substantial increase in risk of low birth weight or preterm delivery in pregnancies following induced abortions, whereas others do not. Most, if not all, of these reports suffer from substantial methodological shortcomings which are, however, equally present in those reports which reveal adverse subsequent effects as in those which do not.

I shall only highlight certain of the more recent publications and thereby point out the disarray in our current knowledge as well as the lack of substantial information regarding the experience in this country.

Two recent studies (Pantelakis, Papadimitriou and Doxiadis, 1973; Papaevangelow et al., 1973) came from Greece and were very similar in design and population studied. They showed a substantial increase in the rate of preterm deliveries in pregnancies following induced abortions. The study by Pantelakis et al. (1973) reported the experience from a large hospital in Athens between 1966 and 1968. During that time, pregnant women admitted for delivery were interviewed about their social class, age, medical and obstetric history, including history of induced abortion. The data about the abortion history in this study were therefore collected at the time of delivery. Approximately 13,000 women were included in this report. There was a two-fold increase in premature births and in stillbirths in women with a prior history of induced abortions while holding the effects of social class constant. The second study (Papaevangelou et al., 1973) was based upon data from a large hospital in Athens for the years 1969–1970. The proportion of preterm deliveries increased in relation to the number of prior induced abortions. Also, mean birth weight decreased as the number of prior induced abortions increased. Among the methodological issues raised by these two studies are the recall bias by interviewing at the time of delivery and lack of consideration of other factors such as smoking and the like among the groups which were compared.

Two studies done in Japan (Roht and Aoyama, 1973 and 1974) came up with negative findings. In one of these (Roht and Aoyama, 1974) a sample of about 3000 women who were approached through a mail questionnaire was obtained from an area in southern Japan. The other (Roht and Aoyama, 1973) consisted of an interview survey of about 600 women. No relationship was found between the history of induced abortion and subsequent spontaneous abortion and low birth weight adjusting for differences in age and parity. Another study from Japan (Muramatsu, 1972), however, reported a positive relationship: that is, an increase in the rate of low birth weight in infants of women with a prior history of induced abortion. This report compared the deliveries of Japanese women with a history of induced abortion to women without a history of induced abortion.

A study, very carefully conducted methodologically, of low birth weight in relation to induced abortion (Hogue, 1975) was based upon a historical prospective investigation of 948 women in Yugoslavia. The study subjects were derived from record reviews at a university hospital. Subsequent pregnancies and their outcomes were identified in these women. Women whose first pregnancy ended as an induced abortion had a significant increase in low birth weight babies in their subsequent pregnancy as compared to women whose first pregnancy did not end in induced abortion. However, there was no difference in the rate of low birth weight among the second pregnancies of women with a prior induced abortion as compared to primiparous women. The author concluded that induced abortion during the first pregnancy did not protect against the increased risk of low birth weight known to be present among first births. Hogue was able to identify considerable underreporting of induced abortion by reference to existing hospital records, pointing to important sources of bias of underreporting if ascertainment of abortion history is obtained by interview.

Another historical prospective study was reported by Harlap and Davies (1975). This project was based upon the Jerusalem Perinatal Study which covered all births in that community. During the interval of 1966–1968, pregnant women were interviewed about their abortion history at the time of the first visit to the prenatal clinic. Data on many other variables known to affect low birth weight were available for analysis. Adjusting for other differences, women with a prior history of induced abortion had a significant increase in the rate of low birth weight.

Finally, Daling and Emanuel (1975) reported a study from Taiwan. The project included births in six hospitals for the years 1965–1968. The abortion history was obtained at the time of delivery. In the analysis, data were adjusted for differences in age, pregnancy order and the presence of prior fetal death. Matched pair analysis showed no difference in the rate of low birth weight or of preterm delivery by history of prior induced abortion.

Hogue (1976) recently discussed in detail the methodological issues which were apparent in these and other studies of adverse medical consequences of induced abortion. These involve the methods of ascertainment of the abortion history and of the study subjects, and also confounding through important covariables which are known to affect low birth weight and prematurity.

There are several studies currently underway in this country of the possible adverse effects of induced abortion on subsequent pregnancy performance. They are mostly prospective in design and are also collecting information on certain confounding variables. In one or two years, information about the risk of low birth weight or preterm delivery in relation to induced abortion should be available based upon the experience from these investigations.

There is little information available on a possible effect of the various methods of contraception on low birth weight. Conceptions occasionally occur in women with an intrauterine device *in situ*. Since these are unwanted pregnancies, many of them are terminated by induced abortion. Among those permitted to continue, a substantial proportion terminate either in spontaneous abortion or in premature delivery (Vessey et al., 1974; Shine and Thompson, 1974; Steven and Fraser, 1974).

Exposure to contraceptive steroids at or around the time of conception or early in pregnancy is associated with a slight increase in risk of congenital malformation (Janerich, Piper and Glebatis, 1974; Nora and Nora, 1974; Harlap, Prywes and Davies, 1975). It is not currently known whether such exposure affects low birth weight or prematurity, although research along this line is currently in progress.

Current family planning practices have substantially reduced fertility rates in many countries. Access and motivation to adopt these practices may vary among different segments of the population. As a result, it is not difficult to postulate changes in reproduction of population groups differing in risk of unfavorable pregnancy outcome which may increase or decrease the rate of low birth weight in the aggregates. Examples of such effects will be briefly highlighted.

Lanman, Kohl and Bedell (1974) compared the rate of low birth weight in six Brooklyn hospitals before and after the introduction of the abortion act in New York City. A reduction in the rate of low birth weight was noted in the year after passage of the act, possibly because of a decrease in high risk pregnancy through an increase of induced abortion among high risk groups.

In Romania, induced abortion has for some years been the main method of fertility regulation. In order to increase the birth rate, government authorities issued a restrictive abortion decree in 1966 which was followed by a dramatic increase in birth rate (Wright, 1975). This increase was also paralleled by a marked rise in the rate of low birth weight. The rate of low birth weight before the restrictive abortion decree came into effect in 1966 was 8.1% and had risen to 10.6% one year later. The rise was most marked for newborns weighing less than 1500 gm. Here the rate changed from 0.5% in 1966 to 1.1% in 1967.

A detailed investigation of the possible effect of various family planning practices on a community in the United States has been provided by Pakter and Nelson (1974). Patterns of reproduction were compared for New York City for 1962-1964, the period before the widespread availability of contraceptive steroids; 1965-1969, the interval which reflects the growing availability of oral contraceptives; and 1970-1972, which is immediately after the liberalized abortion act became effective.

A marked decrease in fertility was apparent between 1965-1970, except in white women under 20 years of age; 1970-1971 showed a further decline in fertility which now also included women under 20 years of age. While out of wedlock births continued to increase through 1969 despite the general availability of contraceptive pills, these began to decline in 1970 with the abortion act. Furthermore, there was also a marked drop in births to women of low socioeconomic status, including those receiving aid to dependent children. The rate of births among women on aid to dependent children dropped from 173 per 1000 in 1962-1965, to 115 per 1000 in 1966-1969, to a low of 72 per 1000 in 1972. The abortion/birth ratio was highest among the youngest women and the older age groups. Paralleling these changes in birth rate and distribution of birth by age and socioeconomic status were reductions in the rate of low birth weight for 1965-1969 and 1970-1971. This decrease in the rate of low birth weight was apparent in all weight interval groups under 2500 gm. The rate of decrease was more marked for non-whites and Puerto Ricans between 1970-1971, and was consistently lower for all three ethnic groups for birth weights under 1000 gm. These data certainly suggest a parallelism which may have causal implications between these altered patterns of reproduction resulting in differences in risk of low birth weight and the widespread use of oral contraceptives since 1965 and the marked increase in induced abortion through the abortion act of 1970. The reduction in low birth weight appears more marked since passage of the abortion act, possibly due to the greater reduction in out of wedlock births and births to young women during this interval.

The experience in Hungary suggest a somewhat different pattern (Czeizel et al., 1970). In Hungary, an increase in low birth weight had been noted for more than a decade. The rate of low birth weight rate had risen gradually from 6% in 1950 to 10.8% in 1967. During this interval, Hungary had relied largely on induced abortion as the main method of fertility regulation. The number of induced abortions rose from 1707 in 1950 to a high of 185,527 in 1967. Part of the change in the rate of low birth weight during this interval was thought to be due to better reporting because of the marked decline in home deliveries which were apparently associated with underreporting of low birth weight.

However, family planning practices seem to account for at least a portion of the increase in low birth weight. Such practices differed among various subgroups of the Hungarian population. The crude birth rate for Hungary in 1960 was 14.4 per 1000; however, for the gypsy population and other low socioeconomic groups, the crude birth rate was as high as 40.9 per 1000. The rate of low birth weight for the population of Hungary in 1960 was around 9%, but for the gypsies it was 15%. As family planning was adopted by the middle class population, the proportion of births from the low socioeconomic groups, including gypsies, increased substantially. This became particularly apparent by observing the shift in the rate of low birth weight among high parity women. The number of births to women at parity 10 and above markedly declined from a total of 2332 in 1953 to 793 in 1967. At the same time, the rate of low birth weight for this high parity group rose from 6.1% to 16.1%. This was due to the much higher proportion of births from women in the low socioeconomic groups among high parity births during the later year.

In addition, two other factors have contributed to the increase in the rate of low birth weight. The adoption of family planning practices has resulted in a higher proportion of first births which made up 50% of all births in 1967. This change alone has been estimated to account for an increase in low birth weight of about 0.5%. Furthermore, for the city of Budapest it has been estimated that approximately 12% of the increase in low birth weight is due to the effects of earlier induced abortion.

The comparison between New York City and Hungary suggests contradictory effects. The reasons for this difference are readily apparent. In New York City, methods of family planning appear to have been available to and used by all segments of the population. In effect, they appear to have been used more frequently by women at high risk. This has resulted in a reduction in low birth weight. The opposite pattern has emerged in Hungary. Women at high risk of low birth weight are now contributing a higher proportion of the total births than before.

Judicious use of family planning practices undoubtedly could have a substantial beneficial public health impact and result in a reduction of low birth weight and prematurity. Aside from the assurance of the availability of methods of family planning to all segments of the population, the motivational factor determines the extent to which different population groups will make use of them. This in turn will affect the reproductive patterns of the various groups, resulting in variable but predictable effects on perinatal outcome, including low birth weight.

TEXT REFERENCES

Czeizel, A.; Bognar, Z.; Tusnady, G.; Revesz, P.: Changes in Mean Birth Weight and Proportion of Low-Weight Births in Hungary. Brit J Prev Soc Med 24(1970)146

Daling, J. R.; Emanuel, I.: Induced Abortion and Subsequent Outcome of Pregnancy. Lancet 2(1975)170

Harlap, S.; Prywes, R.; Davies, A. M.: Birth Defects and Estrogens and Pro-

gesterone in Pregnancy. Lancet: (1975) 682–683

Harlap, S.; Davies, A. M.: Late Sequelae of Induced Abortion: Complications and Outcome of Pregnancy and Labor. Am J Epidemiol 102(1975)217

Hogue, J.: Low Birth Weight Subsequent to Induced Abortion. Am J Obstet Gynecol 123(1975)675

Hogue, J.: Induced Abortion as a Risk

Factor for Later Pregnancies: Methodological Issues in Current Studies. Presented at the 104th Annual Meeting of the American Public Health Association, Miami, Oct. 19, 1976

Janerich, D.; Piper, J. M.; Glebatis, D. M.: Oral Contraceptives and Congenital Limb-Reduction Defects. New Engl J Med 291(1974)697

Lanman, J. T.; Kohl, S. G.; Bedell, J. H.: Changes in Pregnancy Outcome After Liberalization of the New York State Abortion Law. Am J Obstet Gynecol 118 (1974)485

Muramatsu, M.: A Survey of the Effect of Induced Abortion on Weight at Birth. Bull Inst Pub Health 21(1972)127

Nora, J. J.; Nora, A. H.: Can the Pill Cause Birth Defects? New Engl J Med 291(1974)731

Pakter, J.; Nelson, F.: Factors in the Unprecedented Decline in Infant Mortality in New York City. Bull NY Acad Med 50(1974)839

Pantelakis, S. N.; Papdimitrion, G. C.; Doxiadis, S. A.: Influence of Induced and Spontaneous Abortions on the Outcome of Subsequent Pregnancies. Am J Obstet Gynecol 116(1973)799

Papaevangelou, G.; Vrettos, A. S.; Papadatos, C.; Alexiou, D.: The Effect of Spontaneous and Induced Abortion on Prematurity and Birth Weight. J Obstet Gynecol Brit Comm 80(1973)418

Roht, L. H.; Aoyama, H.: Induced Abortion and Its Sequelae: Prevalence and Associations with the Outcome of Pregnancy. Int J Epidemiol 2(1973)103

Roht, L. H.; Aoyama, H.: Induced Abortion and Its Sequelae: Prematurity and Spontaneous Abortion. Am J Obstet Gynecol 120(1974)868

Shine, R. M.; Thompson, J. F.: The in situ IUD and Pregnancy Outcome. Am J Obstet Gynecol 119(1974)124

Steven, J. D.; Fraser, I. S.: The Outcome of Pregnancy After Failure of Intrauterine Contraceptive Device. J Obstet Gynecol Brit Comm 81(1974)282

Vessey, M. P.; Johnson, G.; Doll, R.; Peto, R.: Outcome of Pregnancy in Women Using an Intrauterine Device. Lancet 1: (1974)495

Wright, N. H.: Restricting Legal Abortion: Some Maternal and Child Health Effects in Romania. Am J Obstet Gynecol 121 (1975)246

DISCUSSION

Dr. Susser: Of the papers, how many are talking about induced legal abortions?

Dr. Berendes: The data which I have discussed on the effect of induced abortion on subsequent pregnancy performance involved either induced legal abortions or illegal abortions, depending on the country from which the data were derived. The studies I reported from Greece, Israel and Taiwan involve illegally induced abortions, and as you recall, the data from Greece and Israel show an adverse effect on subsequent pregnancies whereas the data from Taiwan do not. In Hungary, Japan and Yugoslavia, abortions were legal and yet the studies based on the Hungarian experience suggest a pronounced adverse effect of induced abortions whereas the data from Japan and Yugoslavia do not. The fact as to whether the studies were based on legally or illegally induced abortions therefore does not account for the differences in the findings.

Dr. Emanuel: There are some preliminary data from the United States. Janet Daling, who is my coauthor on a previous paper (Daling and

Emanuel, 1975), has done her Ph.D. dissertation research on a similar study among 5000 University of Washington Hospital births, using similar matching techniques. Results so far are very similar to our previous study. Abortion was not related to subsequent abnormal pregnancy outcome. The analysis is not complete, but I think it is complete enough to say that the results are very similar.

I think one might also look a little more at some of the national statistics to get some insights as to what long-term effects abortion may have. For more than two decades, Japan has had about one-million abortions a year and approximately two-million births a year. Yet during that time, birth weight has increased, as Dr. Stanley showed, and infant mortality has plummeted.

In the United States about 700,000 induced abortions were reported to about 3.1 million births in the last year (Center for Disease Control, 1976). This has been going on for several years and American infant mortality statistics are also improving. The future risks reported by some studies of abortion are so fantastically high that if they were true, one would certainly expect to see problems mirrored in national statistics. I think I have to conclude that in some of these countries, standards for performing abortions may be very low. On the other hand, most of the studies relating abortion to subsequent reproductive outcome have not adequately considered maternal characteristics. One might expect some occasional long-term complications to abortion since there are infrequent significant immediate complications. That long-term complications are frequent is not supported by the abundant data now available.

There is, of course, much emotionality connected with abortion, but there is no place in research for such emotionality. It is possible to study the question of abortion and its possible consequences just as objectively as most other problems relating to human health.

Dr. Niswander: I would like to suggest that a major difference between the recent Japanese and American studies and some of the earlier studies is the use of the laminaria tent as a technique to prepare the cervix for the abortion. Laminaria is dried seaweed, which is inserted into the cervix and, by hygroscopic action, swells and dilates the cervix. This is done during the preabortion period. The laminaria provides gradual dilatation, as opposed to a very rapid dilatation of the cervix with instruments. This technique may reduce the risk of subsequent premature delivery. Laminaria is being used rather widely in the western United States. I understand it is still not being widely used in much of the eastern United States; the Japanese, of course, have used it for a long time.

I would also like to ask if there is any information on the results following mid-trimester abortion as opposed to early abortion?

Dr. Berendes: The studies which I have reviewed do not separate out mid-trimester abortions from early abortions. I can therefore not answer your question. I recall, however, a report of a small number of cases from England on hysterotomy as a method of mid-trimester abortion. These data imply an increase in small-for-gestation babies in subsequent pregnancies.

DISCUSSION REFERENCES

Center for Disease Control: Abortion Surveillance, 1974. Department of Health, Education and Welfare, Washington DC, 1976

Chou, W. W.; Crompten, A. C.: The Wounded Uterus: Pregnancy after Hysterotomy. Brit Med J 1(1973)321

Daling, J. R.; Emanuel, I.: Induced Abortion and Subsequent Outcome of Pregnancy. Lancet 2(1975)170

Studies of Prevention
and Intervention

David Rush, M.D.

Prevention and intervention are unlike the preceding issues of this conference, which so far has been concerned with the relationship of specific independent variables to prematurity. I have been asked to comment now on whether these possible causes of prematurity might be made the basis for the design and execution of intervention studies, as a step in developing effective preventive programs. Few current preventive strategies are of proven value, although the medical community has implied to the public and government that if only money were made available, proven techniques stand ready to be applied, with near certainty of success. My judgment is that these techniques are, in general, poorly evaluated, and that if called upon to produce, we could easily fail. And we are not, through our government's research priorities and the work these priorities have generated, likely to be much better off in the near future.

Relating independent variables, around which we cannot efficiently design interventions, to mortality, gestation or birth weight is important, but of limited utility. Such variables include genetic inheritance, social class, race, geography, altitude, maternal height, and to a lesser extent, secular change, maternal age, parity, pregnancy interval and prior pregnancy performance.

These variables define groups at different levels of risk, but do not directly imply strategies that might alleviate risk, for they are either impossible or difficult to change. They may provoke hypotheses that can in turn be made operational, but such hypotheses should still be tested directly, unless they are to stay in the limbo of "likely, but not proven."

We do have at hand a number of hypotheses which could be subjected to controlled trial (which implies no less attention to generating new ones).

It was chastening to review, a decade after publication, the comprehensive review of Abramowicz and Kass (1966), and the monograph edited by Chipman et. al. (1966) which followed a conference like this one that took place 13 years ago. At that conference, Dr. Terris said: "One of the paradoxes of the study of low birth weight is the disproportion between the ample findings of descriptive epidemiology and the meager results of analytic epidemiology. Although a large amount of information available on relative risk in different population groups provides many clues to etiology, the answers remain elusive."

In the same volume (Chipman et al., 1966) Dr. William Silverman, a distinguished perinatal clinician, wrote the following: "While the importance of observational evidence cannot be denied, such evidence should not be expected to replace experiment in untangling the chain of causation. The lack of information of the type which can be obtained only from planned experiment is, in my opinion, the most important weakness in our knowledge concerning the principle problems which contribute to perinatal mortality and morbidity."

Things have not changed that much since Drs. Terris and Silverman made those judgments 13 years ago. I agree with Lewis Thomas (1976) who, in reviewing Ivan Illich's jeremiad against modern medicine, *Medical Nemesis*, cautioned that "medicine has hardly begun as a science, is still at its earliest beginnings." We should be careful not to assert or imply that we know things that we don't.

The *New York Times*, our newspaper of record (hardly a voice of the counterculture), announced last July, on the cover of its Sunday magazine: "A Doctor's Prescription: Avoid Your Annual Physical Checkup." We really don't know if that is good advice, because of our past unwillingness, inability, or lack of foresight to properly evaluate, with controlled trials, the preventive visit to the doctor.

This parallels the gaps in knowledge needed to establish scientific preventive perinatal medicine, because of the same unwillingness to do (and to fund) trials of prevention.

There are a number of issues around which trials could now be mounted. Dr. Emanuel's handout presents a useful list. Dr. Terris (Chipman, 1966) discussed the following descriptive variables 13 years ago (which are all amenable to trial): maternal nutrition; work (for which I also read physical activity and rest, physical fitness and the related set of variables); cigarette smoking; asymptomatic bacteriuria (a specific example of maternal and fetal infection, which should now also include mycoplasma and, if therapies are developed, cytomegalovirus and other viral infections); and heart volume (one of a set of interrelated variables, including plasma and blood volume, red cell and hemoglobin mass and concentration, and vascular perfusion).

I have omitted one of the variables on his list (birth interval, which is theoretically amenable to controlled study, but such study would be awkward), and I would add the issues of prenatal care, maternal education and disposable income. Unemployment and economic stress relate to perinatal mortality, and a trial to alleviate the consequences of unemployment is possible.

We avoid intervention studies for many reasons. We are appropriately conservative about involving patients in trials that are unlikely to be of benefit. Also, such studies are tedious, at times to the point of drudgery, and results are deferred: they neither accelerate the fattening of the academic bibliography, nor do they promptly justify research expenditure.

Our nutritional study (Rush et al., 1974) was described by Dr. Susser. We think it is a good study, but, sadly, there are no others in any western country. Several replications have folded under the pressures mentioned. We were, and are, being castigated for denying the high protein supplement to all the women enrolled. Yet, under controlled conditions, the high protein supplement has been associated with unexpected (and chastening) adverse outcome, which we could not have predicted: this in spite of all the indirect and descriptive evidence that has suggested to our critics that a direct test was not only wasteful of time and money—the benefit was considered a foregone conclusion—but also heartless and immoral.

Consider how little we are going to learn from the massive WIC program, which assumes benefit for prenatal feeding and whose scanty evaluation is focused on process measures rather than on the effect of the food supplements on either the mother or the child.

Where are the other controlled trials of important issues? As far as I know, there is no trial in the United States for the prevention of cigarette smoking in pregnancy. (There has been one in London, by John Donovan, but it is not yet published.)

We are still uncertain about the effects of asymptomatic bacteriuria. A recent report by Brumfitt (1975) found that among those women whose infection had not easily cleared, there were adverse perinatal consequences.

Dr. Kass and his group are continuing their controlled trial of mycoplasma treatment.

For physical fitness, exercise and work, little is known. Räihä et al.'s (1957) studies in Finland on rest during pregnancy for those with small heart volume have not been repeated, and should be, even though others have only been able to find a weak relationship of small heart volume to low birth weight. Räihä did initiate an intervention program, and noted reduction in the incidence of low birth weight and perinatal loss with maternal rest.

Can any of us judge the effect of maternal work during pregnancy? I was asked, in preparation for a recent Supreme Court case, whether pregnancy leave might have explicit health benefits; I could find no direct data. A trial ought to be executed around this issue.

The effects of prenatal care remain controversial. Dr. Niswander mentioned that there have been controlled trials of fetal monitoring, showing little or no benefit. Most clinicians do not accept that this issue needs a controlled trial. Yet, the cost of care using such new and complicated techniques is enormous.

Finally, there are the educational and economic correlates of pregnancy risk. There could be trials of health education in pregnancy. Also, why not a trial, controlled and randomized, of giving pregnant women five dollars a day and letting them do what they will with it? One state's WIC program with which I an familiar supplies approximately 1000 "supplemental" calories a day. No woman could add that much food to her diet, and it therefore becomes an income supplement, freeing money that otherwise would have been spent on food. Why not try a direct income supplement? If health improved, it would be an efficient strategy, compared to the cost of visits to a public clinic.

We ought to refocus our public health enterprise, and controlled trials are an important step towards getting operational public health intervention.

TEXT REFERENCES

Abramowicz, M.; and Kass, E. H.: Pathogenesis and Prognosis of Prematurity. New Engl J Med 275(1966)878-885, 938-943, 1001-1007, 1053-1059

Brumfitt, W.: The Effect of Bacteriuria in Pregnancy on Maternal and Fetal Health. Kidney Int 8(1975)113-119

Chipman, S. S.; Lilienfeld, A. M.; Greenberg, B. G.; Donnelly, J. F.: Research Methodology and Needs in Perinatal Studies. Thomas, Springfield, Ill., 1966

Räihä, C. E.; Johansson, C. E.; Lind, J.; Vara, P.: Heart Volume During Pregnancy with Special Considerations of its Reduction. Ann Paedictr Fenn 3(1957) 65-69

Rush, D.; Stein, Z.; Christakis, G.; Susser, M.: The Prenatal Project: The First 20 Months of Operation. In: Malnutrition and Human Development, pp. 95-125, ed. by M. Winick, Wiley, New York, 1974

Silverman, W. A.: Gaps in our Knowledge of Perinatal Mortality and Morbidity. In: Research Methodology and Needs in Perinatal Studies, pp. 243-250, ed. by S. S. Chipman et al. Thomas, Springfield, Ill., 1966

Terris, M.: The Epidemiology of Prematurity: Studies of Specific Etiologic Factors. In: Research Methodology and Needs in Perinatal Studies, pp. 207-232, ed. by S. S. Chipman et al. Thomas, Springfield, Ill., 1966

Thomas, L.: Rx for Illich. NY Rev of Books. 23(1976)3-4

DISCUSSION

Dr. Terris: In 1968 I did another review and it covered some of the points Dr. Rush mentioned (Terris, 1968). I said that we were now able to make more definitive statements about the role of certain presumed factors in the etiology of prematurity than were possible five years before. Cigarette smoking during pregnancy was clearly associated with prematurity by weight but not by gestation. However, its relation to perinatal mortality was still uncertain. That was true at that point. I think one of the items of progress since then is that we know that it is related to perinatal mortality.

Asymptomatic bacteriuria is definitely not associated with prematurity. That statement is based on an extremely thorough review of every paper that was published, and there was simply no evidence, outside of Kass' own work, for the relationship between asymptomatic bacteriuria and prematurity, according to the data available.

Available evidence did not appear to give firm support to a relationship of prematurity to maternal relative heart volume, work during pregnancy, birth interval and prenatal care. Maternal weight is more clearly associated with prematurity than maternal height. And if you review the literature carefully, you will find that height always disappears as a variable when weight is taken into consideration. The relation with height is a secondary association, not a primary association.

Mothers of prematures tend to have repetitive premature births, but it is not clear whether and to what extent this holds true both for prematurity by weight and prematurity by gestation. I ended this review by saying two things. First, that somehow everyone had forgotten about maternal nutrition and that it was time we did something about it. And secondly, it was time we got away from mixing apples and oranges. We were in great trouble because our definition included infants premature both by gestation and by weight.

Dr. Rush: We do not have an intervention study for smoking to judge whether, if women can be induced to stop smoking, benefit accrues. A recent repetition of Dr. Kass' work on bacteriuria by Brumfitt (1975) has suggested that asyptomatic bacteriuria is not benign. Heart volume is related to vascular volume and maternal weight and height, which are strongly related to birth weight. It is unknown whether (a) blood volume can be changed, and (b) whether the change would, in turn, affect birth weight.

DISCUSSION REFERENCES

Brumfitt, W.: The Effect of Bacteriuria in Pregnancy on Maternal and Fetal Health. Kidney Int 8(1975)113-119

Terris, M.: Epidemiology of Prematurity. In: Proceedings of the National Conference for the Prevention of Mental Retardation through Improved Maternity Care, Washington, D.C., March 27-29, 1968

Classification of Births by Weight and Gestational Age for Future Studies of Prematurity

Howard J. Hoffman, M.A.
Frank E. Lundin, Jr., M.D., D.P.H.
Leiv S. Bakketeig, M.D.
Ernest E. Harley, M.S.

INTRODUCTION

In the past, considerable effort has been spent in attempting to define the degree of maturity and development of the fetus and the newborn baby. The focus has been mainly on birth weight and gestational age, and particularly on the extremes within the distributions, as indicated by terms like prematurity, preterm births, low birth weight, postterm births, small-for-gestational-age, and large-for-gestational-age.

Most definitions and classifications have been based on univariate distributions of birth weight or gestational age. With few exceptions (Yerushalmy, 1967), much less effort has been devoted to the task of devising classifications which consider the interaction between birth weight and gestational age.

This presentation focuses on the importance and usefulness of the bivariate distribution of birth weight and gestational age data, both as a tool in descriptive and analytical studies as well as a basis for the evaluation of classification schemes. Some classification systems are discussed in relation to the bivariate distribution of birth weight and gestational age.

MATERIALS

The analysis to be presented here is based on two sets of data. One data set was obtained from the National Center for Health Statistics and represents information recorded on birth certificates for a 50% systematic sample of single live births, and on fetal death certificates for all single fetal deaths, in the United States in 1968. The study data set consists of resident births which occurred within the District of Columbia and the 36 states that required the date of the last menstrual period (LMP) on the birth certificates. In 1968 several states first required a record of LMP on birth certificates in compliance with the newly-revised standard live birth and fetal death certificates. The following 14 states did not require a record of the LMP in 1968 and are therefore not included in this study data set: Alabama, Arkansas, Connecticut, Delaware, Florida, Georgia, Idaho, Massachusetts, New Mexico, Oregon, Pennsylvania, Texas, Virginia and Wisconsin.

The other set of data represents all single live births in Norway, 1967–1971. This data set was made available through the Medical Birth Registry of Norway. The medical birth registration system was introduced in Norway in 1967. This notification system covers all live births and fetal deaths with gestational age of 16 weeks or more (Bjerkedal and Bakketeig, 1975).

British data from the 1970 survey of live births and perinatal deaths have been included in Table 1 for comparison with the US and Norwegian data sets. Details of this study are presented elsewhere (Chamberlain et al., 1975). In the British study, data were presented based on the certainty of the last menstrual period in the reported date. Because of this opportunity, we have used these data in order to examine to what extent the bivariate distributions of births by birth weight and gestational age are being affected by the validity of the information on gestational age.

Table 1 displays the number and proportion of single live births by known and unknown birth weight (BW) and gestational age (GA) categories for these US, Norwegian and British births. The relatively high rate of predominantly missing gestational age information in the US sample has been discussed previously by Hoffman et al. (1974), where more detailed tables can be found showing the distribution of the unknown data by single week and 500 gm. categories. The potential for bias of these unknown data on the bivariate distributions to be reported in this study has been examined using three different procedures for redistributing the unknowns. These methods revealed no noticeable changes in the contour levels for the bivariate distributions of BW and GA (Hoffman et al., 1974). The proportion of single live births with

Table 1. Number and Proportion of Single Live Births with Known and Unknown Birth Weight (BW) and/or Gestational Age (GA) in the United States, Norway and Great Britain.

	Known BW Known GA	Known BW Unknown GA	Unknown BW Known GA	Unknown BW Unknown GA	Total
I. United States, 1968†					
White					
Male	412,177	97,894	803	525	511,399
Female	389,451	91,897	734	475	482,557
Combined Sex	801,628	189,791	1,537	1,000	993,956
Percent	80.65	19.10	.15	.10	100.00
Black					
Male	64,683	21,639	179	148	86,649
Female	62,754	21,212	171	129	84,266
Combined Sex	127,437	42,851	350	277	170,915
Percent	74.56	25.07	.21	.16	100.00
Non-White, Non-Black					
Male	8,267	2,865	20	29	11,181
Female	7,845	2,797	12	24	10,678
Combined Sex	16,112	5,662	32	53	21,859
Percent	73.71	25.90	15	.24	100.00
II. Norway, 1967–1971*					
Male	161,590	5,035	167	250	167,042
Female	152,534	4,582	164	229	157,609
Combined Sex	314,124	9,717	331	479	324,651
Percent	96.76	2.99	.10	.15	100.00
III. Great Britain, 1970 Survey**					
Singletons,					
LMP Certain	13,408	32	24	0	13,464
All Singletons	15,822	856	29	2	16,709
Percent	94.69	5.12	.18	.01	100.00

†Based on a 50-percent sample of live births from 36 states and the District of Columbia which reported date of last menstrual period (LMP). Gestational ages from 20–52 weeks are included.

*Based on the Medical Registration of Births in Norway. Gestational ages from 16–52 weeks are included.

**Derived from Chamberlain et al. (1975). Gestational ages from 23–48 weeks are included.

known BW and GA was remarkably high in the Norwegian data set, namely 97%. This level of completeness even surpasses the rate achieved in a special study like the British survey.

In both the US and the Norwegian data sets, the analysis is restricted to single live births with known gestational age and birth weight: 945,177 US births and 314,124 Norwegian births. While this number represents 97% of all Norwegian single live births, it represents only 80% of the US single live births in the study data set: 81% of the White births, 75% of the Black births and 74% of the non-White, non-Black births. In 1968 the non-White, non-Black population of births in the study data set consisted of 39% American Indian, 15% Japanese, 11% Chinese, 10% Hawaiian or part-Hawaiian and 25% other. All births for which race was not stated for either parent or child were assigned either to the White or Black race by a method which results in essentially proportionate assignment between the two races (National Center for Health Statistics, 1970).

CONTOURS OF BIRTH WEIGHT AND GESTATIONAL AGE DISTRIBUTIONS

Figure 1 illustrates the contour approach for displaying the bivariate distribution of birth weight and gestational age variables. This figure is based on data for US White single live births, 1968. The contour levels or lines displayed in the figure are a two-dimensional representation of a three-dimensional surface. If gestational age is denoted as the x-axis and birth weight as the y-axis, then the number of single live births corresponding to each x and y may be thought of as the z-axis, which is orthogonal to both the x and y axes. In this figure, each contour level (A,B,C,...,I) represents a specific number or "level" of live births. In all the figures which follow, these contour levels represent a specific proportion of the total live births in each bivariate distribution, as documented in Table 2. Hence, the contour levels represent relative "altitudes" in terms of proportions of live births on the z-axis scale.

All the contour diagrams shown in this report have been derived from tables of counts. In these tables birth weight was grouped by 500 gm. intervals and gestational age by single weeks.[1] The contour diagrams have been obtained by the following procedure: the count in each cell was divided by the total count for the respective tables, excluding births with unknown birth weight and/or gestational age. The proportions in

---

[1] Although gestational age calculated from LMP was tabled in completed weeks (Hoffman et al., 1974) following the international convention, the designation of weeks and tick marks in the figures correspond to the beginning of each week. A scale of corresponding exact days is provided in each figure, also.

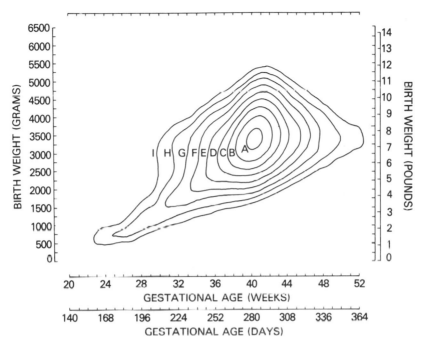

Figure 1. **Contours of Birth Weight and Gestational Age Distribution of U.S. White Single Live Births, 1968.**

each cell were then transformed using natural logarithms. Contour levels were drawn based on a smoothing, spline function interpolation method (Birkhoff and Garabedian, 1968). A standard algorithm is available at the Computer Center of the National Institutes of Health in a graphics package program (Ashbrook and Sande, 1975) for creating these contour plots. Contour levels which were originally drawn by hand using a method described by Tukey (1971) are virtually identical to the contour levels produced by the computer algorithm.

The contour levels shown are equally spaced on the log scale as shown in Table 2. For example, the highest contour level in Figure 1 (labelled "A") expressed in natural log scale is -2.465, which corresponds to a proportion of 0.0850. Since the contour levels shown in Figure 1 are based on a total of 801,628 US White single live births with known birth weight and gestational age (Table 1), the innermost contour level corresponds to approximately 68,000 live births per 500 gm. and single week cell. The next contour level (labelled "B" in Figure 1) is -3.233 in natural log scale and 0.0395 as a proportion. The frequency count for this contour level is approximately 32,000 live births. Contour level "C" corresponds to -4.000 in natural log scale and 0.0183 as a proportion.

Table 2.   Proportions, Natural Logarithms and Logits Corresponding to Contour Levels.

I. Live Birth Contours

Label	Natural Log (LN)	Proportion of Total Count
A*	-2.465	8.50×10^{-2}
B	-3.233	3.95×10^{-2}
C*	-4.000	1.83×10^{-2}
D	-4.768	8.50×10^{-3}
E*	-5.535	3.95×10^{-3}
F	-6.303	1.83×10^{-3}
G*	-7.070	8.50×10^{-4}
H	-7.838	3.95×10^{-4}
I*	-8.605	1.83×10^{-4}

*Alternate contour levels only are shown in Figures 2, 4-10 and 12.

II. Fetal Viability Contours[+]

Order	Logit	Fetal Deaths Per 1000 Births[§]
1 (Innermost)	-6.0	2.5
2	-5.0	6.7
3	-4.0	18.0
4	-3.0	47.4
5	-2.0	119.2
6 (Outermost)	-1.0	268.9

[+] Shown in Figure 11

[§] All products of conception—live births plus fetal deaths—surviving through the first 20 weeks of gestation are included in the term "births."

The frequency count which corresponds to this contour level is approximately 15,000 live births in Figure 1. The outermost contour level (labelled "I" in Figure 1) expressed in natural log scale is -8.606 and 0.000183 in proportion. The corresponding frequency count in the original table was about 150. Thus the outermost contour level in Figure 1 divides the birth weight and gestational age plane into two regions. Outside the boundary formed by this contour level, fewer than 150 live births are expected in each 500 gm. and single week cell. Inside the contour level "I," each cell has a count which exceeds 150 live births.

The contours shown in Figure 1 describe the rate of occurrence of US White single live births, 1968, as a function jointly of birth weight and gestational age. Approximately half of all these births occur in the region inside the "B" contour. The remainder fall outside the "B" contour level and are shown using seven additional contour levels. Since the contours are equally spaced on a log scale, the change in distance between adjacent contour levels indicates the rate of change in the number of births in any given direction. For example, if we draw a vertical line at exactly 40-weeks gestational age, the number of births increases rapidly as birth weight increases from 1500 to 2500 gm. (adjacent contour levels are closely spaced). From 2500 to about 3500 gm., the increase in relative number of births is not so rapid. From about 3500 up to 5500 gm. moving out from the inner contour, the relative number of births decreases, and at an accelerated rate above 4000 gm.

These contour plots are a two-dimensional representation of a three-dimensional "mountain" of births. It is convenient to refer to different portions of the figure with language borrowed from geographical contour maps, as for example, "ridge," "peak," etc. The birth-weight-appropriate-for-gestational-age ridge ascends from about 24 weeks and 500 gm. to the peak of the distribution near 40 weeks and 3500 gm. The rate of increase in the number of births for increasing BW and GA is slow at the lower left end of the ridge but increases as birth weight and gestational age approach nearer to 38 weeks and 2700 gm. At 40 weeks this growth axis bifurcates into a high-weight-at-term ridge and a postterm-average-birth-weight ridge. Alternatively, we could say there is an absence of a ridge in the direction of postterm births with weight exceeding 4000 gm. Another notable feature of this contour plot is the tendency for some births to have weights near 3000 gm. before 37 weeks of gestation. This bulge corresponds to large-for-date babies.

In this configuration a bivariate Gaussian (or normal) distribution is characterized by elliptical contours. In the center of the distribution the contour levels are elliptical in shape. Since a large population of births was used to construct these contours, it is not too surprising, based on knowledge of the limit theorems of probability theory (Cramér, 1946; Karn and Penrose, 1951), that the distribution of births appears Gaussian in this region. However, we shall pay attention also to the departures from the Gaussian distribution elliptical contours in the "tails" and "shoulders" of these bivariate frequency distributions. In the comparisons which follow we shall point out differences both in the center of these distributions and in the extremes.

VALIDITY OF GESTATIONAL AGE FOR CONTOUR DIAGRAMS

Figure 2 illustrates two sets of contours that are superimposed in the same plot. Both are derived from the 1970 survey of British births (Chamberlain et al., 1975). The solid lines correspond to the subsample of women who declared that the recall of their last menstrual period was certain. The dashed lines, however, are derived from all single live births in the survey. Several births with less certain LMP were included in the latter set of contours. In order to reduce the confusion of too many lines in the figure, only alternate contours levels are shown. The levels shown in Figure 2 correspond to those levels marked A, C, E and G in Figure 1.

Although there are many legitimate doubts about the accuracy of the LMP measurement, there have been few large-scale attempts to check

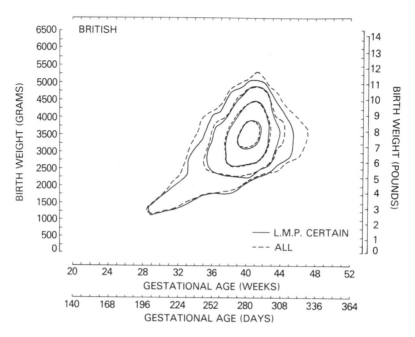

Figure 2. **Selected Contours of Birth Weight and Gestational Age Distributions, by Certainty of Date of LMP, British Single Live Births, 1970.**

its validity. The opportunity afforded by these British data is one of the first direct internal checks available for a large representative sample of single live births. By examining the difference between corresponding contour levels in Figure 2, we can infer that by including all single live births, the two innermost contour levels are not much affected compared with only single live births in which LMP was certain. However, if we compare the outer two sets of contour levels, it is apparent that the "uncertain" LMP births increase the relative number of postterm and preterm births. The effect is somewhat more marked in postterm rather than preterm births. Large-for-date births, although slightly reduced in number, are by no means eliminated by relying on data with a presumably more valid assessment of length of gestation.

In addition to the above comparisons, Hammes and Treloar (1970) have compared a series with extremely accurate LMP determination to vital statistics data derived from recorded LMP dates. Their results showed only slight differences between the two cumulative percent curves representing births by weeks of gestation. Thus our position is similar to that arrived at many years ago by McKeown and Gibson (1951) that gestational age information calculated from LMP, when it is available, is a useful and important measurement for classifying births.

PERCENTILES RELATED TO THE BIVARIATE DISTRIBUTIONS OF BIRTHS

Figure 3 illustrates contour levels and selected percentiles for US White and Norwegian male single live births. The number of US White males used in calculating these percentiles and contours was 412,177 and the number of Norwegian males used was 161,590 (Table 1). The methods used in calculating percentiles from either ungrouped or grouped data have been explained in previous publications (Bjerkedal, Bakketeig and Lehmann, 1973; Hoffman et al., 1974). Tenth, fiftieth and ninetieth percentiles are shown in each of the four plots of the figure. The upper two plots show percentiles of birth weight conditional on known gestational age. The lower two plots show percentiles of gestational age conditional upon known birth weight categories. In each of the four plots there is a solid dot at 37 weeks and 2250 gm. This particular combination of birth weight and gestational age will serve to point out the paradox which exists if one attempts to use both sets of percentiles to classify births.

A priori, why should one prefer percentiles derived by assuming either

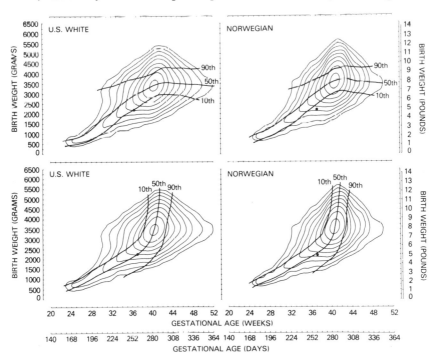

Figure 3.   **Percentiles of Weight by Gestation (top) and Percentiles of Gestation by Weight (bottom), Superimposed on Contours of Birth Weight and Gestational Age Distributions, for U.S. White Single Male Live Births, 1968, and Norwegian Single Male Live Births, 1967–1971.**

known birth weight category or known gestational age category? But when both sets of percentiles are presented, we are faced with a choice. For the birth weight category 2001–2500 gm., 37 weeks (259 days) is the median gestational age (the solid dot falls on the fiftieth percentile) in the US data. However, at 37 weeks, 2250 gm. is on the lower tenth percentile of birth weight. The newborn with this birth weight and gestational age combination is at risk for being in the lower tenth percentile of birth weight, and yet is also at an average gestational age for its birth weight. A similar point can be made for the Norwegian male births shown on the right side of the figure. However, the same combination of gestational age and birth weight falls slightly below the tenth and the fiftieth percentiles respectively where the percentiles are based on Norwegian births, reflecting somewhat heavier births compared to the US population.

Yerushalmy (1967) pointed out the problem of interpretation which arises in using percentiles conditional upon either birth weight or gestational age. The solution he proposed was to treat birth weight and gestational age data as bivariate in order to define high and low risk groups. This proposal for classifying births by birth weight and gestational age uses both variables jointly in defining groups (see Figure 12). Figure 3 confirms Yerushalmy's earlier findings using our own current large data sets. In the figure, percentiles are superimposed on the contour levels of the bivariate BW-GA distributions. A comparison of the two median percentile lines between the top and bottom panels of Figure 3 for US and Norway demonstrates that the two differ markedly above 3000 gm. in weight and 40 weeks of gestational age. As birth weight increases, the median gestational age for each country remains near 41 weeks. On the other hand, as gestational age increases, median birth weight levels off near 3500 gm. Below 40 weeks and 3000 gm., neither fiftieth percentile line coincides with the birth-weight-appropriate-for-gestational-age ridge. The median birth-weight-given-gestational-age line exceeds the ridge, while the median gestational-age-given-birth-weight line is below the ridge.

COMPARISONS BETWEEN POPULATIONS AND ETHNIC GROUPS

On the left side of Figure 4, the contour method is used for comparison of US White, US Black and Norwegian male single live births. The comparison shown in the lower panel between US White and Black births has been presented and discussed previously (Hoffman et al., 1974). US White births are heavier and less preterm than US Black births. The US White and Norwegian comparison in the upper panel extends this comparison. The contours of the Norwegian births bear a

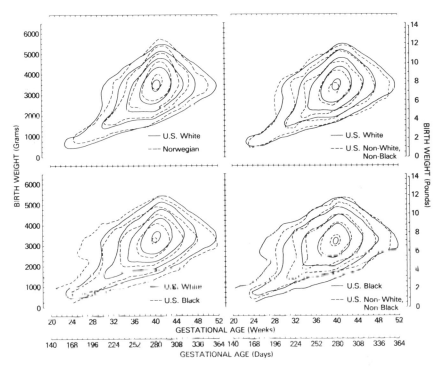

Figure 4. **Contours of Birth Weight and Gestational Age Distributions, U.S. White, Black, and non-White, non-Black Single Male Live Births, 1968, and Norwegian Single Male Live Births, 1967–1971.**

relationship to the contours of the US White births similar to the relationship found between the contours of the US White and Black births. Norwegian mothers show a tendency for delivering heavier and relatively fewer preterm (as well as postterm) infants than their US White counterparts.

The relative concentration of live births weighing 3000–4500 gm. with a gestational age 39–41 weeks is greatest among Norwegians, intermediate in US Whites and least for US Blacks. The proportions of all singletons with this combination of birth weight and gestational age are 58, 49 and 34%, respectively. As a result, the area enclosed by the innermost contour is smallest for US Blacks, intermediate in size for US Whites and largest for Norwegian live births. Since the innermost contour level includes the mode, the size of this contour reflects the concentration of the bivariate distribution about the mode.

The relative shifts in contour levels for the US White, US Black and Norwegian birth comparisons follow the "track" of the gestational age percentiles for fixed birth weight categories as can be seen by comparing them with the lower panel of Figure 3. Although Erhardt et al. (1964)

presented percentiles calculated in this way for a study of different ethnic groups in New York City, it has been traditional in this field to calculate only birth weight percentiles for fixed gestational age categories (Lubchenco et al., 1963; Battaglia, Frazier and Hellegers, 1966). Neither method of constructing percentiles is very effective, however, in illustrating the relative shifts in the underlying BW-GA distributions of US Whites, US Blacks and Norwegians.

The right side of Figure 4 contrasts the US non-White, non-Black male single live births with Whites in the upper panel and with Blacks in the lower panel. Historically, vital statistics data have been reported by race as "White" and "all other" in the United States. Typically, "all other" may be subclassified as Negro ("Black") and other non-Negro in the *Vital Statistics of the United States* volumes. Given this background, the question arises whether the heterogeneous group of non-White, non-Black births would be more similar to the US White or Black births in terms of the BW-GA contour levels. In fact, a mixture of the characteristics of both can be seen in the non-White, non-Black birth contours. The two outermost contour levels (Figure 4, upper right) of non-White, non-Black births are virtually superimposed on the White contour levels instead of the Black. Also, the size of the innermost contour for the non-White, non-Black births is even larger than for White births. Nevertheless, the three innermost contour levels are centered on the same mode as are the Black births. These inner contour levels, which enclose most of the births, are shifted toward lighter and more preterm deliveries compared to the White births. From this standpoint, the non-White, non-Black births are similar to the Black births.

Figure 5 illustrates the differences between Norwegian and US White single live births for each sex, and differences between the two sexes within each population group. As shown earlier by Hoffman et al. (1974) for US White and Black, male and female, there is no apparent interaction in the contour levels between sex and race. The effects contributed by sex and race (and nationality) seem independent, judged by these contours. On the left side of Figure 5, the contour shifts for US White and Norwegian males shown previously in Figure 4 are also found by comparing female births. The right side of the figure shows that males are heavier than females for both US White and Norwegian births.

CONTOURS OF BIVARIATE DISTRIBUTIONS OF BIRTHS FOR MATERNAL AGE AND PARITY GROUPS

Since contours of bivariate distributions have not been widely used in the analysis of variables known to influence birth weight and gestational age, this section will explore shifts in contours using maternal age and

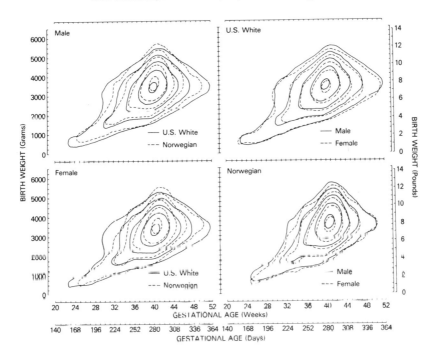

Figure 5. **Contours of Birth Weight and Gestational Age Distributions by Sex for U.S. White Single Live Births, 1968, and Norwegian Single Live Births, 1967–1971.**

parity, two standard demographic variables. The comparison of contour levels permits a flexible means to jointly analyze birth weight and gestational age differences. By using the contour method, one can detect simultaneous shifts in birth weight and gestational age (as in the race comparisons of Fig. 4) as well as a shift primarily in one variable (as in the sex comparisons of Fig. 5).

Figure 6 shows comparisons for five different maternal age groups for first births (parity one) for US White single live births (sexes combined) in 1968. Parity is used here as defined by the National Center for Health Statistics (1970) as the number of previous live births plus the current one; fetal deaths are not included.[2] The solid line contour levels for the maternal age group 19–24 are repeated in each of the four plots contained in Figure 6 in order to provide a standard reference set of contour levels to compare with each of the other maternal age groups. The upper panel of the left side of the figure shows that the contour levels for the maternal age group 25–29 are essentially congruent to the con-

---

[2] This definition is different from clinical terminology (Pritchard and MacDonald, 1976) which includes "viable" births in the definition of parity. "Viable" in this context is not sharply defined, but could be defined operationally to mean 24-weeks or greater gestation.

tour levels for the reference group (maternal age group 19–24). All of the remaining three comparisons show some departures from the solid line contour levels. The maternal age group 18 years or younger shows a tendency for shorter gestational age births compared to the 19–24 age group. Mothers having their first child at 35 years or older have contours which are shifted simultaneously towards lower birth weight and shorter gestational age births. This same tendency is present to a smaller degree in the age group 30–34. For first parity, then, the effect of older maternal age on the contour levels is similar to the effect found in the comparison between the US Black and White births. Births by young primiparous mothers are shifted primarily towards shorter gestational ages rather than lower birth weight. This is the converse of the male-female effect in which birth weight was shifted primarily.

Figure 7 shows the same maternal age comparisons, except that only women having their second live birth (parity two) are included. Comparing Figure 6 with Figure 7 shows that the effect of maternal age on BW-GA contour levels is essentially the same for second births as for first births. The group of mothers 18 years or younger tends to deliver more preterm births than does the next older age group. Also, mothers 35 years or older have relatively more low birth weight, preterm babies than

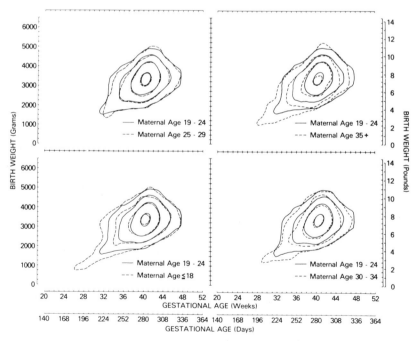

Figure 6. **Contours of Birth Weight and Gestational Age Distributions for First Births (parity one) by Maternal Age for U.S. White Single Live Births, 1968.**

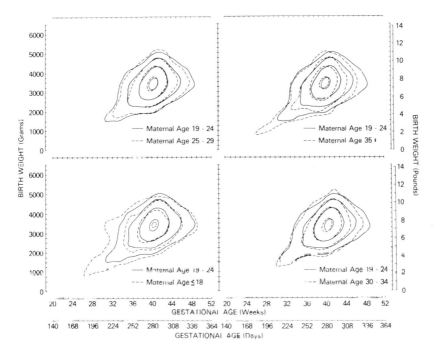

Figure 7. **Contours of Birth Weight and Gestational Age Distributions for Second Births (Parity Two) by Maternal Age for U.S. White Single Live Births, 1968.**

do mothers from 19-24 years. The conclusion which can be drawn is that parity one is not interacting with the extreme maternal ages to produce these results. The increase in preterm and low birth weight births is related more to maternal age than to parity.

Some interaction effects of parity and maternal age can be seen by comparing Figures 6 and 7, although the effects are smaller than the maternal age effects alone. For example, second parity with maternal age 25-29 years is more concentrated around the mode (larger inner contour) than for the standard maternal age group 19-24. This was not apparent in the comparisons for first parity. Another feature that appears in the second parity comparison is the much smaller innermost contour level for maternal ages 18 years or younger compared to the standard maternal age group, 19-24 years. We discussed previously the significance for US White, US Black and Norwegian births of the relative size of the innermost contour level. In this sense, second births to mothers 18 years or younger compared to second births to mothers aged 19-24 years behave in a fashion similar to the US Black/White comparison. Similar plots for Blacks showing maternal age group comparisons by parity (not shown) revealed the same pattern as for young White mothers. Younger mothers delivered more preterm births for both parities one and two. Also, the Black and White contour levels were shifted for each parity and maternal age group in the same manner as the race shift shown earlier (Figure 4).

Figure 8 shows the effect directly of first parity (dashed line) versus second parity (solid line) for four maternal age groups. The fifth maternal age group (30–34) is displayed in the lower panel of the left side of Figure 9. The innermost contour level consistently shows a tendency of more postterm deliveries in first parity compared to second parity births within each maternal age group, except for the maternal age group 18 years or younger. There is also a tendency for second parity births to be heavier than first parity. In contrast to maternal age contour shifts, first and second parity differences do not appear in the two outermost contour levels. Again, this implies that maternal age alone, instead of parity alone, is more related to the occurrence of preterm and low birth weight babies.

Figure 9 shows comparisons between parity two and four other parity groups for one selected maternal age category, 30–34 years. This age group was chosen in order that sufficient numbers of sixth and higher

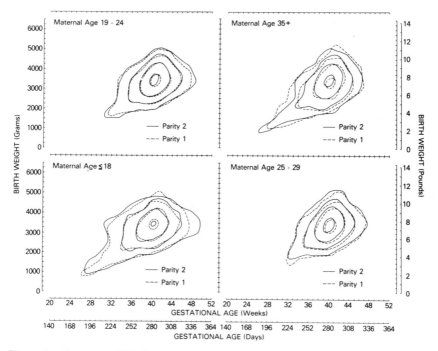

Figure 8. **Contours of Birth Weight and Gestational Age Distributions for First and Second Births (Parities One and Two) by Maternal Age for U.S. White Single Live Births, 1968.**

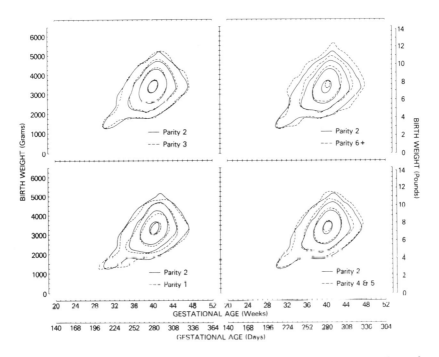

Figure 9. **Contours of Birth Weight and Gestational Age Distributions by Parity for Births of Mothers Aged 30–34 Years for U.S. White Single Live Births, 1968.**

parity as well as first parity births would be available for computing stable contour levels. The gestational age shift noticed in Figure 8 between the innermost contours of first and second parity births is not maintained in the contrast between second and third or higher parities. Thus, the increase in postterm deliveries is an effect which distinguishes first parity births from all other parities.

The differences in contour levels between parity two (solid line), the standard for each panel, and parity six or higher are the most marked. These higher parities are more likely to result in heavier babies than are second parity births. Yet this tendency for increased birth weight is not simply analogous, for example, to the differences between the Norwegian and US White births shown in Figure 5. Note that the portion of the contour levels for birth weights below 2500 gm. does superimpose for second and sixth and higher parities. Also, the innermost contour for sixth and higher parity has shrunk in size. Hence, the suggestion is that babies which at parity two would have been average in size are born much heavier if they were parity six or higher. The whole bivariate distribution has not shifted, as seemed to be the case for the Norwegian and US White comparison. Parities four and five, which have been combined into one group, show the same tendency as do parities six or higher, although not as marked. Another inference which can be drawn from this figure is that parity two or higher does not seem to alter the frequency of low birth weight and preterm births, at least for maternal age group 30–34. Again, this is in contrast to the influences of extreme maternal ages demonstrated previously.

To this point, the data have not shown any major influence of parity on the frequency of low birth weight and preterm births. However, we have not yet looked at the effect of extreme or unusual parity and maternal age combinations. Figure 10 compares a typical parity with a less typical parity for each maternal age group shown. For example, for the maternal age group 18 years or younger, first parity (solid lines) is considered here the typical parity. Third parity (dashed lines), however, is not considered typical for this age group. The effect of this inappropriately high parity-for-age, judged from the contours, is to reduce the number of term live births of average weight. The size of the innermost contour for these third parity births has shrunk dramatically, even when compared to second parity births in this age group (see Figure 7). There is a concomitant increase in low birth weight and preterm births for the third parity births to mothers less than 19 years old.

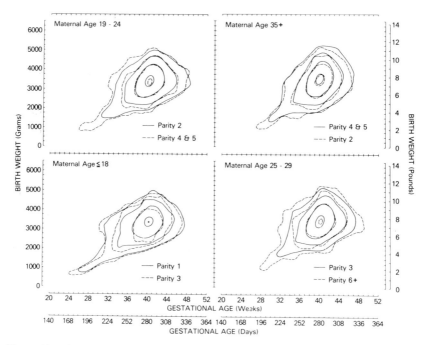

Figure 10.   **Contours of Birth Weight and Gestational Age Distributions for Typical and Less Typical Combinations of Parity and Maternal Age for U.S. White Single Live Births, 1968.**

For the maternal ages 19–24, second parity (solid lines) was chosen as typical, whereas fourth and fifth parities (dashed lines) were chosen as less typical. Again the size of the innermost contour has shrunk for the inappropriately high parity-for-age group compared to the normal parity-for-age group. Again there is an increase of low birth weight and preterm births for the high parity-for-age group.

For maternal ages 25–29, third parity (solid lines) was chosen as typical. Parities six or higher (dashed lines) were considered high for this maternal age group. Again the size of the innermost contour has shrunk for the high parity-for-age group compared to the normal parity-for-age group. There is also an increase in preterm (and some postterm) and low birth weight births.

The upper panel on the right side of this figure shows the maternal age group 35 years or older. Fourth and fifth parities (solid lines) are considered rather typical at this age. Parity two is atypically low for this age group. This comparison is the converse of the other three comparisons in that the less typical parity is low instead of high for age. The size of the innermost contour is not smaller for the inappropriately low parity group. There are, however, more low birth weight babies among second births compared to fourth and fifth parity births for mothers aged 35 and older.

These comparisons have shown that an interaction associated with unusual parity and maternal age combinations can increase the relative proportion of low birth weight and preterm births. In particular, this is true for high parity births to mothers under 30 years old. Otherwise, maternal age alone seems to affect the proportion of low birth weight and preterm births more than does parity by itself.

FETAL MORTALITY AS A FUNCTION OF BIRTH WEIGHT AND GESTATIONAL AGE

Shifts in the contours of birth weight and gestational age distributions have revealed several potentially important differences in comparisons among various population subgroups. A shift in birth weight or gestational age, however, does not necessarily imply a higher risk for mortality or morbidity. In this section we will examine some fetal mortality risks as a function of birth weight and gestational age, using the contour method.

Figure 11 compares the fetal "viability" contours for US White and Black single births, 1968. Previously (Fig. 4), we have shown that Blacks have a higher frequency of preterm and low birth weight births compared to Whites. In this figure we are comparing the risk of a fetal death for given birth weight and gestational age for all products of con-

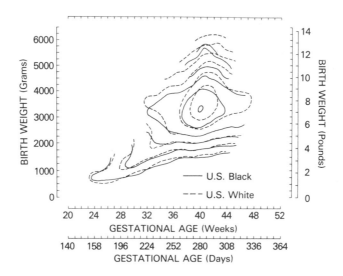

Figure 11.   **Contours of Fetal Viability by Race for U.S. Single Births, 1968.**

ception—live births plus fetal deaths—surviving through the first 20 weeks of gestation.

The method for producing these contours is similar to that explained earlier for the live birth contours. In each 500 gm. and single week cell of the original tables, there is a count, m_{ij}, of fetal deaths and a count, n_{ij}, of the 50% sample of live births. The proportion, $p_{ij} = m_{ij}/(m_{ij} + 2n_{ij})$, of fetal deaths in all products of conception is formed. (Suppose "i" indexes birth weight categories and that "j" indexes weeks of gestation.) The logit transformation, $\ln(p_{ij}/(1 - p_{ij}))$, is used on the proportions in each cell, instead of the natural log transformation used earlier to construct contours based on counts of the live birth distributions.[3] The same computer algorithm is used to compute contours of the fetal viability surface. These contour levels are equally spaced on a logit scale. The only modification to this scheme was that the original fetal death counts were smoothed using counts in neighboring cells of the table before applying the above procedure (see Hoffman et al., 1974). This was necessary in order to eliminate "noise" from zero counts in some cells of the fetal death table. The much larger population of live births made it unnecessary to smooth those counts.

In addition to explaining the method for constructing contour levels

---

[3] The argument for using the logit transform rather than a log transform for proportions is based on a notion of symmetry. Since proportions are bounded by zero and one, an appropriate transform should preserve symmetry around 0.5. For example, 0.9 and 0.1 should be displaced relative to 0.5, by an equal amount after transformation. The logit transform has this property, while a log transform does not.

for fetal mortality surfaces, it is necessary to indicate what each contour level specifies in Figure 11. Numerical values associated with each contour level may be found in Table 2. The innermost contour level (solid line for US Blacks and dashed line for US Whites) represents 2.5 fetal deaths per 1000 products of conception which have survived through the first 20 weeks. The second contour level represents a risk of 6.7 fetal deaths per 1000 products of conception. The difference between each neighboring contour level (for either the solid line or dashed line contour levels) is one unit on a logit scale. The relative risk of a fetal death outcome increased 2.7-fold in moving from the innermost contour level to the next outer contour level. However, the decrease in relative risk of a fetal death outcome is 2.3-fold in moving from the outermost contour level to the next inner contour level. This demonstrates that the change which occurs in moving from one of these fetal mortality risk contour levels to an adjacent one is not constant in terms of the underlying proportions of fetal deaths. This is a feature of logit scale somewhat different from the more familiar logarithm scale. The outermost contour level corresponds to a rate of 269 fetal deaths per 1000 products of conception, or more than one out of every four births.

In the region below 2500 gm. and from 36–40 weeks, which encompasses a large proportion of the small-for-date births, the fetal viability contour levels are almost parallel to the gestational age axis. The outermost contour level, between 36 and 40 weeks, is very close to 1500 gm. The next contour level is very close to 1750 gm. The third contour level is close to 2000 gm.; the next is close to 2250 gm. Also, both sets of contour levels, Black and White, are nearly identical in this region. This finding is equivalent to the statement that each 250-gm. decrement in birth weight, for this range of gestational age, increases the risk of fetal death by one unit of logit risk. Dropping from 2500 to 1500 gm., the risk of fetal death increases about 40 times, from 6.7 per 1000 to 269 per 1000.

Perhaps the most striking feature of Figure 11 is that the contour levels are nearly identical for Whites and Blacks below 2500 gm. Above 2500 gm. White fetal viability contour levels are shifted above the corresponding Black fetal viability contour levels in the weight dimension. Thus a Black birth weighing 4250 gm. at 39 weeks is at the increased risk of 18 fetal deaths per 1000 products of conception which survive through the first 20 weeks of gestation. The risk of fetal death in White births is 6.7 per 1000 at the same weight and gestational age. The increase in relative risk for Blacks compared to Whites in the high birth weight region is consistent with earlier observations (Baumgartner, 1962; Erhardt et al., 1964; Wiener and Milton, 1970) on relative mortality of White and Black births in relation to birth weight.

Overall, higher weight births are at an increased risk to fetal death compared to average weight births in both the White and Black populations. Also, it appears from this figure that the birth weight which minimizes fetal loss for the Black births may be lower than that for the White births.

Figure 11 has shown that for a given high weight, Black births are at an increased risk of fetal death compared to White births. Also, low birth weight babies of Blacks and Whites are at virtually the same levels of risk for fetal death. Previously (Fig. 4), we have observed that Blacks deliver relatively more preterm and low weight births than do Whites. However, this feature of Black births has not affected the fetal mortality risk for any specific combination of low birth weight and gestational age. Instead, there are simply more Black births affected by the high risk associated with being preterm and low birth weight.

These contour comparisons seem to conflict with what some authors have suggested, namely, that Blacks have lower mortality rates compared to Whites for shorter gestational ages. However, this sudy has focused only on fetal mortality. Similar contour diagrams for perinatal, neonatal and infant mortality could be informative on the subject of varying mortality rates by birth weight and gestational age for Whites and Blacks. Also, similar mortality contours could be valuable as a tool in describing differences in perinatal, neonatal and infant mortality between countries. Such a comparison between Norwegian and US births is underway and will be presented elsewhere.

SCHEMES FOR CLASSIFICATION OF BIRTH WEIGHT AND GESTATIONAL AGE

Bivariate contour displays have been used to demonstrate considerable shifts in the frequency distributions of births by birth weight and gestational age both between countries and between ethnic groups within a country. In addition, we have endeavored to show the usefulness of this method of analysis for displaying the effects of variables like maternal age and parity on BW and GA distributions. In the following, a brief discussion will be given of some of the currently used schemes for defining BW and GA groups which have been proposed to facilitate summary comparisons, whether derived from local or international data sources. Contour diagrams are presented in conjunction with each classification scheme shown in Figure 12.

The discussion of classification schemes of birth weight and gestational age is based on a consideration of the relative merits of fixed standards, in which specific cutoffs can be applied separately to birth weight and gestational age data. This choice excludes consideration of the population-specific percentile approach. To use a classification scheme

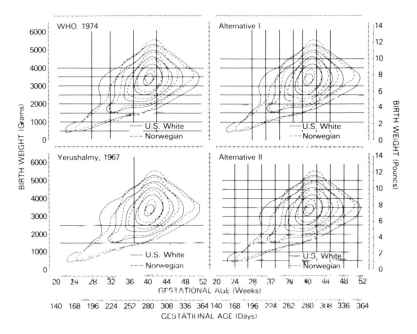

Figure 12. **Classification Schemes for Birth Weight and Gestational Age Superimposed on Contours of Birth Weight and Gestational Age Distributions for U.S. White Single Female Live Births, 1968, and Norwegian Single Female Live Births, 1967–1971.**

based on percentiles normally requires the original ungrouped birth weight and gestational age information, which is another reason for not considering classification schemes based on percentiles.

One of the simplest successful schemes for classifying joint information by birth weight and gestational age has been proposed by Yerushalmy (1967), and this method is shown in Figure 12 superimposed on the contours of two populations: Norwegian female single live births (dashed lines) and the US White female single live births (solid lines). Yerushalmy's classification defines one normal group, namely, births weighing more than 2500 gm. with gestational ages of 37 or more weeks, and four other groups of preterm and/or low birth weight. One of these groups consists of births which are very premature in the sense of weighing less than 1500 gm. Two more groups are established by dividing births with weights between 1500 and 2500 gm. into two groups: those with gestational ages less than 37 weeks versus those with gestational ages of 37 weeks or more. The former of these two groups represents mainly births with birth weight appropriate for gestational age, whereas the group with longer gestations reflects small-for-date babies. The remaining category refers to births greater than 2500 gm. but less than 37 weeks of gestation. This group consists primarily of large-for-date births.

This classification scheme has the fewest number of categories of any illustrated in Figure 12. Yerushalmy's classification is attractive in part because of its simplicity and in part because it treats the data as essentially bivariate in nature. A still simpler classification could be obtained by eliminating the birth weight cutoff at 1500 gm. Then there would be only four categories based on 37 weeks and 2500 gm.

The upper panel of the left side of Figure 12 displays a recent informal proposal of the World Health Organization superimposed on the same set of Norwegian and US White female single live birth contour levels. A report by a WHO working group (1974) suggests categories separately for birth weight and gestational age. For birth weight, the report recommends 500-gm. categories. For gestational age, calculated from LMP, the following grouping is suggested: less than 28 weeks (under 196 days); 28–31 weeks (196–223 days); 32–36 weeks (224–258 days); 37–41 weeks (259–293 days); and 42 weeks (or 294 days) and over.

Implicit in the report is a suggestion that more appropriate cutoffs may exist for a joint birth weight and gestational age classification system. For example, in the report there is a statement that 27 weeks corresponds to 1000 gm. more closely than does 28 weeks. Also, the report suggests that 36 weeks corresponds more closely to 2500 gm. in several data sets than does 37 weeks. Because of past conventions, however, the report chooses not to suggest realignment of already well established international standard cutoffs for gestational age. Nevertheless, the still older definition for preterm births was less than 38 weeks (Dubowitz, 1974). Postterm births are defined as those occurring at 42 weeks and over. Preterm births are classified as early preterm (28–31 weeks) and late preterm (32–36 weeks). Unfortunately, the implication for a joint classification based on these recommendations is that there should be a cutoff at 1750 gm., which agrees with the 32-week cutoff. This is not possible, however, if birth weight is grouped into 500-gm. intervals.

Alternative I, shown in the upper panel of the right side of Figure 12, is a modification of the WHO recommendations. It achieves eight categories each on birth weight and gestational age, using the underlying contour diagrams to guide the selection of cutoffs. As in the WHO report, 28 weeks and 37 weeks are retained. However, three rather than two subdivisions are made on preterm births, which correspond to the three 500-gm. intervals from 1000 to 2500 gm. Term births are split into two groups: 37–38 and 39–41 weeks. The former of the two corresponds with birth weights from 2500 to 3000 gm. Postterm births are also subdivided into two groups: 42–44 and 45 or more weeks. The corresponding cutoff on the weight axis comes at 4500 gm. This modified grid has been used by Bakketeig (1977) to analyze the tendency to repeat birth weight and gestational age in subsequent pregnancies.

Alternative II, displayed in the lower panel of the right side of Figure 12, uses 10 cutoff lines to define 11 groups each for gestational age and birth weight. The principle behind this proposal is that of an equally spaced grid with a rule that 500-gm. birth weight intervals correspond to three-week intervals in gestational age. The only two-week interval from 37–38 completed weeks shown in Alternative I has been eliminated. Recognition that 27 weeks corresponds closely to 1000 gm. and that 36 weeks corresponds well with 2500 gm. has led us to shift each of the cutoffs prior to 37 weeks by one week. Equally spaced grids have several mathematical advantages. For example, simple interpolation formulae can be used to convert equally spaced data to other less regular groupings (Hamming, 1962). Converting irregularly spaced data to other groupings by interpolation methods is much more difficult.

The choice among the four grids displayed in Figure 12 (or grids similar to the ones displayed) should be determined by a variety of competing factors. For relatively small data sets, Yerushalmy's categories may serve well. The choice among the WHO standards and either Alternatives I or II for larger data sets should depend on the subsequent use of the data. Alternative I preserves most of the elements in the WHO recommendations, while Alternative II is perhaps easier to use for analytical purposes.

DISCUSSION

Several previous publications, e.g., the American Academy of Pediatrics (1967), the Second European Congress of Perinatal Medicine (1970), and a recent preliminary report by the World Health Organization (1974), have all dealt with issues of classifying—but more specifically, standardizing—the reporting of births by birth weight and gestational age. All of the above efforts were the result of select committees representing experts with many different points of view. The aim of this study has been to provide some perspective on the nature of the problem of classifying births on the basis of two highly correlated variables, birth weight and gestational age. The principal analytic tool which we have employed is the description of bivariate distributions of births, as a function of birth weight and gestational age, using contour levels.

Contour levels of bivariate distributions of births were used to a limited degree in some early studies of birth weight and gestational age data (Karn and Penrose, 1951; Fraccaro, 1956). Recently, Goldstein and Peckham (1976) have presented contours of neonatal mortality surfaces for British births included in the 1958 British Perinatal Survey. Although the methodology used in constructing contours in the latter study was different from the methods used in this paper and in Hoffman et al., (1974), the overall impression given from their bivariate description of neonatal mortality is rather similar to that shown by the plot of the fetal viability surface in this report. Neither perinatal mortality as a function of either birth weight or gestational age separately, nor conventional percentiles of birth weight for weeks of gestation, convey an impression of the data resembling that based on the bivariate approach. Namely, the contours of the fetal viability surface suggest that it is primarily birth weight and not gestational age which is changing the fetal mortality risk for birth weight below 2500 gm. In this region the contour levels are almost parallel to the gestational age axis. However, a tenth percentile curve would cut across several of these contour levels. This is a finding which we feel deserves the attention of clinicians and research workers who have been using percentiles or other methods for classifying births into different risk categories.

The results demonstrated using contour levels of live birth distributions in this report have many antecedents in the literature of the subject. The contour method of analysis has served to display rather complicated interactions, when they exist, in a tractable manner. Descriptions of the shifts in birth weight and in gestational age by race and sex in the United States have been mentioned previously by Anderson, Brown and Lyon (1943), Taback (1951), Henderson and Kay (1967) and Penchaszadeh et al. (1972), although these researchers were not using contours to describe birth weight and gestational age distributions. When the effects are as strong and relatively simple as they are in the race and sex comparisons, one does not need a trenchant method for discovery.

The advantage of the contour approach in the analysis of births by birth weight and gestational age is perhaps best illustrated in the figures comparing different maternal age and parity groups. Many reports have dealt with the effects of maternal age and parity on, for example, perinatal or infant mortality as the outcome of interest (Yerushalmy, 1938; Karn and Penrose, 1951; Newcombe, 1966; Knox, 1971; Vavra and Querec, 1973; Dott and Fort, 1975; Sandahl, 1975; Johnson, Bjerkedal and Bakketeig, 1977). Some studies (Westphal and Joshi, 1964; Selvin and Garfinkel, 1972) have analyzed the percent of low birth weight or preterm infants in relation to parental age and birth order. However, there are few studies which describe joint birth weight and gestational age effects for combined parity and maternal age groups. MacMahon (1974) has summed up the situation by stating:

> The relations between maternal age and parity, between these two variables and infant mortality, and between them and other variables related to infant mortality risk (such as socioeconomic status)

are complex and so far have defied attempts to isolate their under-lying determinants.

We feel the contour diagrams for maternal age and parity groups shown in this report have demonstrated a way to sort out relationships between these two variables and their interaction with birth weight and gestational age variables in the US data. Nevertheless, explanations for the apparent differences between combinations of parity and maternal age groups shown in this study will have to await new studies aimed at discriminating between competing hypotheses.

We have attempted to avoid suggesting a single classification scheme for presenting birth weight and gestational age data. Rather, our inten-tion has been to suggest some considerations necessary to understand and use alternative classification systems. Our point of view has been to use the bivariate approach to birth weight and gestational age data, as illustrated by the contour diagrams and Yerushalmy's system of classi-fying births. The development of standards based on population-specific percentiles has not been dealt with extensively. Percentile graphs with refinements to take into account parity, mother's height or weight, race and sex of the newborn, etc. have been presented in several publications (Tanner and Thomson, 1970; Bjerkedal, Bakketeig and Lehmann, 1973; Hoffman et al., 1974; Chamberlain et al., 1975). In spite of the large exposure which the percentile method has already had in this field, we have found it fruitful to develop and expound the bivariate approach to birth weight and gestational age data using contour diagrams.

Examples have been given of the utility of contour diagrams for displaying bivariate birth weight and gestational age distributions for births and perinatal events, such as fetal mortality. This method is considered valuable in making international comparisons of vital sta-tistics, not as a substitute for but as a supplement to other valid methods of comparison.

ACKNOWLEDGEMENTS

The authors wish to acknowledge Mr. Robert A. Israel of the National Center for Health Statistics who provided us with computer tapes of the 1968 US births and fetal deaths. Also, the authors wish to express their gratitude to Professor Tor Bjerkedal and his staff at the Medical Birth Registry of Norway, Institute of Hygiene and Social Medicine, Univer-sity of Bergen, for having made the Norwegian data available for analysis.

COMMENT

Tables of the original data used in the construction of the contour diagrams are available from the authors. These tables were newly derived from the actual data on computer tapes provided by the National Center for Health Statistics for the US data. The maternal age and parity comparisons given in this report were not part of the verbal presentation at the workshop.

TEXT REFERENCES

American Academy of Pediatrics, Committee on Fetus and Newborn: Nomenclature for Duration of Gestation, Birth Weight and Intra-uterine Growth. Pediatrics 39 (1967)935–939

Anderson, N. A.; Brown, E. W.; Lyon, R. A.: Causes of Prematurity. III: Influence of Race and Sex on Duration of Gestation and Weight at Birth. Amer J Dis Child 65(1943)523–535

Ashbrook, J. D.; Sande, G.: A User's Guide to the Integrated Plotting Package. Report of the Division of Computer Research and Technology, National Institutes of Health, Bethesda, Md., 1975

Bakketeig, L. S.: The Risk of Repeated Preterm or Low Birth Weight Delivery. In: The Epidemiology of Prematurity, ed. by D. M. Reed and F. J. Stanley. Urban & Schwarzenberg, Baltimore, 1977

Battaglia, F. C.; Frazier, T. M.; Hellegers, A. E.: Birth Weight, Gestational Age, and Pregnancy Outcome with Special Reference to High Birth Weight-Low Gestational Age Infant. Pediatrics 37 (1966)417–422

Baumgartner, L.: The Public Health Significance of Low Birth Weight in the U.S.A. Bull WHO 26(1962)175–182

Birkhoff, G.; Garabedian, H. L.: Smooth Surface Interpolation. J Math & Physics 39(1968)258–268

Bjerkedal, T; Bakketeig, L.: Medical Registration of Births in Norway during the 5-year Period 1967–71. Institute of Hygiene & Social Medicine, University of Bergen, Norway, 1975

Bjerkedal, T.; Bakketeig, L.; Lehmann, E. H.: Percentiles of Birth Weights of Single, Live Births at Different Gestation Periods (Based on 125,485 Births in Norway, 1967 and 1968). Acta Paediat Scand 62(1973)449–457

Chamberlain, R.; Chamberlain, G.; Howlett, B.; Claireaux, A.: British Births 1970. I: The First Week of Life. Heinemann Medical Books, London, 1975

Cramér, H.: Mathematical Methods in Statistics. Princeton University Press, Princeton, N.J., 1946

Dott, A. B.; Fort, A. T.: The Effect of Maternal Demographic Factors on Infant Mortality Rates. Amer J Obstet Gynecol 123(1975)847–860

Dubowitz, V.: The Infant of Inappropriate Size. In: Size at Birth (Ciba Foundation Symposium 27, new series), pp 47–64. Elsevier-Excerpta Medica-North Holland, Amsterdam, 1974

Erhardt, C. L.; Joshi, G. B.; Nelson, F. G.; Kroll, B. H.; Weiner, E. E.: Influence of Weight and Gestation on Perinatal and Neonatal Mortality by Ethnic Group. Amer J Public Health 54(1964)1841–1855

Fraccaro, M.: A Contribution to the Study of Birth Weight Based on an Italian Sample. Ann Hum Genet 20(1956) 282–297

Goldstein, H.; Peckham, C.: Birthweight, Gestation, Neonatal Mortality and Child Development. In: The Biology of Human Fetal Growth, pp. 81–102, ed. by D. F. Roberts and A. M. Thompson. Taylor & Francis, London, 1976

Hammes, L. M.; Treloar, A. E.: Gestational Interval from Vital Records. Amer J Public Health 60(1970)1496–1505

Hamming, R. W.: Numerical Methods for Scientists and Engineers. McGraw-Hill, New York, 1962

Henderson, M.; Kay, J.: Differences in

Duration of Pregnancy. Arch Environ Health 14(1967)904-911

Hoffman, H. J.; Stark, C. R.; Lundin, F. E., Jr.; Ashbrook, J. D.: Analysis of Birth Weight, Gestational Age, and Fetal Viability, U.S. Births, 1968. Obstet Gynec Survey 29(1974)651-681

Johnson, C. A.; Bjerkedal, T.; Bakketeig, L.: Patterns of Perinatal and Infant Death in Norway. In preparation.

Karn, M. N.; Pernrose, L. S.: Birth Weight and Gestation Time in Relation to Maternal Age, Parity and Infant Survival. Ann Eugen 16(1951)147-164

Knox, G. E.: Teenage Mothers. Minn Med 54(1971)701-705

Lubchenco, I. O.; Hansman, C.; Dressler, M.; Boyd, E.: Intrauterine Growth as Estimated from Liveborn Birth-Weight Data at 24 to 42 Weeks of Gestation. Pediatrics 32(1963)793-800

MacMahon, B.: Infant Mortality in the United States In: Mortality and Morbidity in the United States, pp. 189-209, ed. by C. I. Erhardt und J. E. Berlin. Harvard University Press, Cambridge, Mass., 1974

McKeown, T.; Gibson, J. R.: Observations on All Births (23,970) in Birmingham, 1947. IV: "Premature Birth." Brit Med J 2(1951)513-517

National Center for Health Statistics: Vital Statistics of the United States 1968, Vol. 1—Natality, Vol. 2—Mortality (Part A). U.S. Government Printing Office, Washington, D.C., 1970

Newcombe, H. B.: Environmental versus Genetic Interpretations of Birth Order Effects. Eugen Quart 12(1966)90-101

Penchaszadeh, V. B.; Hardy, J. B.; Mellits, E. D.; Cohen, B. H.; McKusick, V. A.: Growth and Development in an "Inner City" Population: An Assessment of Possible Biological and Environmental Influences. I: Intra-uterine Growth. Johns Hopkins Med J 130(1972)384-397

Penchaszadeh, V. B.; Hardy, J. B.; Mellits, E. D.; Cohen, B. H.; McKusick, V. A.: Growth and Development in an "Inner City" Population: An Assessment of Possible Biological and Environmental Influences. II: The Effect of Certain Maternal Characteristics on Birth Weight, Gestational Age and Intra-uterine Growth. Johns Hopkins Med J 131(1972)11-23

Pritchard, J. A.; MacDonald, P. C.: Williams Obstetrics, 15th ed. Appleton-Century Crofts, New York, 1976

Sandahl, B.: Short Term Changes in Still-birth Rates in Sweden, 1965-1971. Acta Obstet Gynec Scand 54(1975)45-48

Second European Congress of Perinatal Medicine: Working Party to Discuss Nomenclature Based on Gestational Age and Birth Weight. Arch Dis Child 45 (1970)730

Selvin, D.; Garfinkel, J.: The Relationship between Parental Age and Birth Order with the Percentage of Low Birth-Weight Infants. Hum Biol 44(1972)501-510

Taback, M.: Birth Weight and Length of Gestation with Relation to Prematurity. JAMA 146(1951)897-901

Tanner, J. M.; Thomson, A. M.: Standards for Birth Weight at Gestation Periods of 32 to 42 Weeks Allowing for Maternal Height and Weight. Arch Dis Child 45 (1970)566-569

Tukey, J. W.: Exploratory Data Analysis, Vol. 3, Limited Preliminary Edition. Addison-Wesley, Reading, Mass., 1971

Vavra, H. M.; Querec, L. J.: A Study of Infant Mortality from Linked Records by Age of Mother, Total-Birth Order, and Other Variables, United States, 1960 Live-Birth Cohort. Vital and Health Statistics, Series 20, No. 14, DHEW Pub. No. (HRA) 74-1851, National Center for Health Statistics, U.S. Government Printing Office, Washington, D.C., 1973

Weiner, G.; Milton, T.: Demographic Correlates of Low Birth Weight. Amer J Epidem 91(1970)260-272

Westphal, M. C.; Joshi, G. B.: The Inter-relationship of Birth Weight, Length of Gestation, and Neonatal Mortality. Clin Obstet Gynec 7(1964)670-686

World Health Organization, Scientific Group on Health Statistics: Methodology Related to Perinatal Events, Report, pp 1-32. WHO Document ICD/74.4, Geneva, 1974

Yerushalmy, J.: Neonatal Mortality by Order of Birth and Age of Parents. Amer J Hyg 28(1938)244-270

Yerushalmy, J.: The Classification of Newborn Infants by Birth Weight and Gestational Age. J Pediatr 71(1967)164-172

DISCUSSION

Dr. Rush: In Figure 4 would you explain what it means when the contour is further left.

Mr. Hoffman: It means that there are relatively more Black babies that are preterm (also low birth weight) compared to White babies.

Dr. Susser: Well, perhaps another explanation may be that contours should be perfectly circular or elliptical without showing any departure from symmetry. What is the basis from which you move?

Mr. Hoffman: To answer the question let me mention that in a classic paper Karn and Penrose (1951), fitted contour levels to birth weight-gestational age data. What they actually did was to fit a bivariate Gaussian or normal surface which forced the contours to be ellipses. The contours in Figure 1 were constructed without using any such parametric model. They are in fact smooth interpolations based on the original data. Hence there is no requirement that the contours appear elliptical.

Prof. Meyer: Is that a frequency distribution?

Mr. Hoffman: These are merely contours of bivariate frequency distributions of live births as a function of birth weight and gestational age.

Dr. Hardy: If you had the ideal situation, would the contours resemble a bull's eye target?

Mr. Hoffman: Let me mention again that these are derived from tables of log transformed frequency counts. If one drew contours based on the original data without first taking log transforms then more contour levels would appear in the center region, simply because most births occur there. This is precisely the region where the contour lines appear as nearly perfect ellipses in Figure 1. In this restricted region of the bivariate surface the Gaussian, or normal, distribution fits well. The log transform of the data, however, makes it possible to delineate several contour levels in the tails, or extremes, of the bivariate distribution.

Prof. Meyer: It seems to me that our future work will benefit greatly if we can all agree now to use the new ICD definitions (9th revision). In these, the word "prematurity" is no longer used. Instead, they have defined "low birth weight" as under 2500 grams (instead of under 2501 grams) and "preterm" as less than 37 completed weeks of pregnancy (less than 259 days). It is a great step forward to consider birth weight and gestation separately, as the risk factors may be different, and the implications are also different.

The risk of preterm delivery is worse the earlier the delivery occurs, with no survivial before 20 weeks, and with increasing possibility of survival with time up until term. The low weight and high risk of these babies is secondary to the fact that they have had too little time to grow. Because most of the fetal deaths occur early in gestation and deliver sometime soon after death, these babies are preterm and are low weight because of this and probably also because of whatever caused the death. For these babies we should study the causes of death in utero and the causes of preterm delivery, and we are not primarily interested in the birth weight or the growth rate. About two thirds of the Ontario study deaths were in this group.

In term babies without malformations we are primarily interested in factors causing low birth weight, and we know that there is a wide range of mortality risk for small babies. If we think in terms of an optimum weight for each baby, this optimum would vary with maternal size, race, sex of child, altitude, maternal smoking, and many other factors. I think we want to know how the factors that result in lower than optimum birth weight are also causing increased mortality and to look for possible interventions in these areas. In other words we will make progress by taking account of the fact that 2500 grams does not define risk without other information, and that known causes of birth weight below this level may vary from benign to lethal.

Another important area of study is to follow up children of known birth weight to see whether there are long-term effects of factors that reduce birth weight but do not cause death. The same should be done for surviving children who were delivered preterm.

Dr. Stanley: Obviously many studies have got to be done again using different outcomes, both gestation and birth weight.

Dr. Rush: There are methodologic problems which are implicit in this study. One follows from the observation of Milner and Richards (1974) that at all early gestations there is a bimodal distribution of birth weight; the heavier mode is at constant weight, while the lighter mode changes and is heavier with advancing gestation, until it merges at term with the first mode. The heavier mode is surely due to error, either advertent or inadvertent. Also, the earlier the gestation, the more that the overall mean of the bimodal distribution is affected by error, both because the mean of the higher mode contributes more, and the number of subjects in the higher mode is relatively larger.

Mr. Hoffman: May I respond to that comment before you go on to the next one? I think that is not a flaw actually in the bivariate approach. I think the bivariate approach allows you to look at the structural ridge separately from the ridge that you are pointing out as the high weight for preterm delivery. Also I am not quite sure—I don't feel that I know—that all of that is due to error. I think that I would be much more struck, if you look at Figure 1, if the contribution of the large-for-dates ridge was confined primarily to a region near 3000 grams and 28 weeks in gestation. Actually the ridge contributes substantially to births near term, and it is really impossible to decide whether those are real or misclassified babies.

Dr. Susser: 2000 grams and 20 weeks—it is impossible.

Mr. Hoffman: Those are very small numbers, but we are talking about the general tendency. Are all of those babies due to error? I am not willing to say that, and I think there are several here who do not feel that all the reported gestational ages contributing to the large-for-dates ridge are in error.

Dr. Hardy: Well, I think that certainly many of those babies are due to error, but when we looked at this in terms of outcome for the babies in the upper mode and compared their outcome with babies of similar weight but 38 weeks gestation, we found that the babies of lower gestation in this upper mode had an outcome that was less favorable than the controls.

It is my opinion that the upper mode represents a mixture of babies who are truly large-for-dates and babies who are misclassified.

Dr. Rush: I disagree. Otherwise the distribution wouldn't be bimodal, but would be skewed. We know there are social correlates with misreporting. Also, misreporting, whatever the origin, identifies a group which might be predicted to be at higher risk for developmental abnormality, either because of illegitimate birth (with a motive to consciously change dates) or for a variety of reasons, such as lower educational level.

There is yet another problem. If one is using multivariate analysis (this doesn't apply to the contour analyses) results may be misleading when one variable is measured with higher error than another: wrong conclusions can be reached.

Gestations reported in vital statistics may mislead us if we are interested in the functional significance of gestational length. We need special data sources to judge this issue.

Dr. Alberman: I find it very worrying. I just wanted to say that the British data showed exactly what Janet Hardy said, that error or no error, the second mode at the earlier weeks always have a higher mortality.

Dr. Stanley: They may contain women who bleed early in pregnancy whose offspring also have a higher mortality.

Prof. Meyer: I wonder if we could discuss whether we are creating more confusion than clarity in analyzing birth weight and gestation jointly instead of separately. Even though there are probably more errors in gestation than in birth weight, I think you are better off looking at how each acts alone.

Dr. Rush: Since there is interaction among these variables (the error is not linear, but is larger at shorter gestations), birth weight and gestation should be considered simultaneously.

Dr. Terris: I take exception. There is no reason why you can't treat them separately. There is always observed error, and there is error in the choice of cases and controls. You will have some errors here. They will be rather small compared to your whole series.

Prof. Meyer: I don't see how looking at them together improves the error. It is there whether you look at them one at a time or together. I think it is easier if you look at them separately.

Dr. Susser: How do you handle the error? Milner and Richards (1974) used the rule of excluding all beyond two standard deviations. If you want to make the limit two and a half or three that is all right too since this would exclude values that are clearly not viable biologically.

Mr. Hoffman: It is necessary to stress what Dr. Bakketeig's data has shown that the delivery of an infant large-for-dates defines a group of women who have an increased risk for repeating subsequent large-for-date babies.

Dr. Bakketeig: If you look at Table 2 in my paper you will discover 845 mothers whose first births weighed between 3000 and 4000 grams and had a gestation age between 34 and 37 weeks. Of these mothers 8.9 percent produced a preterm 2nd birth, which indicates a significant tendency of repeating preterm birth.

Dr. Rush: Look at your far left column of the same table. You show data for 16 to 28 weeks gestation, and there is clear bimodality where in the first mode the mean is under 1000 grams and in the second mode the mean is between 3000 and 4000 grams, where you have 35 individuals. Now, if you all want to work with that as biologically possible, you are more than welcome to.

Mr. Hoffman: Actually, the point is what use are you going to make of these data? Should you arbitrarily begin to exclude data? I feel that one should report all the data collected in a uniform system. You will notice that we are not trying to attach an interpretation in this region since there are no rates calculated in the cells under 31 weeks and above 2000 grams. We are not trying to attach an interpretation there at all, but neither are we going to hide the data from you.

Dr. Rush: Of that group, about a fifth of the total are probably in error. If you were not looking at the bivariate distribution here, a high proportion of the women in the group delivering with gestations less than 31 weeks would have reported physiologically impossible data.

Mr. Hoffman: Right and that is why looking at the bivariate surface prevents you from falling into the trap.

Dr. Rush: It certainly seems a useful technique.

Dr. Alberman: I would like to say one thing and that is in many years of experience in looking through obstetric records the cardinal sin that an obstetrician can commit, as far as I am concerned, is to cross out the reported LMP. I have seen this time and time again. The LMP written in as reported by the woman and crossed out by the obstetrician, saying too small for dates, must be four weeks out. If we can beg obstetricians at least to keep the original LMP and perhaps record their impression of an LMP as well, this might clear up some of our problem.

Dr. Chase: I would like to raise a question, and maybe Dr. Placek can answer this. Has the National Center for Health Statistics looked at what difference this one gram change might make. I have seen many birth certificates with exactly 2500 grams written on them.

Dr. Placek: I just now checked Vital Statistics of the United States, Volume 1, Natality (1976), and our definition of low birth weight is 2500 grams or less instead of less than 2500 grams.

Dr. Chase: Actually in New York State we used under 2500 grams as the lower class before 1950. When WHO came out with their definitions of 2500 grams or less in 1950, New York State changed to the same WHO definitions that are used in the national data. It sounds like WHO is backtracking to something that existed before 1950. But, I am wondering about what statistical effect this has when one has a clump of births that are exactly 2500 grams, which were in the low birth weight class and which are now no longer going to be in the low birth weight category.

Dr. Placek: Mr. Heuser, the Branch Chief of the Natality Statistics Branch of the National Center for Health Statistics, can provide an answer.

Mr. Heuser: I don't think that this is going to be as much of a problem as it could have been. Because most of the birth weights are recorded in terms of pounds and ounces and then converted to grams, I don't believe there will be much shift one way or the other. If the majority of the weights were reported in grams, then there would be a bigger potential for this.

Dr. Chase: What percentage of the birth weights on the United States certificates are in pounds and ounces?

Mr. Heuser: I think it is close to 97 or 98 percent.

Dr. Chase: This is another statistical factor, then. About 97 percent of the weights are recorded in pounds and ounces and converted mechanically to grams. The conversion is from a coarser grouping to a finer grouping, which may be troublesome.

Dr. Davies: In Jerusalem, 0.8 percent of all births are recorded as 2500 grams. This is part of the reason that I had a hand in changing the WHO definition.

Dr. Mellits: I wish to address some possible problems and statistical considerations, and where possible to suggest solutions. In the previous discussion a lot has been said about bimodality and I disagree with some of the observations that have been made. Accepting that there is some error in reporting of LMP, it has also been shown conclusively that much of the data in the second mode is not, in fact, reporting error. This mode does not superimpose with the smaller mode four weeks later in gestation or on any general mode of the next distribution of four weeks off. There are differences in mortality and morbidity between the modes and these differences remain after controlling for socioeconomic conditions.

Some of the bimodality is reporting error and some could be biological. The separation of causes is not the important consideration. We should not be so concerned with definitions of prematurity *per se*, but should be concerned with what we are using them for. I would much rather see us concentrate on dimensions of outcome that we are interested in. All of us are concerned with mortality, so we could certainly start there. I suggest definitions of basic descriptor variables of interest, for example, birth weight and gestation, possibly race and sex, perhaps placental weight, perhaps more, in terms of where these outcomes of interest change.

For example, if the perinatal and/or neonatal death rates are examined as a function of birth weight, there is a steep descending line, which "breaks" or discontinues and then flattens out. In White infants that break, or flattening out, is at approximately 2500 grams. In Blacks it is not. In Blacks it is somewhat earlier, 2000 to 2250 grams, perhaps. Therefore, if one were to make an empirical or operational definition of prematurity based on the neonatal mortality rate then the prematurity rate for Blacks and Whites would be defined separately. In the data that I displayed earlier on placental weight, we looked at prematurity defined at 2500 grams. The data for Blacks was re-examined based on 2000 grams and intermediate levels. However, the results based on the two different cutoffs were similar. The bimodality question illustrates my belief that often we get too involved with methodology and definitions, and sometimes lose the real essence of what we are trying to accomplish.

Dr. Reed: The question that is important to us as researchers is what we need in the future to keep this clear. There will always be the lumpers and there will always be the splitters. But Dr. Bakketeig has shown that birth weight is the best predictor of future birth weight and that gestation is the best predictor of preterm delivery. I think it is therefore very apparent that, no matter which recommended cutoff points are used, both birth weight and gestation should be obtained. The decision to analyze them separately or together can depend upon the nature of the study.

Dr. Stark: Somewhat along the same lines, I would like to make a plea for reporting all of the data in a distribution and then use any rules and cutoffs that you like. But please report it all.

DISCUSSION REFERENCES

Karn, M. N., Penrose, L. S.: Birth Weight and Gestation Time in Relation to Maternal Age, Parity and Infant Survival. Ann. Eugen. 16(1951)147

Milner, R. D. and Richards, B. (1974) An Analysis of Birth Weight by Gestational Age of Infants Born in England and Wales, 1967 to 1971, the J. of Obstet. and Gynaecol. of the Brit. Comm., 81, 956-967

National Center for Health Statistics: Vital Statistics of the United States 1972, Vol 1—Natility. U.S. Government Printing Office, Washington, D.C., 1976

Descriptive and Analytic Studies of Etiology

Milton Terris, M.D.

I can't help remarking that I was surprised and pleased when I walked into this room to find the portrait of my hero, Joseph Goldberger, overlooking the conference table. Goldberger was undoubtedly the greatest epidemiologist ever produced by the United States. He worked with Rosenau on influenza and with Anderson on typhus fever. It was Goldberger who conquered pellagra in a series of classical studies, and this was done without benefit of discriminant function analysis, multiple regression or other fancy methods.

Now the basic characteristics of the Goldberger approach were as follows. On the issue of multiple causation versus the search for key factors, Goldberger always went for the jugular, a key rule in epidemiology which some people tend to forget. Of course, there are multiple causations, both in the infectious and the noninfectious diseases. The trick is to go for the key factors. This is what Goldberger did, as you know, very successfully.

Secondly, Goldberger was a master of experiment. I think some of you may know that he solved the problem of pellagra first by experiment and then by observation, reversing the general procedure in epidemiologic work. In his experiments with patients in asylums in Georgia and in childrens' orphanages, he was able to show that he could prevent pellagra by nutrition. Also, he was able to produce pellagra by means of a deficient diet among volunteers in the Rankin prison farm.

The third point about Goldberger, which was true of most of his generation and certainly of the people in the Hygienic Laboratory whose portraits you see on the walls of this room, was that he never separated off epidemiology as an esoteric discipline divorced from clinical medicine and from the laboratory sciences. As a matter of fact, when he studied the seven cotton mill villages in South Carolina, it was his staff that made the rounds and made the diagnoses.

Also, he did a lot of work in the laboratory. It was his group that discovered that black tongue in dogs was the analogue of pellagra in humans. He also did a tremendous amount of routine and unglamorous work trying to determine the anti-pellagra action of different foods, first using humans and then dogs with black tongue.

Fourthly, he never separated epidemiology from public health. This is a very common error, particularly in the United States at this time when epidemiologists are becoming more and more academic and more and more divorced from the problems involved in reducing the burden of illness and death in the population.

Goldberger made numerous proposals to improve agriculture in the South, such as diversification and other changes. He fostered the use of brewer's yeast and other pellagra-preventing foods. He conquered pellagra not because he thought about it as an academic exercise, but because in 1914 the Surgeon General ordered him to go down South and find out what caused pellagra and what could be done about it. He did very well indeed in following his orders.

I am using this discussion of Goldberger's work as an introduction because I think it is pertinent to what we are doing here. I am going to cover just a few of the many issues raised during the workshop, but first I want to raise the question of multiple causation versus looking for key factors.

I think it is extremely important that we don't get fixated on multiple causation, which has the psychological and philosophical effect of saying: well, we have a disease with 20 different causes; isn't that nice! I think we have to look instead for the key factors. They may not be there, but this is what our orientation has to be.

The main emphasis, therefore, has to be, not on global descriptive studies, although they play a useful role, but on two kinds of analytic studies: retrospective or case history studies on the one hand, and prospective or cohort studies on the other. The prospective studies should include not only observational investigations, but also experimental studies in the Goldberger tradition. These are the approaches where the emphasis must be placed, rather than on the demographic studies which are producing much the same information obtained from similar studies done 20 years ago.

On the question of the definition of prematurity, I disagree very strongly with those who say that it is not important. When I worked on cancer of the cervix or other cancers, I more or less knew what I was dealing with. But in the case of prematurity, we are dealing with an unfortunate definition. It is, as you know, a definition of convenience; WHO adopted it because there was no other measure available. It took a while before it was realized that the last menstrual period could be used to obtain a fairly good approximation of the period of gestation.

I think we ought to draw the logical conclusion, just as WHO has done, and that is to stop talking about prematurity. We have two entities to deal with, and let us separate them once and for all. Let us study the causes of preterm birth (the term WHO is using), regardless of the weight of the infants involved. And let us also study the causes of low birth weight in so-called normal children, in children born at term. Let us then see what the findings will be.

I am convinced that practically all of the studies, including mine, have to be done over again because they included apples and oranges—preterm infants and low weight term babies—in the single category of prematurity. What we have to do, and I hope the Institute will help us, is to reanalyze our data, where possible, and to carry out new studies, where required, in order to determine which factors belong with which entity, which are related to preterm birth and which are related to low birth weight in mature infants.

I am not too worried about observational error. If you have a case-control series on preterm birth that includes 800 infants and there is a 10% error in definition of the case, that is not so bad. There is error in every epidemiologic study, indeed in every scientific study, and we should accept this fact. If we have factors that are really involved in the etiology of these conditions, they will show up despite the error.

Another point I would like to make is that we have to tie in with the laboratory sciences, with pathology, with physiology, with biochemistry, both here at the Institute and in the university centers. We have to stop talking about these etiologic factors as though they exist in the sky. If they are indeed etiologic, then they operate through some kind of bio-logical mechanism. And we ought to be working with the people who study these mechanisms. The investigations of the effects of tobacco and of altitude have led us in this direction, and I believe we ought to do the same thing with regard to other problems.

Finally, I want to mention a number of things that I consider impor-tant. I think there is a need for intensive study of repeaters. Much will be learned from looking at repeaters in both the preterm and the low-birth-weight term infant groups.

I believe maternal weight before and during pregnancy, which was emphasized by a number of the speakers, is an area we ought to look into more thoroughly, and not by ourselves but with the laboratory scientists and the clinicians.

I found the point raised today on the role of hypertension to be very interesting, and I was surprised that there was so little reaction to it. Among other things, this might help explain at least some of the black/white differences in prematurity rates.

The report of low prematurity rates in American Indians is an important clue which ought to be followed up to see whether it is true and, if so, what there is about American Indians that might explain this finding.

Need for Future Epidemiologic Research: Studies for Prevention and Intervention

Irvin Emanuel, M.D.

Contemporary clinicians and biomedical scientists feel increasingly constrained in proposing and applying new treatments, even though they may appear rational. Part of the hesitancy relates to new government regulations, to medicolegal litigations and to a recent accumulation of examples in which new, and at the time, logical therapeutic regimes were instituted only to later prove worthless, harmful or even disastrous.

The proceedings of the Sixty-Ninth Ross Conference on Pediatric Research (Moore, 1976) are entitled *Iatrogenic Problems in Neonatal Intensive Care.* In his keytone address to the Conference, Sydney Gellis presents a list of historic therapeutic misadventures to which infants have been subjected in the name of good medical care. The list includes, inevitably, retrolental fibroplasia related to high incubator oxygen tension, thyroid cancer related to X-irradiation of "status thymicolymphaticus," and the gray baby syndrome related to chloramphenicol therapy. The volume then goes on to present a variety of contributions by other workers relating to additional difficulties associated with neonatal intensive care. Parenthetically, as of yet there is probably no compelling evidence for the efficacy of modern neonatal intensive care in terms of reducing neonatal mortality or improving postnatal development. Moreover, it is rather difficult to determine what constitutes neonatal intensive care in many of the papers which claim benefits, and procedures and equipment are rapidly changing.

There are also stories of medical technological developments which have adversely affected pregnancy outcome, the most glaring example of which was thalidomide.

Because of some of these misadventures, there is increasing concern that developments in medical technology not be prematurely applied on a population basis before they are adequately tested. Any technological development which might be expected to influence birth weight and its related hazards, of course, should be properly tested. The story presented by Susser and Stein about their prenatal supplementation study gives us some further cause for concern.

The value of many animal models in studies of pregnancy outcome (Emanuel, 1976) is questionable, although it appears that certain primate models (Sackett et al., 1974) should have considerable utility. Ultimately, however, human problems must be studied in humans. The question is how can this best be done?

The usual strategy of epidemiology involves a progression of approaches, from descriptive studies to analytic studies to experimental or intervention studies. Intervention studies are of necessity relatively uncommon in most problems in which epidemiologists are interested, and a greater reliance is placed on what have been called "natural experiments."

There are several possible reasons for the sparsity of intervention studies in the control of prematurity. First, many of the established risk factors, such as maternal age, birth order and socioeconomic status, are of a very general nature. Since the specific biologic significance of these risk factors is not known, it is difficult to devise very specific interventions. Second, there is, in this country at any rate, rather poor communication between obstetricians and epidemiologists, and obstetricians are poorly represented among epidemiologists, in contrast to such medical specialties as pediatrics and internal medicine. Third, the nature of some possible intervention techniques is probably such that randomized clinical trials might be difficult.

There are at least two reasons for performing intervention studies of any sort: 1) to better delineate etiologic factors and mechanisms, and 2) to develop permanent programs and solutions for health problems. These two reasons should be kept in mind in considering the pursuit of any intervention study.

Even though evidence may be overwhelming in analytic studies in supporting the plausibility of a given casual factor, there is additional comfort to be derived from further substantiation from intervention studies. Obviously, some kinds of experimental studies are inappropriate when the factor involved is toxic. For instance, if a given drug, such as thalidomide, appears to damage the fetus, hopefully no one would dream of doing an intervention study which involved giving the drug at various stages of human pregnancy and then carrying the pregnancy to term. On the other hand, one might attempt an intervention study in which pregnant women are encouraged to stop smoking, or to stop drinking alcoholic beverages, for instance.

With respect to the problem of prematurity, there are at least two kinds of intervention studies to be considered: 1) those that prevent conception and/or completion of pregnancy in high risk women, and 2) those that alter prenatal risk factors in such a way that a normal pregnancy outcome is enhanced.

It seems probable that procedures or processes which prevent births to populations of high risk women, or those which produce healthier mothers, also reduce the frequency of abnormalities in babies being born. Sir Dugald Baird, at this conference and elsewhere (1975), has described some of the social processes which seem related to improved pregnancy outcome. The social processes are not easily subject to intervention studies, but some programs and procedures which influence the social processes may be. Dr. Berendes brought up the possibility that liberalized abortion may be partly responsible for improving pregnancy outcome. Again, intervention studies of abortion would not be feasible.

This workshop has comprehensively covered the epidemiology of prematurity. Various correlates of low birth weight and premature gestation have been proposed or demonstrated. The appendix lists most of these established or possible factors and suggests possible intervention techniques which might conceivably influence these factors and thereby reduce prematurity. I emphasize the word "conceivably," since for many it is quite questionable what effect some interventions will have. Nevertheless, most of these possible interventions are rational, and have been either proposed already or are suggested by the results of various studies. Some, of course, are conjectural but, nevertheless, probably rational. I want to emphasize that most of the risk factors are nonspecific. Since the underlying mechanisms are not known, it is difficult to propose scientific interventions.

Socioeconomic status is commonly a factor in a variety of health problems, including prematurity and other problems of pregnancy outcome (Emanuel, 1976). The mechanisms by which social status influences pregnancy outcome remain more or less obscure. Some of the most usual presumptions of mechanisms relate to suboptimal nutrition and lack of prenatal care. Possibilities for intervention studies in these two areas will be discussed later. Of the other listed interventions to counteract the possible effects of deprived social circumstances, one might be reasonably amenable to some sort of clinical trial; that is, an income supplementation program. The rationale for such a study involves the presumption that an increase in income will lead to an improvement in habits which bear on pregnancy outcome. These habits would include those relating to nutrition, health care and personal hygiene. Actually, there have been several experimental programs of income supplementation in different cities in this country, including Seattle, but to my knowledge none has tried to measure the effects on pregnancy outcome. However, there is probably little evidence that merely increasing purchasing power will change habits in such a way that they will immediately and directly influence maternal and child health. For instance, it was found that federal food stamps have failed to improve the nutrition of the poor (Clarkson, 1975). In a study of Filipino rice farmers, my colleagues and I found no relationship between per capita family income and either fetal, infant and preschool mortality or growth of preschool children (Taylor et al., in press). Dr. Garn has shown that income is not related to low birth weight in the Collaborative Perinatal Project. Health problems related to socioeconomic factors seem rooted more deeply than mere availability of financial resources.

In most of the entries in the appendix, education is listed as a possible intervention technique as regards virtually all the factors related to low birth weight. The question may be asked: What kind of education, given at what time of life?

It is of interest that in the Maryland study by Rosenwaike (1971), no differences in low birth weight rates related to time of onset of prenatal care were found for mothers who were college graduates. This suggests that the total pattern of living habits may be more important than some specific behaviors. Various attempts at sex education have not seemed to be very successful in preventing teenage pregnancy (Jekel, 1975; Goldsmith et al., 1972). In spite of the fact that it appears likely that one important basis for the socioeconomic relationship is the general living habit pattern, it might be worthwhile to attempt to develop very specific educational intervention trials and to test their efficacy in reducing low birth weight and other related problems.

At this time it must be concluded that the real meaning of the socioeconomic relationship is for the most part obscure, and intensive investigations into behavior patterns and the social biology of poverty may be rewarding.

It can likewise be said that the biological meaning of the relationship of maternal age and birth order to birth weight is also obscure and awaits further elucidation. As mere availability of financial resources is probably not the crucial aspect of the socioeconomic relationship, it is clear that mere availability of contraceptive techniques and abortion is not the total solution in influencing the maternal age, birth order, pregnancy spacing and illegitimacy relationships. Factors other than availability of contraception are involved in many conceptions in high risk groups, such as the very young and the unmarried (Abernethy, 1974; Dickens et al., 1973). Nevertheless, clinical trials making contraceptives easily available to persons at high risk for unwanted pregnancy might be worthwhile. In trials such as this, and others as well, the ethical designation of a randomized control group may be difficult.

Long ago, Baird and his colleagues in Aberdeen proposed that childhood factors were important in later influencing reproductive outcome (Baird, 1952, 1962, 1964). Virtually all the work done in this important area has been done in the United Kingdom (Illsley, 1955.) This work has important implications in terms of possible interventions, one of which is that it may not be possible to erase all the damage done to the maternal organism during the previous period of growth and development. If this is the case, then concentration on interventions during the reproductive years is not sufficient, and greater concern for the total life history of mothers, such as the conditions which affect health at different ages, including infancy and childhood, will be required. It is impossible to test directly the effects of interventions which affect child health on future reproductive preformance, and any possible effects must be surmised from other kinds of studies. A possible consequence of better defining the role of childhood factors may be a greater realization of the urgency of giving increased attention to problems of child health, and the realization that the improvement of pregnancy outcome is a long-term process which may not easily respond to interventions during pregnancy alone.

Dr. Garn has proposed that maternal fat-free weight is important in determining fetal size, and this attribute is probably not very amenable to intervention during pregnancy. Drs. Placek and Niswander have shown that underlying maternal medical conditions also increase the risk of low birth weight, and some of these do not respond well to intervention during pregnancy.

There have been a number of studies of the relationship between nutrition and nutritional supplementation and pregnancy outcome. There seems little question that extreme deprivation, as in the hunger winter in the Netherlands and the siege of Leningrad, is related to reduced birth weight (Smith, 1947; Antonov, 1947; Stein and Susser, 1975). What is less clear is the value of supplementation to pregnant women of more or less adequate nutritional status and habits (Bergner and Susser, 1970). The paper at this conference by Susser and Stein raises additional questions about nutrition during pregnancy and pregnancy outcome.

Trials of nutritional supplementation, however difficult to conduct, are more straightforward than trials designed to change nutritional habits. On the other hand, the nutritional supplements sometimes used are not those which are either present or desired in the diets of the recipients. Furthermore, it appears unlikely that some supplements, even if successful, will be permanently adopted as a practice of pregnant women. Scrimshaw (1974), in another context, has questioned the value of feeding programs in the long-term solution of nutritional problems of developing countries where, of course, low birth weight and other related problems are of great importance. A problem in feeding programs relates to the assurance that the food reaches the person in question in the right quantity and frequency.

Another possible type of nutritional intervention study involves education of children and adults, or counseling during pregnancy, providing we really knew exactly what kind of education is needed. The effects of educational practices are difficult to measure. Pregnancy counseling involves more than the attempt to optimize food habits, although it is conceivable that studies could be designed which control for everything but nutritional counseling.

It is appealing to contemplate the improvement of problems of reproductive outcome by medical technology and intervention. There have been a number of studies, reviewed by Dr. Stanley, which attempt to study the efficacy of prenatal care. Little more needs to be said about this subject. It seems clear that studies of maternal care seeking behavior as a measure of prenatal care received leave much to be desired. Such studies cannot easily deal with the problem of self-selection. Further, they cannot deal with specificity and variability of actual care procedures employed. If the role of prenatal and obstetric care in the prevention of problems of pregnancy is to be understood, specific care procedures must be studied. It would seem that intervention studies have a role to play in this regard.

Various government programs have been developed from time to time which are proposed to improve pregnancy outcome, such as the Maternal and Infant Care Program. There have been several reports claiming significant improvement in pregnancy outcome resulting from this program (Chabot, 1971; Gold, 1969; Morton, 1970), none involving adequate study design and, to my knowledge, no pilot project was set up to adequately test effectiveness.

Such government programs are justifiable on the basis of humane considerations. Good intentions, however, are not sufficient to solve problems. Problems must be defined before possible solutions can be formulated. Proposed solutions must be tested for efficacy, and not just offered on the basis of the conventional wisdom. Proposed programs should be those which are feasible for translation to entire populations. Ineffective or insufficient programs have the danger of luring us into a sense of false security, while the problems persist.

The list of possible intervention techniques in the appendix indicates that, with few exceptions, rather complex processes are involved. Only in a few instances do the techniques involve simple procedures to be performed by health care personnel or the mothers. Randomized intervention studies of most of them are difficult; some would be impossible. The list, I'm sure, is by no means exhaustive, but will hopefully help to illustrate the complexity of the problem. Prematurity, like most health care problems, has multiple interacting etiologic factors, and there is no "philosopher's stone" to prevent its occurrence. To control any single factor is not apt to result in a marked and rapid reduction in rate. Like many other health problems, prematurity will be gradually reduced through the combined action of social, cultural and economic forces, together with contributions from medical and behavioral science and practice. Until we have some better understanding of underlying mechanisms, it is unlikely that we will consciously reduce the problem very much. Rather than attempting non-specific intervention programs, it is probably time to develop collaborative enterprises among obstetricians and other clinicians, epidemiologists, biostatisticians and other basic and behavioral scientists in a concerted effort to unravel the mysteries of the relationships covered in this conference.

APPENDIX

Factor (Established or Presumed) Related to Prematurity	Possible Intervention Technique
1. Socioeconomic status	Improve income
	Improve nutrition
	Prenatal care
	Improve education
	Change role of women
2. Inadequate prenatal nutrition	Nutritional supplementation
	Improve education
	Alter food habits
	Increase income
3. Maternal childhood factors	Improve maternal and child care
	Improve public health practices
	Improve child nutrition
	Stabilize economic conditions
	Foster upward social mobility
	Parent educational programs

4. Inadequate prenatal care	Improve education of mothers
	Improve education of physicians, nurses and midwives
	Improve distribution of prenatal care
5. Pregnancy spacing	Education
	Contraception
	Induced abortion
	Change role of women
6. Maternal age	Improve education
	Contraceptive practices
	Induced abortion
	Change role of women
	Prolongation of gestation
7. Birth order	Improve education
	Contraceptive practices
	Induced abortion
	Change role of women
	Prolongation of gestation
8. Unmarried state	Contraception
	Education
	Induced abortion
9. Toxic substances	Discontinue use of toxic substances (e.g., cigarettes, alcohol)
	Education
10. Maternal infections	Development and testing of vaccines
	Improve personal hygeine
	Pregnancy isolation
	Treatment of maternal infections
11. Toxemia of pregnancy	Improve nutrition
	Improve prenatal care
12. Ethnic group	
13. Genetics	?

TEXT REFERENCES

Abernethy, V.: Illegitimate Conception Among Teenagers. Am J Publ Health 64 (1974) 662-673

Antonov, A. N.: Children Born During the Seige of Leningrad in 1942. J Pediatrics 30 (1947) 250-259

Baird, D.: Preventive Medicine in Obstetrics. New Eng J Med 246 (1952) 561-568

Baird, D.: Evironmental and Obstetrical Factors in Prematurity, With Special Reference to Experience in Aberdeen. WHO Bull 26(1962)291-295

Baird, D.: The Epidemiology of Prematurity. J Pediatrics, 65 (1964) 909-924

Baird, D.: The Interplay of Changes in Society, Reproductive Habits, and Obstetric Practice in Scotland between 1922 and 1972. Brit J Prev Soc Med 29 (1975) 135-146

Bergner, L.; Susser, M. W.: Low Birth Weight and Prenatal Nutrition: An Interpretative Review. Pediatrics 46 (1970) 946-966

Chabot, A.: Improved Infant Mortality Rates in a Population Served by a Comprehensive Neighborhood Health Program. Pediatrics 47 (1971) 989-994

Clarkson, K. W.: Food Stamps and Nutrition. American Enterprise Institute for Public Policy (Evaluation studies), Washington, D.C., 1975

Dickens, H. O.; Hartshorne Mudd, E.; Garcia, C.; Tomar, K.; Wright, D.: One Hundred Pregnant Adolescents, Treatment Approaches in a University Hospital. Am J Publ Health 63(1973)794-800

Emanuel, I.: Problems of Outcome of Pregnancy: Some Clues from the Epidemiologic Similarities and Differences. In: Birth Defects: Risks and Consequences, ed. by S. Kelly, E. Hook, D. T. Janerich, and I. H. Porter. Academic Press, New York, 1976

Gellis, S. S.: Keynote Address: The Problem in Historical Perspective. In: Iatrogenic Problems in Neonatal Intensive Care, Report on the Sixty-Ninth Ross Conference on Pediatric Research, ed. by T. D. Moore. Ross Laboratories, Columbus, Ohio, 1976

Gold, E. M.; Stone, M. L.; Rich, H.: Total Maternal and Infant Care: An Evaluation. Am J Publ Health 59 (1969) 1851-1856

Goldsmith, S.; Gabrielson, M. O.; Gabrielson, I.; Mathews, V.; Potts, L.: Teenagers, Sex and Contraception. Family Planning Perspectives 4 (1972) 32-38

Illsley, R.: Social Class Selection and Class Differences in Relation to Stillbirths and Infant Deaths. Brit Med J 99 (1955) 1520-1524

Jekel, J.; Harrison, J. T.; Bancroft, D. R.; Tyler, N. C.; Klerman, L. V.: A Comparison of the Health of Index and Subsequent Babies Born to School Age Mothers. Am J Publ Health 65 (1975) 370-373

Moore, T. D.: Iatrogenic Problems in Neonatal Intensive Care, Report on the Sixty-Ninth Ross Conference on Pediatric Research. Ross Laboratories, Columbus, Ohio, 1976

Morton, J. H.: Experiences with a Maternity and Infant Care (MIC Project). Am J Ob and Gyn 107 (1970) 362-368

Rosenwaike, I.: The Influence of Socioeconomic Status on Incidence of Low Birth Weight. HSMHA Health Reports 86 (1971) 641-649

Sackett, G. P.; Holm, R.A.; Davis, A.E.; Fahrenbruch, C. E.: Prematurity and Low Birth Weight in Pigtail Macaques: Incidence, Prediction, and Effects on Infant Development. Symp. 5th Cong. Intl. Primat. Soc., 189-205, 1974

Scrimshaw, N. S.: Myths and Realities in International Health Planning. Am J Publ Health 64 (1974) 792-798

Smith, C.: Effects of Maternal Undernutrition upon the Newborn Infant in Holland (1944-1945). J Pediatrics 30 (1947) 229-243

Stein, Z.; Susser, M.: The Dutch Famine, 1944-1945, and the Reproductive Process: Effects on Six Indices at Birth. Pediatric Res 9 (1975) 70-76

Taylor, C. A.; Emanuel, I.; Morris, L. N.; Prosterman, R. L.: Child Nutrition and Mortality in the Rural Philippines: Is Socioeconomic Status Important? J Trop Ped Envir Child Hlth, in press

Closing Discussion

Dr. Stanley: One of our important tasks is to consider the kinds of studies that you all think might be worthwhile to do, taking into account what has been said by the previous three or four speakers and also looking at the review of the epidemiology of low birth weight or preterm delivery that was presented earlier.

Dr. Terris started by saying that he thought that prospective and case-control studies of mothers at risk of preterm and low birth weight infants would be of interest, and Dr. Emanuel made an interesting point about animal models for prematurity, of which I think there are very few. There have been some very elegant experiments coming out from Oxford concerning fetal initiation of premature labor which related to endocrine levels. This ties in nicely with Dr. Terris' idea of getting back to clinical and laboratory studies and tying in with those as well.

Prof. Meyer: There are a number of really good existing data sets such as the Collaborative study and the British study, in which certain things haven't been looked at. We have been working with the Ontario Perinatal Mortality Study and have looked, for smokers and non-smokers, at the incidence of high risk complications like bleeding, abruptio placentae, placenta previa and ruptured membranes. I think that some of the existing data sets could be reexamined very easily just to corroborate these findings.

Then I would think the next step that we want to take is to use these data sets for case-control studies. For example, the cases could be people with bleeding, and we would study them as if we had gone out and collected them and looked at all the characteristics that we have, including obstetric factors, maternal age, smoking and whatever else is there. Then as a control for this, we could use the whole population. Other case groups that could be examined using these large data sets might include "repeaters," those mothers who have a past history of spontaneous abortions, fetal loss or neonatal loss. Still others might be those with a tendency to premature rupture of membranes, preterm delivery or low birth weight deliveries.

I think this type of approach to existing data sets, each of which has different types of information, would save a lot of time, trouble and money and would give us insight into what kind of case-control studies using new data would be worthwhile to do. I also think that future prospective studies should study very intensively the mothers identified as having high risk of a preterm baby of low birth weight. These could be compared with a sample of total births, studied in the same way.

Dr. Davies: In Jerusalem in our perinatal studies over the last 12 years, we have recorded something like 60,000 deliveries, You can't be born in Jerusalem without getting onto our record, onto our record-linked data bank.

We looked at the problem of the risk of starting one's reproductive career with an abortion. We have taken those whose first pregnancy ended in abortion and those whose first pregnancy ended in delivery, and found they are different people. If you really want to do a case control, you have to control for the hundred variables that you know about, realizing that there are at least 5000 variables you don't know about.

So I would support very strongly the reanalysis of existing data. I would suggest that one should examine how the cases differ from the total population, and then look at as many differences as you want to measure, as many variables as you want to measure.

I am very worried about the controls. Even if you have two, three or four controls, one might have spurious differences because of intervening variables that haven't been looked at. It is really a general methodological problem.

Prof. Meyer: The population control is what I was suggesting to get around these problems. For many variables, the group can be compared with the whole population of births to see how they differ. For special tests, a sample of total births could be used, and should work much better than any attempt at matching.

Dr. Hardy: David Mellits and I are looking at birth weight/gestational age relationships in the Collaborative Perinatal Study data. We are doing this in a longitudinal fashion, considering antecedent characteristics which relate to birth weight and gestational age, the effect of concomitant variables such as placental size and, finally, the long-range outcomes with various birth weight/gestational age combinations.

We are doing this in a rather systematic fashion, first addressing in a univariate way the descriptive characteristics which affect birth weight and gestation. Then we are moving into the more complex interactions between numbers of variables, and we are in the throes of determining or divising an index variable, which we can then use as a continuous variable in relation to outcome.

One of the important things we can do is to consider the repeat pregnancies. There are about 8000 or 9000 of these. In a number of subgroups the data from women who had a small baby with their first pregnancy can be examined to determine their risk of having a small baby in their second pregnancy; then those who had a small second infant can be separated from those who did not, and the variables which may characterize one group versus another can be determined.

The objective in looking carefully at this really wonderful body of data has been to try to devise a number of practical tools. Can one develop a risk index that could be used by a pediatrician when a baby is born to assign a relative risk of bad outcome later on? Could one perhaps devise a way of defining sets of characteristics which would help the obstetrician when the lady walks in for her first prenatal visit?

Another important opportunity, I think, is the development of hints which can lead to more basic types of research or to follow-up studies that can elucidate mechanisms.

Dr. Mellits: In the repeat pregnancies or in any segment of this population, we could run a matched case-control type of study, controlling on those variables which we feel may influence outcome but which we cannot manipulate. Then, in fact, we can examine in our data base those variables which are alterable in order to suggest what interventions may be indicated for properly designed clinical trials.

Dr. Friedman: Regarding the high risk in black and poor mothers, do we know what it is about those high risk mothers who don't produce premature infants? Do we have any information about the mother that produces the premature baby and the mother who doesn't, even though they supposedly come from the same background?

Dr. Stanley: Following on from that, I think we must be prepared to accept the fact that a lot of factors are involved in preterm delivery in Norway. These in-depth studies need to be repeated in other areas, for example, with the American Indians and possibly the Australian aborigines and so on, because they obviously are going to be different in each case.

I think it is essential that in major government programs in the perinatal area (where you people, I assume, get called in on consultation), there ought to be epidemiologists in those research groups and in the study sections at the time when these are being planned so that there is some sense that these represent an experiment. The ones that have been done so far are bad experiments, and they could, without skirting some of these so-called ethical issues, be done much better. I think it is terribly important for those of us who possibly bridge the clinical and the social services or social programs and the epidemiologic world to try to live in all these worlds simultaneously.

Dr. Mellits: I have a suggestion for a different study that hasn't been suggested yet out of these large data sets. We have an opportunity for second generation studies. In the perinatal project some of the index children are 14 and 15 years old and having babies of their own. We have an excellent opportunity for the study of juvenile pregnancy, and also for second generation studies in general.

Dr. Susser: Yes, one of the points that I was going to make relates to that. Sir Dugald Baird's work in Aberdeen assumed that nutrition in the current pregnancy wasn't the critical variable, and pointed to the alternative hypothesis that a more likely critical variable was nutrition in the maternal generation.

No systematic effort has been made, as far as I know, to approach this problem through the appropriate analytic tool, which would be cohort analysis. I am talking about a completely structured comparison of the full panoply, if you like, of cohort and periodic analysis through time with all the useful data that are available. It needs thinking about and hasn't been, as far as I know, fully exploited.

Dr. Baird: The diet factor is rather important, and you know more about this than most of us. In the Aberdeen experiment the thing was to find out what people were eating and to analyze what they did. A substantial number were discarded because they couldn't read or write and so on, and these are the people with the trouble.

Dr. Susser: I think that we should try to refine our analysis of birth weight as an index or as a pathway, whatever it may be. A natural way of doing it is in gestation by weight categories. One thing that recurs in all data sets ever since Karn and Penrose (1951) and possibly before is the existence of an optimum birth weight, as Dr. Morton mentioned earlier. Above the optimum stage of gestation and the optimum birth weight, mortality rises. I have never seen any systematic study of that area.

In the approach to refining and elaborating the birth weight variable and its meaning, I think that we ought to follow the lead that Newton Morton gave us this morning and use a logical structure of variables. Such a structure demands of one that hypotheses are made explicit: what birth weight means; what the consequences of birth weight are, whether in mental growth or overall mortality or in very specific kinds of mortality?

Dr. Hardy: I would like to suggest one more variable for this kind of trial. I wonder whether exercise may not be an important variable, and whether this is a reason why Chinese babies in rural Taiwan are so much larger than Baltimore babies. The Chinese women work hard in the fields throughout pregnancy.

Dr. Emanuel: I think that we can almost always tap more information from existing data and learn more from different kinds of analysis. But I would like to reinforce what Dr. Daniel Seigel and other members of the audience said, namely, that we need some new variables. We can continue to study and analyze the same tired old variables and we will probably learn from doing so. However, I don't think that we are really going to get very far until we go off in new directions.

With few exceptions, such as smoking, we have no direct link to causation, or even something that hints at a direct mechanism. We know well enough that prematurity is related to social class, but most poor women do, in fact, have good babies. We know about the relationship of prematurity to maternal age and parity, but in fact, most younger and older mothers and most primigravidas also have healthy babies.

I think we have to do something similar to what has been suggested, and that is, for example, to compare poor women who have good babies to poor women who have premature babies. Similarly, we might compare well-off women who have premature babies to well-off women who have healthy babies. The real question is: What variables should we use for these comparisons? I think that to some extent we are at the stage of a fishing expedition. Some of the variables should relate to reproductive physiology and biochemistry. Others might be less direct, perhaps relating to maternal physiological aging. We have suggested that maternal biological aging may be a factor in some kinds of abnormal reproductive outcomes (Emanuel et al., 1972). In any event, I don't think we are going to get very far unless we attempt some new approaches which may help to unravel the meanings of the non-specific relationships which have already been established.

I think that with respect to prematurity, we are much further removed from direct lines of causation than was the case for pellagra or the case for the Broad Street pump. Therefore, the chances for success using non-specific interventions for prematurity do not seem very probable.

Dr. Janerich: Valadian and Reed at Harvard had some longitudinal data on nutrition, and I think they showed that the protein intake around the time of puberty was related to the birth weight of the offspring. These were prospective studies and the techniques were pretty good.

Dr. Alberman: I don't think we have enough good international data on birth weight. Also, one of the things we must start doing is separating out the birth weight babies for whom we think we know the cause (where there is an obvious maternal condition) and concentrate on the ones where the causes are not clear.

Mr. Hoffman: I wish to make a point in line with what Drs. Emanuel and Susser have mentioned before. I am not only interested in what happens below 2500 grams and before 37 weeks and in what happens above 4500 grams. But I am also interested in that region in between where the most striking effects may well occur as a result of any intervention trial. I think we have to look particularly at the middle of the distribution where most of the births are if we wish to assess the benefit of an improved outcome as measured by reductions of morbidity or mortality.

Dr. Stein: I suggest that an intervention trial of smoking and birth weight would be of value. We don't know how to stop people from smoking, but the evidence seems to show that if we could do so during pregnancy, it would do something. We also have a strong idea that if we stopped them smoking for a long time, it would do other things for them as well.

Dr. Rush: I differ with Dr. Emanuel. I think trials are possible now, and if we cannot now design intervention trials, then our descriptive and analytic research ought to be aimed towards the time when we can.

When we reviewed the literature on smoking and perinatal mortality several years ago, the excess perinatal mortality of the offspring of smokers was about 30% greater than non-smokers (Rush and Kass, 1972). I am not aware of any other variable for which an intervention could be mounted with potential benefit of this magnitude. Also, there is a very strong interaction of smoking with social status. In the British Perinatal Mortality Study population, the excess mortality among smokers in social classes four and five was 45%, but only 13% in classes one and two (Butler and Alberman, 1969).

The role of infection is important and should be reviewed, as should activity, work and physical condition. Although Pomerance, Gluck and Lynch (1974) found no relationship between pregnancy outcome and physical condition, it is hardly a closed issue, in part because the methodology to assess physical fitness is so poor.

We are uncertain about the benefits that accrue from prenatal care. Obstetric care has become more and more expensive, while we have almost no data on how effective new, highly sophisticated diagnostic and therapeutic techniques are. Yet these new procedures are amenable to controlled study.

Dr. Reed: Let me respond by focusing on this one question: Should we plan studies of a single variable, like smoking, or should we put together half a dozen that we have mentioned here and try intervention studies on all at once?

Dr. Davies: One possibility would be to develop a number of hypotheses for testing and to try to test them simultaneously on the various bodies of data which exist and see if they are biological truths or peculiar to one particular place.

Let us talk about two main groups. Of course, birth weight goes up with parity. Immigrants who come from North Africa have babies which are higher than the Israeli mean. And immigrants who come from Asian countries have babies lower than the mean. Now, the daughters of those immigrants who are born in Israel, that is the grandchildren, come close to the Israeli mean. We can explain why people coming from India or Yemen or poor countries who have better food and health care show a rise in their birth weight. We have great difficulty explaining why there was regression to the mean of those who came, let us say, from Morocco and Algiers.

There are two things that I should tell you about, because you can then see a hypothesis and we can test it. First, the fashion was to prefer fat ladies, so the North African ladies from Morocco are very fat and they have big babies. The husbands of their daughters prefer thinner ladies, so about half of this difference can be explained using a multivariate analysis on the basis of prepregnancy weight. Another half can be explained on the basis of out-marriage; that is, it seems that the North African heavy-baby mothers marry light-baby fathers and they are similar in the middle. But much more of the variance depends on the mother than on the father. Now, if a whole series of hypotheses were about genetic and prepregnancy weight diet, one could perhaps test these in other populations.

The second point is about the high risk. Can you give a risk factor to a lady who comes into the obstetrician's consulting room? The answer is that, if she is at very high risk, yes. We have done this for the very high risk group where the risk of perinatal mortality is around, let us say, 10% or more. Then using 15 different variables, one has a sensitivity of about 16% and a specificity of about 90%. But given the kinds of populations which we have in our country and which you have in this country, you have to examine everybody because of high risk.

Dr. Baird: It seems to me that if we were going to follow this question of weight changes in pregnancy and composition of the woman as far as height and weight are concerned, we really need to be aware of the work that is now being done on sheep and other animals on the whole question of nutrition. There are some different genetic types in regard to nutrition, and I wonder if humans are similar?

Prof. Meyer: Everyone seems to think that an intervention trial of smoking would be a good thing. It is clear that smoking reduced birth weight. I am not so impressed with how bad it is for a term baby to weigh 150–200 gm. less because the mother smokes, but I am impressed with the fact that smokers have a significant increase in certain complications such as abruptio placentae, placenta previa, premature rupture of membranes and bleeding not otherwise specified both early and late in pregnancy. We found this in the Ontario study, and similar findings have been published from Cardiff (Andrews and McGarry, 1972), Paris (Goujard et al., 1975), Birmingham (Lowe, 1959) and New Haven (Lubs, 1973). If these findings are corroborated by data from the British study, and if everyone in this room is convinced that maternal smoking will double the incidence of these complications, which are very serious and have high risk of perinatal loss, then we should be able to get a clearer message across to the obstetricians. Perhaps they would then ask about the smoking habits of women who come in with bleeding or with early rupture of membranes. When they become convinced, then I think we will have the means for an intervention trial.

Dr. Rush: Mortality was 20% or so higher among smokers in the Ontario Study.

Prof. Meyer: It was more than that, but that is going from 2–3%. I mean, it is true that most people have good babies. What you need to do is to ask why this woman gets in trouble when she smokes and that one does not.

Dr. Terris: We have to think through the reasons for having an intervention trial. And I am not at all sure I am hearing the right ones.

The reason for an intervention trial is that you are not sure of the result or people are not accepting the data which you now have. This is why the nutrition trials were done—because we weren't sure that it would make any difference, and indeed it didn't.

With smoking, on the other hand, do we really need a trial? I would guess that at this point there is very little doubt in anyone's mind that smoking has a bad effect on the infant. It causes excess morbidity and mortality, and if that is true, what do we need a trial for? What we need is a big educational program directed at obstetricians and at the general public, so that they know it is not only lung cancer and emphysema, but it is also what happens to the baby. That is what I would do. And if the Institute wants to be useful, let it not run a trial but let it go out to the public and to the profession and publicize this fact which many people do not know.

Regarding other trials, I am inclined to think that we ought to look at each issue and decide whether we need a trial. For instance, this may be a foolish idea, but I think we might run a variation of the nutrition trial and get women to gain weight during pregnancy, which is supposedly one of the factors. That is a relatively easy one to do. Let us see what happens on a case-control basis.

Dr. Mellits: I thought that the reason presented for why you need a smoking trial was not to reiterate that there is an effect of smoking, but to see if there is an effect of stopping smoking, or if you can in fact effect a change.

Dr. Terris: In the case of cigarette smoking and lung cancer, there were no trials. The decision was made on the basis of the weight of evidence, which was all observational, not experimental, to counsel the public not to smoke. It seems to me the same really applies here; I don't know anyone who would stand up and say "I don't believe this," not with the data that is already available.

Dr. Rush: There has been extensive study among psychologists about stopping smoking, and those who voluntarily stop smoking are very different in many factors from those who keep going. I am convinced that a trial should be done, but the real problem is the technology for intervening effectively and to facilitate people's stopping of smoking; this is an area where we have felt most weak. But our reading of the necessity of the trial is different. The trial is very important to do.

Dr. Stanley: I wonder if we can't combine those problems into one trial, testing the method used to see if this is successful in stopping smoking as well as looking at the smoking effect. The control group would receive no smoking advice, and you would have a group to which you gave your smoking advice. Now, the ones who didn't comply could be looked at separately from the ones who did, as well as lumping all the treatment group together to code the effect of the total smoking program.

Dr. Susser: There is a lot of pessimism about intervention in relation to smoking. The pessimism arises from the short-term trials of health education over the last 15-20 years which showed either no effect on smoking habits, or a very small effect and a rapid reversion to old habits. The smoking phenomenon is deeply embedded in the social context— economically, socially, politically and also psychologically. But we do in fact see changes in relation to smoking habits. There is a social movement that is manifesting itself in a change in smoking habits throughout the society. I fear an attempt at an intervention trial because of this. We don't have the technology to translate effort directed at individuals into population effects.

Dr. Stein: I think the evidence that we have is fragmentary at which point in pregnancy stopping smoking makes a difference in birth weight. It is quite important because the earliest that you will get women in is the first visit to the prenatal clinic, and it may be important to have women stop smoking then or it may be important to stop smoking before then. I think we do need a trial to know that.

Secondly, I think Dr. Susser is wrong. It may be that during pregnancy women will take upon themselves certain alterations in drinking and exercise habits for the sake of the offspring, whereas they may not want to change their total pattern of smoking. I don't think that we have to wait, from the frequency point of view, for these grand societal changes. I think we might be able to apply the therapeutic measure during pregnancy with more success.

Prof. Meyer: I don't personally think that anybody is going to be able to do an intervention trial or stop anybody smoking in the face of the advertising and the whole campaign that the industry is putting on. I think that if the obstetricians became convinced that certain women are getting into trouble because they smoke and made them stop, and observed the effect, that kind of evidence would be of value. We need to cooperate with the clinician who is with the patient. Also we need a lot of physiological and biochemical studies of high risk women. I think that would be much more productive than putting money into some kind of intervention trial which has all these problems in it and from which we might not achieve very much. You know, we want to be convincing to the public and I think we have to try to get at the most important things first. I doubt whether we are ready for an intervention trial yet.

Dr. Morton: I want to go back to the idea that high risk groups are desirable to work with, both for studying etiology and for intervention, and that repeaters are one way of selecting a high risk group.

Geneticists do this to a considerable degree. They call repeaters "multiplex families" and non-repeaters" simplex families," and there are many cases where this has led to understanding of etiology. But there are obvious problems. One is that a woman with two children who were both premature is more of a repeater than one with 12 children of whom two were premature. This raises some questions as to whether repeaters are a good way to define high risk groups.

People in mental retardation have had this approach. Linus Pauling designed an elaborate study of repeaters for mental retardation which unerringly led to selection of sociofamilial cases where the genetic factors are polygenic and the nongenetic factors are social. If you are looking for simple causes, you couldn't find a less rewarding group to study.

The other problem is that if you go to the existing studies and try to pick out repeaters, the presenting symptom was a pregnant woman. Now you are redefining the presenting symptom as a repeater for prematurity, and I am not sure the right information was collected to explain these cases. Finally, a lot of information is available now about repeat abortions due to trisomy and the fact that there is a great specificity for this. Whether these overlap the moribund children who die immediately after birth has not been mentioned here, but it is possible that they do. It has not been terribly well studied. Here is a category of cases where the appropriate intervention is probably elective amniocentesis and abortion because the child is not viable under present techniques.

I think all of these experiments with familial, with repeater events, should be considered in designing any sort of intervention study or etiological study using repeater women.

Dr. Stanley: I believe that Dr. Bakketeig has some ideas about the maternal complications of pregnancy which might be repeated in each pregnancy.

Dr. Bakketeig: In our repeater study we have not yet looked into the tendency of repeating such conditions as medical complications which might predispose to low birth weight. However, even if we expect some of the tendency of repeating low birth weight to be caused by repeating conditions such as placenta previa and abruptio placentae, the major part of the general tendency to repeat birth weight and gestational age can hardly be explained this way.

Dr. Rush: Repeaters may be a poor group to study, because they are likely to maximally manifest non-environmental causes of low birth weight or preterm delivery, minimizing the real role of environmental causes.

When Dr. Kass and I studied the pregnancies of a mixed racial group, low birth weight and pregnancy loss were more predictable from past pregnancy experience in the whites than the blacks. This suggested that, with lower social status, fewer of the poor outcomes were caused by inherent physiological problems and more by adverse environmental conditions, which would be less likely to be constant between pregnancies.

Dr. Stanley: I disagree with your point about repeaters being a bad group to study, because one can actually look at those who do repeat and those who don't repeat, as well as, look at the factors within repeaters which may be important. Is it, in fact, maternal complications, or is it something else? One shouldn't exclude factors just because we can't change them.

Dr. Mellits: I think you are talking about two different types of repeaters. The study of repeat pregnancies on a stated data base is fine. What was being properly argued against was repeat low birth weights. We should study the repeat pregnancies in the large data bases, not necessarily repeat bad outcomes, but second pregnancies existing in the same study base. I think that is what is meant by repeaters.

Dr. Reed: As maternal weight gain during pregnancy is one of the strongest correlates of infant birth weight, what do you think of a simple trial that would focus upon proper weight gain?

Dr. Susser: Well, we get into a problem there. If you take the data from the Dutch experience and from the New York intervention study, I think that to reconcile the results one must recognize that, above a threshold level of nutritional intake, not much happens in relation to the baby's weight and other dimensions. Effects are seen below the threshold. The threshold is less, I suppose, than the nutritional intake of 90% or more of the population in the United States. One must search out very special high risk groups to find women whose caloric intake is low enough to influence their birth outcome.

Dr. Terris: If you scrambled your data and just looked at weight of the child and weight gain of the mother, was there a relationship?

Dr. Rush: Yes.

Dr. Susser: I think that what we are dealing with was suggested by Angus Thompson nearly 20 years ago. He found a relationship between caloric intake, maternal weight and birth weight in his data. He did partial correlations, and although I think he failed to eliminate plausible alternative explanations of the correlations, he was probably right in the end after all. He thought that the relation between calories and birth weight disappeared by partial correlation because it was explained by maternal weight, and that the causal pathway was maternal size leading to increased caloric intake and big babies, maternal size being the common cause. That is probably the situation with nutrition above the threshold barrier. Big mothers eat more and have bigger babies.

Prof. Meyer: I wonder if we could get a general consensus on how important birth weight is, because I have my doubts about it in a lot of ways. Does everybody think that every baby should be bigger, or that weighing less than 2500 gm. is always bad? I think that there is a tendency to put a value judgment on birth weight that I don't really think is justified.

Dr. Rush: Mr. Hoffman's data contribute to the issue. They showed that optimal birth weight for blacks is different from whites, and that black mortality was lowest not at 3500 gm. but at about 3250 gm., rising for higher birth weights.

Dr. Alberman: In England roughly 6% of births 2500 gm. or less account for 60% of the deaths.

Prof. Meyer: How many are preterm?

Dr. Alberman: Two-thirds.

Prof. Meyer: Talk about term births only. It is not fair to talk about preterm births. They die because they are preterm.

Dr. Rush: There is, however, a strong gradient of higher mortality with lower birth weight at all gestations.

Dr. Janerich: The increasing rate of induction notwithstanding, the gradient of increased risk associated with higher weight births is still there, at least the last time I looked at New York data and this was within the last 12 months. So I think really what you have to say is not how important the birth weight is or how much of a shift we get in the dangerous ranges for each one of these risk factors.

Dr. Susser: There is one important point which isn't given a dramatic place in our study of the Dutch famine. We went to great lengths to relate prenatal famine exposure to subsequent mortality. We did that because there was an immense infant mortality—decimation is the precise term— during the summer following the famine, across the whole country. We can certainly relate the prenatal exposure to subsequent infant mortality up to three months of age increasingly from about seven days to 90 days.

Now, a good part of that could be accounted for (and I have to say "could" be accounted for, not "was" accounted for) by the decline in mean birth weight for the affected cohorts. Unfortunately, we didn't have individual birth weights for each death. But if one analyzes by monthly cohort, mean birth weight accounted for about half the mortality. Now, it could probably account for a good deal more because the birth weight cohorts and the mortality cohorts were not strictly coincident, so that some of the effect was certainly suppressed. So we found a pretty convincing relationship between depressed nutrition, depressed birth weight and subsequent viability.

Prof. Meyer: Couldn't you be having parallel effects of starvation?

Dr. Susser: The stillbirth rate was not related to the famine exposure in the third trimester, nor to any degree was the first day death rate. These rates were in fact related to some kind of exposure in the first trimester. Also, there were two different syndromes of low birth weight: one related to third trimester exposure and to peak mortality after the first week of life, and another related to first trimester famine exposure and first week mortality and thus not related to the decline in birth weight. Yes, there were some parallel relationships and we certainly didn't explain them all anyway.

Speaker: I would like to make a point. The question was asked whether weight is really important, and the answer was in terms of mortality. I don't think this is the most important thing. I think you have to ask yourself how the central nervous system is functioning and if the child is growing, rather than if the child is dead or alive.

Dr. Stanley: This opens another range of topics! At the moment, the evidence seems convincing that neonatal care in these very low birth weight infants improves mortality, but its effect on long-term morbidity, especially neurological development, is a very worrisome problem.

Dr. Morton: Twenty years ago Lionel Penrose said that "the majority of so-called premature infants are perfectly normal, though small, like adults of short stature." I think nothing we have heard so far would tell us whether moderately high birth weight is a symptom of fetal health or a cause of postnatal viability. The predictive value of birth weight does not necessarily signify that it is causal. We need to distinguish between healthy and unhealthy babies of low birth weight.

Dr. Rush: The relationship of birth weight to viability changes as the fetus and infant mature. Birth weight predicts very well the chance of surviving the neonatal period, while social status and other factors relate only through their effect on birth weight. As the infant gets older, other factors, particularly health services (preventive and therapeutic), become the major determinants of survival, along with nutrition and other environmental factors.

Dr. Davies, don't North African Jews in Israel have surprisingly high birth weight, given their stature and social status, and isn't their perinatal survival surprisingly good?

Dr. Davies: Yes.

Dr. Rush: Whatever the origin, whether genetic or environmental, birth weight predicts neonatal mortality. It would be more valuable to know about neurological integrity, but such data are not routinely available.

Dr. Stanley: There are several points that have been raised during the conference which I would like to comment on before we adjourn.

The concept of "optimum" birth weight for gestation was brought up several times. Obviously our interest in low birth weight and preterm delivery is because of the large proportion of infants with these attributes who die or get sick. Studies are needed which will elucidate factors affecting mortality and morbidity in infants in similar birth weight/ gestation categories and help to explain why some die or get sick and others do well.

The fascinating and exciting concept of repeater studies that are possible with some of larger data sets should be followed up by those who have access to these data sets and results compared between them.

The effects of smoking in pregnancy, low birth weight, preterm delivery and perinatal outcome need further study. We need to know the long term detrimental effects of smoking, and the reasons for them. Are they due to the low birth weight of the baby, its relative immaturity or directly to toxicity during pregnancy? The relationship of smoking, abruptio placentae, placenta previa, premature rupture of the membranes, preterm delivery and respiratory distress syndrome need elucidation. We need to know what risk factors interact with smoking to produce these complications and the consequent increases in perinatal loss and morbidity. Trials of anti-smoking advice are needed to determine their effectiveness in pregnant women, the effect of cessation of smoking on the outcomes mentioned and at what month of pregnancy is cessation of smoking still effective.

Dr. Reed: I also have been making a few notes during the conference which summarize some of the major needs for future directions.

Under the heading of the Search for the Causes of Prematurity many participants expressed the feeling that we have been doing descriptive studies of the same variables over and over. Part of the problem is that prematurity is not a simple disease caused by one agent. We have heard reports which show that a great variety of factors can increase the risk of prematurity, including those with biological explanation such as infections, diet and smoking, as well as life style variables such as education, ethnic group and social status. It is my personal belief that this latter group reflects the quality of "caring," that is whether or not a person is concerned about what happens to them or not. If you care about yourself and your baby you do the right things, and of course whether you care or not depends upon all these conditions of life. At the present time we do not know how to solve problems which include a complex interaction of life styles and a multitude of biological variables, but there are some specific sets of interaction which can be delineated. These include:

1. The interaction of smoking, alcohol consumption and blood pressure with special concern for the differences between black and white groups.

2. Analysis of the factors associated with repeated low birth weight or preterm deliveries in the same mother, with concern for both genetic and environmental factors such as occupation, exercise and diet.

3. Comparisons of both high and low risk population subgroups for both causative and protective factors.

4. The interaction of prenatal maternal weight, weight gain and type of diet among women of different physical types.

5. Examination of the role of prenatal care with specific emphasis upon what obstetricians and related health personnel do about prevention of such factors as smoking, alcohol consumption and poor diets.

Under the heading of Prevention of Prematurity I think that there was a clear concensus that we do not have to wait until we have a complete understanding of the pathophysiology of prematurity in order to alter its occurrence. Indeed, several participants suggested that the lack of progress in this area is due to the lack of intervention studies which demonstrate whether or not it is possible to prevent prematurity through manipulation of the known risk factors. The specific risk factors mentioned most commonly included smoking, malnutrition, hypertension, maternal infections, excess alcohol consumption, poverty and teenage pregnancies. Intervention studies of such factors could be carried out among high risk groups in a number of different types of communities. Such an approach would call for a reordering of priorities for research funds; yet a constant theme throughout this conference has been that the time and the need for such a reordering has come.

In conclusion, I think that this has been an extremely worthwhile conference and on behalf of the Institute I wish to thank each of you for your contributions.

DISCUSSION REFERENCES

Andrews, J.; McGarry, J. M.: A Community Study of Smoking in Pregnancy. J. Obstet Gynecol Brit Comm 79(1972)1057–1073

Butler, N. R.; Alberman, E. D.: Perinatal Problems. Livingstone, Edinburgh, 1969

Emanuel, I.; Sever, L. S.; Milham, S. Jr.; Thuline, H.: Accelerated Aging in Young Mothers of Children with Down's Syndrome. Lancet 2(1972)361–363

Goujard, J.; Rumeau, C.; Schwartz, D..: Smoking During Pregnancy, Stillbirth and Abruptio Placentae. Biomed 23(1975)20–22

Karn, M. N.; Penrose, L. S.: Birth Weight and Gestation Time in Relation to Maternal Age, Parity and Infant Survival. Ann Eugenics 16(1951)147

Lowe, C. R.: Effects of Mother's Smoking Habits on Birth Weight of their Children. Acta Obstet Gynecol Scand 50(1971)83–94

Lubs, M. L. E.: Racial Differences in Maternal Smoking Effects on the Newborn Infant. Am J Obstet Gynecol 115(1973) 66–76

Pomerance, J. J.; Gluck, L.; Lynch, V. A.: Physical Fitness in Pregnancy: Its Effect on Pregnancy Outcome. Am J Obstet Gynecol 119(1974)867–876

Rush, D.; Kass, E. H.: Maternal Smoking: A Reassessment of the Association with Perinatal Mortality. Am J Epidemiol 96(1972)183–196

Index